Clinical Ethics in Anesthesiology

A Case-Based Textbook

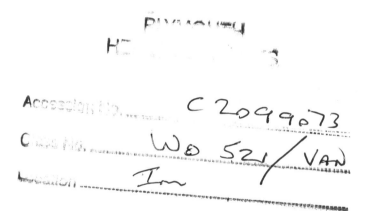

PLYMOUTH

H~ ~S

Accession No. C 2099073

Class No. WO 521/VAN

Location Im

Clinical Ethics in Anesthesiology

A Case-Based Textbook

Edited by

Gail A. Van Norman

Co-editors

Stephen Jackson

Stanley H. Rosenbaum

Susan K. Palmer

DISCOVERY LIBRARY
LEVEL 5 SWCC
DERRIFORD HOSPITAL
DERRIFORD ROAD
PLYMOUTH
PL6 8DH

CAMBRIDGE
UNIVERSITY PRESS

CAMBRIDGE UNIVERSITY PRESS
Cambridge, New York, Melbourne, Madrid, Cape Town, Singapore,
São Paulo, Delhi, Dubai, Tokyo, Mexico City

Cambridge University Press
The Edinburgh Building, Cambridge, CB2 8RU, UK

Published in the United States of America by Cambridge University Press, New York

www.cambridge.org
Information on this title: www.cambridge.org/9780521130646

© Cambridge University Press 2011

This publication is in copyright. Subject to statutory exception
and to the provisions of relevant collective licensing agreements,
no reproduction of any part may take place without
the written permission of Cambridge University Press.

First published 2011

Printed in the United Kingdom at the University Press, Cambridge

A catalog record for this publication is available from the British Library

Library of Congress Cataloging in Publication data
Clinical ethics in anesthesiology : a case-based textbook / [edited by] Gail A. Van Norman;
   co-editors, Stephen Jackson, Stanley H. Rosenbaum, Susan K. Palmer.
      p.   cm.
   Includes bibliographical references and index.
   ISBN 978-0-521-13064-6 (pbk.)
   1. Anesthesiology–Moral and ethical aspects.   I. Van Norman, Gail A.   II. Title.
   [DNLM: 1. Anesthesiology–ethics. WO 221]
   RD82.C548 2011
   174.2′9796–dc22   2010027381

ISBN 978-0-521-13064-6 Paperback

Cambridge University Press has no responsibility for the persistence or
accuracy of URLs for external or third-party internet websites referred to in
this publication, and does not guarantee that any content on such websites is,
or will remain, accurate or appropriate.

Every effort has been made in preparing this book to provide accurate and up-to-date
information which is in accord with accepted standards and practice at the time of publication.
Although case histories are drawn from actual cases, every effort has been made to disguise the
identities of the individuals involved. Nevertheless, the authors, editors and publishers can make no
warranties that the information contained herein is totally free from error, not least because clinical
standards are constantly changing through research and regulation. The authors, editors and
publishers therefore disclaim all liability for direct or consequential damages resulting from the
use of material contained in this book. Readers are strongly advised to pay careful attention
to information provided by the manufacturer of any drugs or equipment that they plan to use.

This book is dedicated to Melvin F. Van Norman (1920–2006), a pilot and flight instructor, who said that a good teacher listens to the question that is asked, hears the questions that didn't get asked, and answers the questions that should have been asked.

Contents

Contributors

Louise B. Andrew MD, JD, FACEP
American College of Emergency Physicians
Founding President, Coalition and Center for Ethical
Medical Testimony

Jane C. Ballantyne MD, FRCA
Professor of Anesthesiology and Critical Care,
Penn Pain Medicine Center,
University of Pennsylvania,
Philadelphia, PA, USA

Sadek Beloucif MD, PhD
Department of Anesthesiology and Critical Care
Medicine, Avicenne University Hospital, France

David Clendenin MD
Associate in Anesthesia, Children's Hospital Boston
and Instructor in Anaesthesia, Harvard Medical
School, Boston, MA, USA

Maliha A. Darugar MD
MA Candidate, Medical Humanities and Bioethics,
Northwestern University, Feinberg School of
Medicine, Chicago, IL, USA

Joanna M. Davies MB BS, FRCA
Associate Professor of Anesthesiology and Pain
Medicine, University of Washington School of
Medicine, Seattle, WA, USA

Michael DeVita MD
Executive Vice President of West Penn
Allegheny Health System
Former Professor, Critical Care Medicine and
Medicine, University of
Pittsburgh, PA, USA

Denise M. Dudzinski PhD MTS
Associate Professor, Department of
Bioethics and Humanities, University of
Washington School of Medicine,
Seattle, WA, USA

Bernice Elger MD
University Center of Legal Medicine of Geneva
and Lausanne, Switzerland

Monica Escher MD
Pain and Palliative Care Consultation,
Division of Clinical Pharmacology and Toxicology,
Geneva University Hospitals,
Geneva, Switzerland

Joel E. Frader MD, MA
Professor of Pediatrics, and Medical Humanities and
Bioethics, Northwestern University Feinberg School
of Medicine, Chicago, IL, USA

Kelly Fryer-Edwards PhD
Associate Professor, Department of Bioethics and
Humanities, University of Washington School of
Medicine, Seattle, WA, USA

James Giordano PhD
Director of the Center for Neurotechnology Studies,
Potomac Insitute for Policy Studies, Arlington, VA;
Research Associate of the Wellcome Centre for
Neuroethics, and Uehiro
Centre for Practical Philosophy,
University of Oxford, UK

Allen Gustin MD FCCP
Assistant Professor, Anesthesiology and Pain
Medicine, University of Washington, Seattle,
WA, USA

Rebecca M. Harris
MA Candidate, Medical Humanities and Bioethics,
Northwestern University, Feinberg School of
Medicine, Chicago, IL, USA

Gerhard Höver PhD
Moraltheologisches Seminar, Rheinische
Friedrich Wilhelms Universitat,
Bonn, Germany

Steven K. Howard MD
Associate Professor of Anesthesia,
Stanford University School of Medicine,
Palo Alto, CA, USA; Patient Safety Center of Inquiry,
VA Palo Alto Health Care System

Carl C. Hug Jr, MD, PhD
Professor of Anesthesiology, Emeritus,
and Faculty Affiliate, The Center for Ethics
Emory University, Atlanta, GA, USA

Samia Hurst MD
Institute for Biomedical Ethics,
Geneva University Medical School,
Switzerland

Steven Jackson MD
Chief of Staff (retired), Department of
Anesthesiology, and Chair of the Bioethics
Committee, Good Samaritan
Hospital San Jose, CA, USA

Nancy S. Jecker PhD
Professor, Department of Bioethics and
Humanities, University of Washington School of
Medicine, Seattle, WA, USA

Jonathan D. Katz MD
Clinical Professor of Anesthesiology, Yale University
School of Medicine, New Haven, CT, USA

Joseph Klein MD
Fellow, Critical Care Medicine, Dept of
Anesthesiology and Pain Medicine
University of Pennsylvania, Philadelphia, PA, USA

W. Andrew Kofke MD, MBA, FCCM
Professor and Director of Neuroanesthesia, and
Co-Director of Neurocritical Care, University of
Pennsylvania, PA, USA

Ruth Landau MD
Professor of Anesthesiology and Director of
Obstetric Anesthesia and Clinical Genetics Research,
Department of Anesthesiology, University of
Washington Medical Center, Seattle, WA, USA

Craig D. McClain MD
Senior Associate in Anesthesia, Children's Hospital
Boston; Assistant Professor of Anaesthesia,
Harvard Medical School
Boston, MA, USA

Alex Mauron PhD
Professor, Institute of Biomedical Ethics,
Geneva, Switzerland

Kelly N. Michelson MD, MPH
Assistant Professor, Pediatrics,
Division of Critical Care,
Northwestern University Feinberg
School of Medicine, Chicago, IL, USA

Cynthiane J. Morgenweck MD, MA
Associate Clinical Professor of Bioethics,
Center for Study of Bioethics
Medical College of Wisconsin, WI, USA

William Notcutt MB ChB, FRCA, FFPMRCA
Consultant in Pain Medicine and Anaesthesiology,
James Paget University Hospital, Great Yarmouth,
Norfolk, UK

Michael Nurok MD, PhD
Anesthesiology and Critical Care Medicine,
Faculty member, Center for Bioethics, Brigham
and Women's Hospital; Faculty, Department of
Social Medicine, Harvard Medical School,
Boston, MA, USA

Susan K. Palmer MD
Staff Anesthesiologist and Patient Safety Committee
Chair, Oregon Anesthesiology Group (OAG),
Former Professor of Anesthesiology and Professor
of Preventive Medicine, Faculty Program in Medical
Ethics and Law, University of Colorado Health
Sciences Center, Denver, CO, USA

Joan G. Quaine MD
Associate in Anesthesia, Children's Hospital Boston,
and Instructor in Anesthesia, Harvard Medical
School, Boston, MA, USA

Michael A. Rie MD
Associate Professor Anesthesiology/Critical Care
Medicine, Associate Scholar in Ethics, Department
of Anesthesiology, University of Kentucky School of
Medicine, Lexington, KY, USA

Stanley H. Rosenbaum MD, MA
Professor of Anesthesiology, Internal Medicine and
Surgery, Director, Section of Perioperative and Adult
Anesthesia, and Vice Chairman for Academic Affairs,
Department of Anesthesiology, Yale University School
of Medicine, New Haven, CT, USA

David M. Rothenberg MD, FCCM
The Max S. Sadove MD Professor of Anesthesiology,
Associate Dean for Academic Affiliations
Director, Division of Critical Care Medicine
Rush Medical College, Chicago, IL, USA

Robert B. Schonberger MD, MA
Fellow in Cardiac Anesthesiology
and Clinical Research,
Dept of Anesthesiology, Yale University School of
Medicine, New Haven, CT, USA

Mark D. Siegel MD
Associate Professor, Department of Internal
Medicine, Pulmonary and Critical Care Section,
and Director of Medical Critical Care,
Yale University School of Medicine,
New Haven, CT, USA

Jeffrey H. Silverstein MD, CIP
Professor, Vice-Chair for Research,
Anesthesiology; Associate Dean for Research,
Mount Sinai School of Medicine

Murali Sivarajan MD
Professor, Anesthesiology and Pain Medicine,
University of Washington, Seattle, WA, USA

Karen Souter MD
Associate Professor, Department of Anesthesiology
and Pain Medicine, University of Washington,
Seattle, USA

Thomas Specht MD
Chair, California Society of Anesthesiologists'
Committee on Physicians' Health and Well-Being

Andrea Trescot MD
Professor, Department of Anesthesia
and Pain Medicine, University of Washington,
Seattle, WA, USA

Gail A. Van Norman MD
Professor of Anesthesiology and Pain Medicine and
Adjunct Professor of Biomedical Ethics, University of
Washington, Seattle, Washington, USA

A.M. Viens BA, BPhil
School of Law, Queen Mary, University of London,
Queen Mary Centre for Medical Ethics and Law,
London, UK and Joint Centre for Bioethics,
University of Toronto, Canada

Elizabeth K. Vig MD MPH
Assistant Professor, Medicine,
Gerontology and Geriatric Medicine
University of Washington and VA Puget
Sound Health Care System, Seattle, WA, USA

David B. Waisel MD
Senior Associate in Anesthesia, Children's Hospital
Boston, and Associate Professor of Anaesthesia,
Harvard Medical School, Boston, MA, USA

Clarence Ward MD
California Society of Addiction Medicine

James M. West MD, MA
Clinical Assistant Professor, Human Values and Ethics
Assistant Professor, Anesthesiology
University of Tennessee Health Science Center
Memphis, Tennessee, USA

Richard L. Wolman MD, MA
Professor, Department of Anesthesiology, University
of Wisconsin School of Medicine and Public Health,
Madison, WI, USA

Steve Yentis BSc MBBS FRCA MD MA
Consultant Obstetric Anaesthetist, Chelsea and
Westminster Hospital, and Honorary Senior Lecturer,
Imperial College London, London, UK;
Editor-in-Chief, *Anaesthesia*

Foreword

The medical profession has had, virtually since its inception, codes of behavior and rules of conduct encompassing the physician's obligations to patients, colleagues and society. Classic versions of the Hippocratic Oath include exhortations to "do good," "avoid harm," and "remain free of intentional injustice," three of the classic principles that are cited as the core of the moral practice of medicine even to this day. Modern medical practitioners have significant power, social importance and financial impact that affect nearly everyone's lives. Medical practice crosses national boundaries, cultural enclaves and systems of spiritual beliefs. A fundamental challenge to the modern physician is achieving balance among patient values and needs, societal costs, and professional standards and codes. Given the vast range of medical need, cultural beliefs and available resources, this challenge to practitioners of all medical specialties globally is daunting.

Anesthesiologists and Bioethics

While the moral foundation of medical practice has been long recognized, the *study* of bioethics is relatively new in the history of medicine, having solidified in the late 1970s. Ethical issues are common to all medical specialties, but the specialty of anesthesiology has been at the forefront of bioethics, being among the first historically to raise critical moral questions. In 1957, Pope Pius XII was invited to address the International Congress of Anesthesiologists about such fundamental issues as whether the use of artificial respiratory equipment was required in even hopeless cases, whether the physician was under obligation to remove such therapy if such withdrawal will result in imminent patient death, and whether permanently comatose patients can be considered dead even before circulation has ceased. John J. Bonica, first chair of Anesthesiology at the University of Washington in Seattle was an early advocate for labor analgesia, at a time when religious institutions considered pain relief for laboring women morally controversial. He was later honored by Pope John Paul II "for contribution to the improvement of the welfare of people worldwide." Henry Knowles Beecher MD, first chair of the Massachusetts General Hospital, famously exposed breaches of the Nuremberg Code in human research being conducted in the United States, leading to the establishment of human subjects review boards. He later chaired the Ad Hoc Committee of the Harvard Medical School that offered a definition of brain death, paving the way for withdrawal/withholding of life-sustaining care at end-of-life, and facilitating developments that made vital organ transplantation possible.

The clinical practice of anesthesiology includes many of the thorniest problems in medical ethics. Anesthesiologists practice in operating rooms involving care that has profound impact on patients' lives at a time when their ability to participate in decision-making may be severely limited. Many anesthesiologists practice in intensive care units, where end-of-life decision-making occurs, including withdrawal and withholding of life-sustaining therapies, resuscitation and do-not-resuscitate orders, and initiation of vital organ transplantation. Anesthesiologists are involved in obstetrical care, where the interests of mothers and fetuses may not always be aligned. They are experts in the treatment of acute, chronic, oncologic and palliative pain. They are researchers, authors and editors of medical journals. They are on the front lines in caring for the casualties of war and natural and man-made disasters. It is no surprise therefore that anesthesiologists have posed some of the most troubling ethical questions confronting modern medicine.

Ethical Theory

The classical style of medical practice until well into the 20th century was paternalistic. Doctors did what they considered best for patients, and patients usually complied. Such paternalism was derived from 'virtue-based' ethics, in which the physician was assumed to be a virtuous person with inherent qualities of competence, sincerity, and altruism, and who would naturally know what was correct for the patient.

In parallel with the rise of individualism, and political activism surrounding human rights, the discipline of bioethics has increasingly emphasized respect for the definition, integrity and autonomy of persons. This has been expressed in bioethics as an emphasis on appropriate consent free from moral, economic, politic, scientific, or social pressures. Medicine is too often practiced as a predominantly technical pursuit, however, and the education of physicians in the art of communication with patients has lagged behind the demands of society. Physicians are accustomed to explaining medical conditions to their patients, but the quality of their conversations concerning the patient's functional status, values or fears is often poor or even non-existent.

Medical practice that minimizes the core of human interactions could be seen as a breach to patient dignity. As patients, we would certainly not like to be treated by physicians who are lacking concern for the humane components of medicine. A respectful and proper way of practicing medicine therefore should lead us not only to concentrate on the *hows* of performing ours tasks, but also on the *whys* that govern our care to unique individuals.

In this regard, growing attention has been paid to the ethical dimensions of medical care, and how we can improve the fulfillment of our duties to patients. The publication and wide acceptance of *Principles of Biomedical Ethics* by James F. Childress and Tom Beauchamp more than thirty years ago was certainly a cornerstone event for what became an authentic discipline. They described cardinal ethical principles (*Autonomy, Beneficence, Nonmaleficence* and *Justice*) that are now routinely discussed and debated among medical professionals.

Although there is general acceptance of these principles as being foundational to ethical medical care, the exact *prioritization* of these principles is not as clear or accepted. Ask virtually any physician in the United States about the order of importance of these ethical principles, and the answer will be "Autonomy first, then Beneficence, Nonmaleficence and Justice." However, if we consider French-speaking textbooks, these principles are usually presented in a different order: Beneficence, Nonmaleficence, then Autonomy and Justice. Among certain Pacific Island cultures, where community values receive more emphasis than individual needs, *autonomy* might not be recognized as an ethical principle at all.

What could be the cause of these differences? In the case of the French physician, has there been difficulty or lag in shifting from a purely paternalistic logic to a contract-based logic? Or a cultural-based reluctance to consider autonomy the dominant relevant principle? Are Pacific Islanders "backward" in placing autonomy low and communitarianism high on the list of important principles? Accordingly, an excessive attention to the principle of respect for autonomy has the potential to prevent us from striving for humanism, philosophy, and spirituality—and thereby promoting a true *therapeutic alliance* between the physician and the patient.

The aims and limits of beneficence are well known. Though intended to protect the vulnerable, and ensure justice, a "beneficence" that is disrespectful of autonomy is unfair, representing a throwback to the paternalism of the past. However, there is a growing realization that over-attention to autonomy which is not imbued with beneficence is also unfair. We, as health care professionals, have an obligation to respect the common good, with a fair balance between empowerment of patients and the concepts of beneficence and nonmaleficence.

In an opinion on education in medical ethics, the French National Ethics Advisory Committee (available at http://www.ccne-ethique.fr), indicated four legitimate reasons for a "disquiet" in the field of bioethics, linked to:

- a depersonalizing effect of specialization, that might limit true chances of personal relationships between the patient and his/her physician,
- a relative eclipse of the clinical side of medicine because of the increasing technology of medicine,
- an emerging form of "excessive legalism" with judiciarisation of the relationships, a symptom of poor quality of communication, as "respect for patients is no longer dependent on the individual virtues of the doctor; it is commanded by the need to observe the law",
- and finally, side effects of apportioning health care, with a need for an ethical reflection linked to the attention for collective accountability of health care expenses.

Ethical concerns, though not limited to these questions, should be seen as an opportunity to share, in harmony, a common understanding of medicine among physicians and their patients. Among the values that are at the core of bioethics, promoting dignity, with its tensions between means and ends is of special interest.

The Concept of Dignity and Medical Ethics

Dignity is a concept not restricted to the medical field. It encompasses good manners and morals. For a politician, it might mean putting national above personal interests, although it cannot be restricted to a battle between "my" autonomy and the collective interests of a group. Human dignity is a complex concept that many believe is the very core of bioethics. It is present in numerous international texts such as the Universal Declaration on the Human Genome and Human Rights (1997), or the Oviedo convention, but can be found as early as in the opening of the Preamble of the 1948 Universal Declaration of Human Rights of the United Nations ("*Whereas recognition of the inherent dignity and of the equal and inalienable rights of all members of the human family is the foundation of freedom, justice and peace in the world*"), as well as in its first Article ("*All human beings are born free and equal in dignity and rights. They are endowed with reason and conscience and should act towards one another in a spirit of brotherhood.*").

Dignity however is difficult to define. Like the cardinal principles of bioethics, it is rooted in practical grounds (preventing abuses) but it is also aiming for a clear respect for principles and values. Dignity is somewhat ambiguous, as it can be understood to be:

- a *quality* (dignitas) attached to a rank or an official position (dignitaries);
- a *general principle* protecting the sovereignty of humans. Dignity here, seen as humanity (i.e. what behavior I expect from my fellow human), would be taken as the concept of equal dignity of all humans;
- an *individual claim* defined by the person itself, that can be used to request new "rights." In this regard we will each have a personal or cultural idea of what dignity is. Special requests have for example been claimed by persons requesting a right to "die with dignity", because they believe that their dignity is now lost and that consequently they have the "right" to obtain euthanasia.

Dignity, furthermore, is a characteristic that *cannot* be suppressed. Even if we consider the horror of Nazi concentration camps, the prisoners held there--although they were inhumanely treated--did not loose their human dignity.

One of the difficulties (and beauty) of the concept of dignity, is that it possesses all of these various meanings. Taken as a general principle, it infers that it is a collective or community characteristic to be protected against external aggressions. But it also represents an individual claim--a means to promote the individual's conception of liberty.

Thus, in human interactions, and in medical practice, there is tension between the good (or dignity) of the group versus the good (or dignity) of a single individual. In this respect, if we consider the four cardinal bioethics principles, would the concept of dignity be more aligned with the *autonomy* of the individual, or the *justice* of the group? If justice is defined as *the promotion of dignity* (with the goal of first promoting equity and equality of chances, and then fighting against discriminations), we find a harmonious agreement that is valid with the different theories of justice, whether the theory be procedural (libertarian), utilitarism ("classic" economic reasoning), egalitarism of primary goods (as expressed by John Rawls), egalitarism of "capabilities" (as expressed by Amartya Sen), or even elitism of merit.

Promotion of human dignity plays out differently in different cultural settings. Comparing Western and Eastern philosophy, the classic: "I think, therefore I am", could be transposed for Eastern philosophers to: "*You are*, therefore I am". An understanding of these differences can be very useful in light of a trans-cultural approach to medical care. To enhance understanding between physicians and patients, we must discuss and promote the idea, not only of simple information and communication, but of true and mature dialogue about our differences. And dialogue is not enough. It is merely a means, a tool towards the goal of ensuring relationships and bonds between us.

Dignity is a "human common denominator" in the promotion of peace and harmony. It encompasses the usual means of communication of culture (through Art, Science, or Prayer), but avoids the accusation that could have been made against culture of not furthering integration ("...*culture does not unite. It identifies, therefore it divides as much as it assembles. The word is ambiguous*" says Alain Lamassoure, member of the European parliament).

In the philosophic understanding of bioethical principles in the practice of medicine, issues are probably more complex even than imagined. Although progress could mistakenly be seen as ever increasing control over life, *authentic* control is knowing where to stop and think about what *ought* to be done, and not just what *can* be done. The beauty of a mature, ethical practice of medicine is that it unites humans while respecting cultural specificities of individuals, by taking reference in our common humanity and through the promotion of dignity.

This textbook attempts to explore many of the issues that confront the modern anesthesiologist, even when those issues cause great uneasiness. They include the variability of autonomy (in vulnerable persons), and respect for autonomy (via consent) in medical practice, along with ideals of communitarianism (in Native American culture). End of life issues include not only concepts of death (e.g. brain death) and turning off bioprosthetic devices, such as pacers and ICDs, but the idea that physicians play a role in understanding and promoting humane legislation to protect dignity at end-of-life. Cultural differences are examined in the management of pain in addicted patients. Critical research issues are discussed, including new and more global concepts concerning the "rights" and interests of animals in research and our obligations to them, as well as the problem of unethical publication practices. Issues of considerable discomfort are scrutinized, such as physician participation in torture, disaster and military triage, and lethal injections of prisoners.

All are presented from the perspective of anesthesia practice in all of its breadth, and by a wide range of experts from Canada, Europe and the United States. Some questions have clear answers that are already incorporated widely into practice. For other questions, the answers are not as evident. For still others, anesthesiologists may not have widely adopted correct moral behaviors, even when there is global consensus about what such behaviors should be. For all, the exploration of moral questions occurring in anesthesia practice involves consideration and balance of the ethical principles of medicine—respect for patient autonomy, beneficence, nonmaleficence and justice—in the promotion of human dignity, for our patients as well as for ourselves.

Sadek Beloucif, France
Gail A. Van Norman, United States

Preface

Anesthesiologists have broad representation in private and academic clinical practices, clinical and laboratory research settings, intensive care units, palliative care facilities, pain treatment centers, journal review boards, and expert panels charged with legislative initiatives and practice guidelines, to name a few. Ethical questions abound in all walks of anesthesia practice; this is abundantly clear to the editors of this book, all of whom have been members and/or chairs of the American Society of Anesthesiologist's Committee on Ethics since its inception in the early 1990s*. The committee receives a steady flow of communications from anesthesiologists seeking answers to questions, wanting someone to vent their frustrations to, and/or asking for reassurance that they "did the right thing." It is moving testimony to the importance ethical principles hold for most members of the specialty.

But while the importance of physician understanding of ethical principles in the practice of medicine is almost universally recognized, few resources exist specific to anesthesia practice or the issues facing anesthesiologists in other settings. This textbook respectfully follows the footsteps of such books as Draper and Scott (*Ethics in Anaesthesia and Intensive Care*, Butterworth-Heineman 2003), and Scott, Vickers and Draper (*Ethical Issues in Anaesthesia*, Butterworth-Heineman, 1994).

While the ethical issues facing anesthesiologists are a numerous and varied as anesthesia practice itself, some general themes emerge. We considered issues roughly (and admittedly artificially) divided into 6 categories. In Section 1 (Informed consent and refusal), common issues such as Do-not-resuscitate orders, and the Jehovah's Witness patient are covered as are more controversial issues, such as anesthesiology involvement in female circumcision. Maternal-fetal issues

are explored in the context of "Ulysses directives" and maternal demand for cesarean section delivery. Consent issues in non-Westernized cultures where autonomy may not be the dominant principle are reviewed. In Section 2 (End-of-life issues), withholding and withdrawing treatments includes considerations of discontinuing cardiac assist devices, organ transplantation issues such as donation-after-cardiac death (DCD) and the legislative efforts of anesthesiology experts, and euthanasia. Section 3 (Pain management) includes different considerations in management of addicted patients in the UK and US settings. In Section 4 (Ethical issues in research and publication), controversial topics concerning the treatment of animals and animal rights are included, as are the relatively new debates around quality improvement initiatives as research, and the pivotal roles of authors, editors and reviewers in publishing medical information. Dealing with the addicted or disabled provider, sleep deprivation, industry gifts to physicians, disclosure of errors to patients, and physician conscientious objection are covered in Section 5. Section 6 concerns anesthesiologists in their roles and duties within the state: expert testimony, response to disasters, ethical issues in the military, torture, and physician involvement in lethal injection of prisoners.

Physicians are educated in their art by study and contemplation, but also, if not primarily, by involvement in and discussion of cases and their management. Highly abstract analyses of ethical issues is not always well understood or received because physicians deal in real-life situations, and seek both practical understanding and advice. For the most part, we have tried to imitate and emphasize the case-based nature of medical education throughout the book. Chapters begin with a case example. By reading the case and subsequent discussion, the authors have attempted to discuss the major issues and principles involved in each case. Where possible, they have proposed some example resolutions, and a list of important points close each chapter. While it is not possible to anticipate the entire

---

* This contents of this book are not a product of the American Society of Anesthesiologists and does not, except where noted by references in the text, represent official policies, guidelines, or statements of the American Society of Anesthesiologists.

scope of complexity of ethical issues that might present in any one case, it is our goal that the discussion fosters thoughtful reflection and aids the physician in future case management.

Because even among Western countries, the perspectives on ethical controversies in medicine are not always in agreement, we have purposefully sought authors from different nationalities, educational backgrounds, and practice experiences to provide international breadth to the book. Whenever possible, resources are cited regarding management in both US and European settings.

The chapter discussions are not meant to provide an exhaustive list of references for each and every issue—to do so would add unnecessarily to the volume of the book, and distract from the main purpose, which is both philosophical and practical discussion. Where needed, we have supplied in the References at the end of each chapter any key resources. Other important, but non-cited readings are included in a "Further reading list" to aid readers in expanding their knowledge of specific topics. In both of these lists, those readings felt to be especially helpful, historic, or even controversial are highlighted with an asterisk.

I would like to personally acknowledge all of the wonderful people who contributed so substantially to the creation of this book. Stephen Jackson and Susan Palmer introduced me to the discipline of medical ethics through their brilliant and compassionate teaching and leadership. Stanley Rosenbaum has been the intellectual and ethical foil, and wonderful friend that all students should be as lucky as I was to find early in their studies. Not only has each been a teacher and friend to me for many years, each has worked tirelessly to write, edit, and provide "moral" support throughout the production of this book. Sadek Beloucif has graciously and patiently providing insights about the different perspectives in Western medical ethics. A host of learned authors and ethics experts willingly and generously contributed their time and effort—many of them meeting last-minute requests and short deadlines to provide chapters and changes. They all have my heartfelt thanks.

From Cambridge University Press, thank you also to Nick Dunton, who embraced the idea, and to Deborah Russell, Laura Wood, Rachael Lazenby, Nisha Doshi and Mary Sanders, who kept it going, to Jonathan Ratcliffe who didn't complain about all of the changes, and everyone of the wonderful production staff who made this book possible.

Gail A. Van Norman MD
Seattle, WA USA
Summer, 2010

Section 1

Consent and refusal

DISCOVERY LIBRARY
LEVEL 5 SWCC
DERRIFORD HOSPITAL
DERRIFORD ROAD
PLYMOUTH
PL6 8DH

Informed consent: respecting patient autonomy

Gail A. Van Norman

The Case

Allen, a 35-year-old man, presents for colectomy after a 20-year history of ulcerative colitis. He does not appear nervous, but is animated and friendly. His sister explains that Allen has developmental delay and is also fearful of needles. He has permitted the nurse to start an intravenous drip. Discussion of an epidural for anesthesia and analgesia with Alan will take extra time, and the anesthesiologist is also concerned that he may not have the necessary self-control to cooperate with an epidural. She decides to discuss only general anesthesia and patient-controlled analgesia with the sister.

Moral imperatives for informed consent in Western medicine and medical research are founded in the ethical principle of respect for patient autonomy. The term "autonomy" comes from the Greek *autos (self)* and *nomos (rule)*. Originally used to describe political self-governance, "autonomy" also has come to be associated with individuals. This concept of self-determination has attained a powerful vocabulary in Western culture, evoking debates over liberty, privacy, free will, rights and responsibilities. Freedom to choose one's destiny is a prominent Western ideology. There is broad moral and legal consensus that this freedom is essential when such choices involve medical treatment.

Of the four "foundational" principles in medical ethics – beneficence, nonmaleficence, respect for autonomy, and justice – the principle with the strongest influence in the United States is respect for personal autonomy. Many ethical questions in US medical practice will be answered by asking foremost what the patient *wants*, and not necessarily what the physician, family, or culture believe is *best*. Respect for autonomy is a key principle in other Western nations as well, but it is usually weighed against the other three principles. Thus, the same ethical question may be answered in other Western countries by asking not only what the patient *wants*, but also what is *best* for them according to their family, society, and reasonable medical resources. Non-Western cultures often depart almost completely from an "autonomy"-based ethic of informed consent, and resort to a more "collectivist" decision-making model, in which families and groups make decisions together, based on obligations to care for one another, concepts of preservation of harmony, and values of group interdependence. (A summary of cultural aspects of medical decision-making in Pacific Islander and Asian cultures can be found in Table 1.1, and a detailed account of Native American medical decision-making is explored in Chapter 13).

Many countries have codified patients' rights to be informed and to give or refuse consent regarding medical treatments (Table 1.2).

Although the Nuremberg Code is often cited as the origin of the modern physician's obligation to obtain informed consent, legal precedents enforcing patients' rights actually predate Nuremberg. In France, legal requirements for consent were established in 1910, and were reinforced by the French Supreme Court in 1942.[1] In the United States in 1914, the case of Schloendorff v. Society of New York Hospital established that "Every human being of sound mind and adult years has a right to determine what shall be done with his own body."[2]

Autonomy

Informed consent involves the concept of "personal autonomy" – a patient's ability to make choices – and "autonomous choice" – whether an autonomous patient's choice is made freely. Respect for patient autonomy involves not only ethical obligations to respect patient choices, but also obligations to *promote* both patient autonomy and autonomous choice.

Clinical Ethics in Anesthesiology: A Case-Based Textbook, ed. Gail A. Van Norman, Stephen Jackson, Stanley H. Rosenbaum and Susan K. Palmer. Published by Cambridge University Press. © Cambridge University Press 2011.

Table 1.1. Values emphasized in medical decision-making in some non-western cultures*

Japanese	• Collective family interests take priority over individual interests • Harmony must be preserved • The family is responsible to care for elders • Caring for parents must be done with deep feelings of gratitude and happiness • Shintoism is prominent – mention of death is taboo, discussing terminal illness may cause *kegare*, or spiritual contamination
Chinese	• Confucian concepts of harmony, unity, survival of the family • Hierarchical family relationships • Elders treated with respect and protected from bad news • Discussing illness or death may cause it to happen
Vietnamese	• Concept of karma and fatalistic attitudes towards illness and death • Individuals do not control their lifespan, advance directives are de-emphasized • Saying "no" to a physician may be disrespectful and could create disharmony
Filipino	• Filial piety • Illness may be "deserved," and seeking health care may be a "last resort" • Deference to the physician out of respect
Hawaiian	• Acceptance of medical condition • Western medicine is seen as autocratic • Holistic approach to health problems and collective decision-making
Samoan	• A specific decision-maker is designated • A chief may be asked to listen to the case and offer judgment • Mistrust of Western medicine • Traditional Samoans do not want to be asked preferences, desiring instead a directive physician.

Summarized from: McLaughlin, L.A. and Braun, K.L. (1998). Asian and pacific islander cultural values: considerations for health care decision-making. *Health and Soc Work*, **23**(2), 116–26.

Autonomous persons

The terms "capacity" and "competence" are both used to describe a group of capabilities necessary for decision-making. In the US, "capacity" usually is used by medical experts to describe functional capabilities, and "competence" is a legal term. In the United Kingdom, the usage is reversed, and "competence" usually refers to functional capacity, while "capacity" is a legal term.[3] In this chapter the terms are used interchangeably.

Capacity is a "threshold" element in informed consent. Without the ability to make decisions, a person is not autonomous. Capacity is task specific: patients may be fully capable of making medical decisions even if they are unable to care for themselves in other ways. Capacity waxes and wanes depending on many factors such as the patient's medical condition, psychological state, level of stress, and ability to orient to unfamiliar surroundings. Although any diagnosis of compromised mentation can interfere

with competence, *no* diagnosis in a conscious patient invariably identifies incompetence. The presence of memory impairment, dementia, or mental illness, for example, does not prove a lack of capacity to make medical decisions.

Physician paternalism and bias pervades assessments of patient competence. Patients are often referred for competency evaluations simply because they refuse medical advice, although such refusals are not generally evidence of incapacity.[4] In one study, noncompliant patients comprised almost two-thirds of referrals for competency evaluations, yet they were only slightly less likely than compliant patients to be judged incompetent by consultants. Patients who discharge themselves against medical advice from hospitals have a somewhat higher prevalence of alcohol abuse than the general population. However, studies have found that such actions are more often related to insurance status and lower income, or factors such as race (which might be associated with mistrust of physicians or

Table 1.2. Summary of patient rights to informed consent by country*

Country	Right to informed consent	Right to refuse treatment	Right to have written advance directives followed	Presumed consent in emergency situations if incapacitated	Therapeutic Privilege allowed	Patient can waiver right to know
Australia	√	√	√	√	√	√
Belgium	√	√	√	√		
Bulgaria	√	√ – must be in writing		√	Not recognized	√
Canada[11]	√	√	√		Controversial in common law[12]	
Cyprus	√	No explicit right to refuse	√	√	√	
Czech Republic	√	√			√ – at physician discretion	No express "right not to know"
Denmark	√	Only to refuse blood products, or if in a terminal condition	√ – only in specific circumstances		Illegal since 1998	√
Estonia	√	√		√	Not recognized	
Finland	√	√		√		
France	√	√				
Greece	√	√		Physician can override pt wishes		√
Hungary	√	√	√	√		√
Italy	√	√		√		
Israel[13]	√			√		√

Table 1.2. (Cont.)

Country	Right to informed consent	Right to refuse treatment	Right to have written advance directives followed	Presumed consent in emergency situations if incapacitated	Therapeutic Privilege allowed	Patient can waiver right to know
Japan[14]	√ physician must inform patient or family				√	√
Latvia	√	√		√		
Lithuania	√	√		√		√
Luxembourg	√	√		√		
Netherlands	√	√	√	√		
New Zealand[15]	√	√		√		√
Poland	√	No provision				
Portugal	√	√	No explicit rule, but would be acceptable under other laws	√	√	
Slovakia	√	√	√			√
Slovenia	√	√	√	√	√	√
South Africa	√	√				
Spain	√	√	√	√		√
Sweden	√	√				
UK[16]	√	√	√	√	√	√
United States[17]	√	√	√	√	√	√

* Obtained from the Centre for Biomedical Ethics and Law unless otherwise noted http://europatientsrights.eu and http://www.kuleuven.be

Spaces were left blank when there was no explicit provision in law according to the Centre for Biomedical Ethics and Law at the time of access to the website on March 1, 2010. Reader should note that provisions may nevertheless be implicit in other laws or regulations.

perceptions of disrespectful treatment) than to decisional incompetence.[5]

Physicians frequently judge patient competence based on their perception of the quality of a patient's decision. A recent study of physicians' attitudes toward patients who refuse cancer therapy found that physicians often regarded such decisions as "irrational," and therefore reflecting mental aberrations.[6] Such judgments place the physician's own values, prejudices, and perceptions about medical treatment and quality of life before those of the patient, and do not reflect appropriate respect for patient autonomy. The same study found that patients refuse medical therapy based on personal values and experience more than on medical facts alone. Most experts believe that quality of life measures are at least equal in relevance to medical outcomes in determining if treatment results meet patient needs.

In general, competence to make medical decisions is adjudged to be present when the patient meets four criteria: they can communicate a choice, understand the relevant information, appreciate the medical consequences of the decision, and reason about treatment decisions (see also Chapter 4). These criteria generally can be assessed in pre-operative conversations with patients, and do not usually require expert consultation. When there is conflicting evidence about patient competence, however, a formal evaluation may be helpful.

The anesthesiologist in our introductory case made a hasty judgment about whether Allen was capable of participating in a complete discussion of options for his anesthesia care. An actual conversation with Allen would have revealed to her that he is employed, and lives independently – although these circumstances do not guarantee he has capacity for medical decision-making. When asked, he says that he needs to have surgery because of his sick intestines, and that he understands that he could get cancer if he does not have the operation. He also hopes that the surgery will reduce his pain and diarrhea. He does not fear anesthesia; he has been through several operations before without problems. Because of his religious beliefs he does not fear death. Allen appears to be an autonomous person with capacity to decide – or at least participate to a great degree – in decisions about his care, and should be given a complete description of his options in language aimed at his level of understanding.

Temporary incapacity

Many common clinical factors, both temporary and permanent, can impair the capacity to make medical decisions. Examples include severe pain or anxiety, intoxication, head injury, organic brain disease, developmental delay, and young age. Criteria for capacity in such patients, however, are no different from in any other situation. Physicians have ethical obligations to promote autonomy by treating patients to restore capacity if possible. Anxious patients or those suffering from pain ideally should have anxiety and pain treated *prior* to informed consent discussions, because they may then be better capable of listening to options, discussing information, and making decisions. Patients retain autonomy even with premedication if they are able to meet the four criteria cited above. Withholding such treatment until a consent form is signed is cruel, probably coercive, and may cause such consent to be legally invalid as well.

If delaying surgery allows a patient suffering from a temporary incapacity to recover competence in a time frame such that the surgery is still meaningful, the surgery should be postponed. If an emergency surgery cannot be delayed for a patient with temporary incapacity, then the physician may need to locate a surrogate decision-maker, or proceed without consent in the best medical interests of the patient.

Autonomous choices

Three conditions must be met in order for an act (or choice) to be autonomous: a person must act with *intention*, with *understanding*, and *without controlling influences*.

Intention

Ethical theory regarding "intention" is complex, but generally speaking intentional acts require "planning," although not necessarily reflective thought or strategy. We do many things intentionally but without thought, such as reaching for a glass of water in order to drink, scratching an itch, or turning a page in a book.

Unintentional acts can result from accidents or habitual behavior, or even as a byproduct of an intentional act. Imagine that Mary presents with flank pain suggestive of a kidney stone. Her physician orders an intravenous pyelogram (IVP). After administration of the contrast agent and IV fluid, increased urine output washes the stone into the bladder. The IVP is negative, but Mary's pain is resolved. The physician intended to run the test to diagnose the cause of her pain and he intended to appropriately treat the condition responsible for it. Both things happened. The test was run according to plan, but pain relief occurred because of an unintended side effect of the test. Mary's pain relief was the result of an accident and not a result of intention, even though the outcome of the accident and the intended outcome of the physician's plan are the same.

Patients are asked explicitly and implicitly to consent to both intentional and unintentional acts by physicians. Intentional acts are broadly categorized as those acts that result in the expected outcomes. Unintentional acts are those acts that result in outcomes that are not expected or not desired, such as side effects, accidents, and medical catastrophes. When autonomous patients consent following adequate information about both the *known and intended*, and *known possible-but-unintended* outcomes of treatment (and they are not manipulated or coerced), then they can be said to have *intended* to consent to the potential unintended consequences of treatment. It would be difficult to assert that a patient *intended* to consent to outcomes about which they were not informed. A patient who is inadequately informed is therefore *not* making an autonomous choice because intention is a requirement for autonomous choice. Adequate information is key to promoting patient autonomy, but what constitutes "adequate information"?

What the physician must disclose

It was not until the mid twentieth century that a legal obligation to *inform* patients prior to obtaining consent was established. In Salgo v Trustees of Leland Stanford Hospital[7] it was found that physicians must discuss risks and alternatives to treatment, as well as describe the procedures and their consequences. This finding was reinforced in Canterbury v Spence in 1972, which determined:

> … it is evident that it is normally impossible to obtain a consent worthy of the name unless the physician first elucidates the options and the perils for the patient's edification.[8]

Physicians argued that the courts had imposed an impossible burden: explaining *all* of the possible risks and outcomes of procedures would be tantamount to providing the patient with a medical education. Patients were neither knowledgeable, nor educable to the level of detail needed to make "competent" medical decisions. Subsequent court findings disagreed. In Harnish v Children's Hospital Medical Center, the duty to inform patients was further clarified:

> A physician owes to his patient the duty to disclose in a reasonable manner all significant medical information *that the physician possesses or reasonably should possess* that is *material* to an intelligent decision by the patient whether to undergo a proposed procedure.[9] [italics added]

Without knowing exactly what information is "material" to a patient, one potential strategy could be to simply recite as many relevant medical facts as possible to obtain consent and avoid liability later on. With regard to patient decision-making, however, it is important to understand that **not all medical facts are material ones and not all material facts are medical ones.** Patients base decisions on a number of matters, only some of which are medical facts. They also consider the potential medical and nonmedical outcomes of the treatment in the context of their lives, personal values, and personal experiences, as in the following scenario:

Ann and Sarah, each 39 years old, have a 1.5 cm breast cancer. Both are weighing the same options: lumpectomy with adjunctive chemotherapy, or mastectomy with chemotherapy. Each treatment is associated with similar cure rates. Ann decides to undergo lumpectomy based on her priorities of minimizing surgical recovery and disfigurement, as well as her confidence that the chance of recurrent cancer is small. Sarah also worries about disfigurement, but is more concerned about cancer recurrence because her mother died of breast cancer after protracted treatment and significant suffering. She requests bilateral mastectomies to ease her fears of experiencing bilateral cancer. Relatively few of the medical facts are actually material to either woman's decision – and even thought the facts are the same in each case, the decision is not. The presence of cancer, recurrence rates, and the potential cure rates of each type of proposed surgery are material to both women. Potential disfigurement from the surgery is also material to both – and this becomes decisive for Ann. But for Sarah, other nonmedical issues, such as her experience of her mother's death and how it affected her perceptions and fears about breast cancer and cancer treatment, are both material and decisive.

An exhaustive presentation of nonmaterial medical information not only dilutes medical information that is essential to a patient's decision, but also potentially neglects "non-medical" information that is also critical to the patient's decision. Physicians are expected to discuss the proposed treatment and reasonable alternatives. Common risks should be discussed because they are likely to occur and the patient should be given a chance to consider those possibilities. Nausea and vomiting, pain, dental damage, sore throat, and adverse drug reactions are examples of some common risks that might be discussed. Serious risks, even if rare, should be disclosed because such serious harm may be material to the patient's decision. Stroke, blindness, major cardiac events, cardiac arrests, and death are examples of serious risks that could be addressed. Physicians should also attempt to discover what other issues are germane to the patient: asking the patient about their questions, fears and special concerns may uncover other questions that are important to clarify.

Autonomous choice: the effects of coercion, manipulation, and persuasion

Even when acting with intention and understanding, autonomous persons can make nonautonomous choices. The bank teller who is forced at gunpoint to hand over money is an autonomous person, but she is being forced by the robber to make a choice against her will – to give up the money or risk being killed. *She* is autonomous, but her *choice* is not. She acts both with intention and understanding, but is under the irresistible power of a controlling influence. In the informed consent process, physicians have ethical obligations to avoid controlling influences that invalidate autonomous choice.

Coercion

Coercion occurs if one person both *intentionally* and *successfully* influences another by making a believable threat of harm that is sufficiently severe such that the other person is unable to resist acting to avoid it. Because it controls the other person's actions and usurps autonomy, coercion is unethical. Even if it is not successful, attempting to coerce someone demonstrates a lack of respect for patient autonomy and is unethical.

Not all threats are coercive. For a threat to be coercive, the threatened person must understand it, believe that it will be carried out, and be unable to resist it. Threatened harms can include physical, psychological, social, legal, and financial harms, among others. Perceptions about what constitutes a believable threat and sufficient harm are subjective and vary from person to person – some threats are universal enough to

coerce almost any persons, while others are selective enough to only coerce a few. Furthermore, *circumstances* that restrict personal choice are not "coercive," because circumstances are not persons and cannot have intentions. A patient who requires surgery to relieve a bowel obstruction is confronted with few viable choices and therefore is not entirely "free", but a choice to undergo surgery can still be autonomous, because within the framework of the circumstances the person can act with intention, with understanding, and without being controlled by the will of other persons.

Coercion is not uncommon in anesthesia and surgical practice. Consider Mr. Forrest, an 85-year-old man with metastatic colon cancer, who has a large bowel obstruction, severe pain and discomfort, and requires palliative surgery. He has requested a do-not-resuscitate (DNR) order because of his terminal disease. Mr. Smith sincerely hopes to survive his surgery, but he understands that death is a risk. He knows that both his age and his diagnosis make his prospects of surviving a cardiac arrest grim. Furthermore, he believes that death under anesthesia, while not his *intended* goal, would be an acceptable and possibly humane outcome, and he consents to it. But the anesthesiologist refuses to proceed unless Mr. Smith rescinds his DNR order, even though cardiopulmonary resuscitation (CPR) is not integral to treating bowel obstruction *per se*. The anesthesiologist is presenting Mr. Smith with a credible threat of harm, and she certainly is capable of carrying out that threat by preventing surgery that will relieve Mr. Smith's pain. The threat is sufficiently severe that Mr. Smith ultimately is controlled by it and agrees to rescind his DNR status. The anesthesiologist has intentionally and unethically coerced him into accepting a treatment he does not want (CPR) and likely will not need, in order to obtain treatment that he both wants and does need (bowel resection). (For a more detailed discussion of DNR orders in the operating room, see Chapter 2.)

Persuasion

Persuasion is a noncontrolling (resistible) form of influence in which one person *intentionally* and *successfully* uses reason to induce another person to freely and willingly accept the beliefs, intentions, and actions of the persuader. Persuasion is an integral part of informed consent as, for example, when the anesthesiologist recommends epidural anesthesia over general anesthesia for an elective Cesarean section, due to the advantages of maternal–infant bonding immediately after birth, the possibility of epidural narcotic analgesia for postoperative pain relief and a perception of decreased risks to mother from pulmonary aspiration. For such a recommendation to qualify as persuasion and not manipulation, it must present accurate and balanced information, and must be resistible by the patient (that is, the patient can choose not to follow the recommendation).

Persuasion is entirely ethical. Patients expect physicians to make rational recommendations about medical treatments and alternatives. In fact, physicians may even be held legally liable and morally culpable if they do not at least attempt to persuade their patients to consent to treatments that are medically indicated.

Manipulation

Between persuasion and coercion lies a group of influential behaviors included under the broad definition of "manipulation," including indoctrination, seduction, deception, omissions, and lies. In general, manipulation strategies work by either altering actual choices provided to patients, or by altering patient's perceptions of their choices.

The degree of control exerted by manipulation (and therefore the degree to which manipulation interferes with patient autonomy) ranges from inconsequential to completely controlling. Not all attempts at manipulation succeed, but many if not all manipulative strategies involve deception, either through false or misleading information or omission of key facts. Manipulation is therefore unethical whether it is successful or not, because it both violates ethical obligations of veracity (telling patients the truth) and disrespects patient autonomy.

In the case introducing this chapter, the anesthesiologist has engaged in manipulation by not describing the benefits and risks of epidural anesthesia and analgesia, even though it is a common anesthetic alternative. Had she discussed this option, she would have discovered that Allen in fact had opted for an epidural for previous bowel surgery, and had done well. By omitting the discussion in order to meet her own goals, she has altered Allen's actual choice, since Allen would probably have chosen to have an epidural if he knew it were possible.

Now, suppose instead that a patient who is a heavy smoker presents for total knee arthroplasty. The anesthesiologist wants to do a subarachnoid block (SAB). She does discuss both general anesthesia and SAB. However, she states that "spinal anesthesia is much safer in for knee replacements," and "spinal anesthesia is much safer in smokers." This is an example of manipulation by creating a false perspective of the patient's choices. There is no strong evidence that SAB is safer for most surgeries or safer in smokers, and the statement inaccurately portrays the comparative risks and benefits of these two anesthetic options. Once again, this anesthesiologist has attempted to manipulate the patient, and has disrespected the patient's autonomy.

Therapeutic privilege and waiver of informed consent

Two exceptions may exist to the rule that competent patients must have risks disclosed to them: the concept of therapeutic privilege and the idea that competent patients may waive their rights to be informed.

In evoking therapeutic privilege, physicians argue that it is ethical to withhold material information from patients in whom such disclosures would cause unacceptable harm, thus causing the physician to violate the ethical principle of nonmaleficence (avoiding harm). Accepting this general argument without restriction, however, is a prescription for paternalism. If the definition of "unacceptable harm" is framed too broadly, then physicians could conceivably justify withholding almost any information, because such disclosures are laden with at least some stress for most patients. Physicians even could use it as an excuse to "control" the decisions of patients whom they feel might refuse therapy after a full disclosure. If unacceptable harm is defined very narrowly as harm that causes the patient to become emotionally, psychologically, or intellectually incapable of making a decision, then therapeutic privilege does not technically violate the principle of respect for autonomy because full disclosure would render the patient nonautonomous anyway. The courts have recognized the risk of physician paternalism, and have reinforced the legal emphasis on respect for autonomy:

> The physician's privilege to withhold information for therapeutic reasons must be carefully circumscribed … for otherwise it might devour the disclosure rule itself. The privilege does not accept the paternalistic notion

that the physician may remain silent simply because divulgence might prompt the patient to forego therapy the physician feels the patient really needs. That attitude presumes instability or perversity for even the normal patient, and runs counter to the foundation principle that the patient should and ordinarily can make the choice for himself.[10]

Waiver of disclosure by the patient is conspicuously different from therapeutic privilege. An autonomous patient may decide intentionally, with understanding, and without controlling influences by others, to waive their rights to have medical information, or may decide to have the facts disclosed to someone else, such as a family member. Because their choice is an autonomous one, respecting such decisions respects patient autonomy, and is consistent with ethical practice. Legal ramifications of patient waiver have not, however, been clearly resolved in case law.

Key points

- The ethical principle of respect for patient autonomy is firmly grounded in western ethical principles valuing individual freedoms.
- Capacity, or competence, is a threshold element necessary to being an autonomous person: patients have capacity to make decisions if they can communicate a choice, understand the relevant information, appreciate the consequences of the decision and can reason about their decision.
- Physicians have ethical obligations to respect patient autonomy, and to promote autonomy when competence can be restored in a time frame that still renders the medical treatment meaningful.
- Disclosure is not required to be comprehensive: rather, ethical and legal disclosure discusses the treatment, reasonable alternatives, common risks and serious risks, as well as anything the physician knows or reasonably should know is material to the patient in making their decision.
- Coercion and manipulation are unethical because they violate the principle of respect for patient autonomy, and because manipulation often involves deception and violates physician obligations of veracity.

- Persuasion does not manipulate or control patient choice, and is consistent with ethical physician behavior.
- Therapeutic privilege and waiver of consent are possible exceptions to informed consent, but only under very restricted circumstances.

References

1* Moumjid, N. and Callu, M.F. (2003). Informed consent and risk communication in France. *BMJ*, **327**(7417),734–5.

2 Schloendorff v. Society of New York Hospital, 211 N.Y. 125, 105 N.E. 92 (1914).

3 Chalmers, J. (2008). Capacity. In *The Cambridge Textbook of Bioethics*, ed. Singer P. Cambridge, UK: Cambridge University Press, pp. 17–23.

4 Mebane, A.H. and Rouch, H.B. (1990). When do physicians request competency evaluations? *Psychosomatics*, **31**, 40–6.

5 Ibrahim, S.A., Kwoh, C.K., and Krishnan, E. (2007). Factors associated with patients who leave acute-care hospitals against medical advice. *Am J Public Health*, **97**(12), 2204–8.

6 van Kleffens, T. and van Leeuwen, E. (2005) Physicians' evaluations of patients' decisions to refuse oncological treatment. *J Med Ethics*, **31**,131–6.

7 Salgo v Leland Stanford, etc. Bd. Trustees, 154 Cal. App.2d 560.

8 Canterbury v Spence, 1972, 464 F.2d 772 (DC Cir. 1972).

9 Harnish V Children's Hospital Medical Center (1982). 387 Mass. 152, 429 N.E.240.

10 Canterbury v. Spence., 464 F.2d 772 (D.C. Cir. 1972).

11 Health Care Consent Act, 1996. S.O. 1996, Chapter 2, Schedule A. Canada. (last amended 2009).

12 Cote, A. (2000). Telling the truth? Disclosure, therapeutic privilege and intersexuality in children. *Health Law J*, **8**, 199–216.

13 Israel Patient Right's Act, 1996.

14 Akabayashi, A. and Slingsby, B.T. (2006). Informed consent revisited: Japan and the US. *Am J Bioethics*, **6**(1), 9–14.

15 Information and Consent. Medical Council of New Zealand. 2002. www.mcnz.org.nz.

16* General Medical Council Guidance for doctors. Consent: patients and doctors making decisions together. 2008 GMC, UK.

17 US case law; see chapter text.

Further reading

Appelbaum, P.S. (2007). Assessment of patients' competence to consent to treatment. *New Eng J Med*, **357**, 1834–40.

Badcott, D. (2005). The expert patient: valid recognition or false hope? *Med Health Care Philos*, **8**(2), 173–8.

Bird, S. (2004). Does my patient have capacity to consent to treatment? *Aust Fam Physician*, **33**(8), 638–9.

Council of Europe. Convention for the protection of human rights and dignity of the human being with regard to the application of biology and medicine: Convention on human rights and biomedicine. CETS no.: 164. Full text available at: http://conventions.coe.int/Treaty/Commun/QueVoulezVous.asp?NT=164&CL=ENG.

Earle, M. (1999). The future of informed consent in British common law. *Eur J Health Law*, **6**, 235–48.

Faden, R. and Beauchamp, T.L. (1986). *A History and Theory of Informed Consent*. Oxford, UK: Oxford University Press Inc.

General Medical Council Guidance for doctors. Consent: patients and doctors making decisions together. 2008 GMC, UK. http://www.gmc-ul.rg/static/documents/consent/Consent_2008.pdf

Green, D. and MacKenzie, C.R. (2007). Nuances of informed consent: the paradigm of regional anesthesia. *HSS J*, **3**(1), 115–18.

Hedayat, K.M. (2007). The possibility of a universal declaration of biomedical ethics. *J Med Ethics*, **33**, 17–20.

McLaughlin, L.A. and Braun, K.L. (1998). Asian and pacific islander cultural values: considerations for health care decision making. *Health and Soc Work*, **23**(2), 116–26.

2 Informed refusal – DNR orders in the patient undergoing anesthesia and surgery and at the end-of-life

David M. Rothenberg

The Case

A 67-year-old male with oxygen-dependent COPD requires a series of electroconvulsive therapies (ECT) for severe depression refractory to medical therapy. The patient has consented to general anesthesia with mask ventilation for these procedures, but refuses endotracheal intubation irrespective if it might be life-sustaining in the event of respiratory or circulatory arrest. As such, he requests that a do-not-resuscitate (DNR) order be enacted and remain in place during the perioperative period and throughout the entirety of his hospitalization.

In 1960, cardiopulmonary resuscitation (CPR) was introduced to clinical practice and was intended to apply to those patients in whom their hearts were considered "too good to die." Unfortunately, the more liberal use of CPR in patients with hearts essentially "too poor to live" prompted ethical consideration of when CPR should be withheld, thus averting the situation whereby death, rather than life, was delayed.

The DNR order is founded on the ethical principle of respect for individual autonomy and the legal doctrine of informed consent. Autonomy to make one's own decisions regarding medical therapy is not a modern day concept. Indeed, John Stuart Mill proposed this idea in his 1869 treatise *On Liberty* in which he stated, "Considerations to aid his judgment, exhortations to strengthen his will, may be offered to him, even obtruded on him, by others; but he himself is the final judge. All errors which he is likely to commit against advice and warning, are far outweighed by the evil of allowing others to constrain him to what they deem his good."[1]

The doctrine of informed consent was defined by Justice Benjamin Cardozo in the case of *Schloendorff v Society of N.Y. Hospital*.[2] In this case a young woman, who consented only to a gynecological examination under ether anesthesia, was instead furtively subjected to uterine surgery. Justice Cardozo of the New York Court of Appeals described the wrong committed as a "trespass," emphatically stating "Every human being of adult years and sound mind has a right to determine what shall be done with his own body." A competent patient's refusal of treatment, including the request to refuse potentially life-sustaining therapy, must be honored. However, individual autonomy is not a legal or moral absolute and can be superceded by the state's rights to protect innocent third parties (e.g., minors), prevent suicide, and maintain the integrity of the medical profession. Concerns about maintaining the integrity of the medical profession and the individual integrity of physicians are often invoked in discussions of futility as it applies to a patient's DNR order.

The theory of medical futility originated in the ancient philosophical teachings of Plato and was later espoused by Hippocrates, who stated that, in general, the role of medicine "is to do away with the sufferings of the sick, to lessen the violence of the diseases, and to refuse to treat those who are over-mastered by their diseases, realizing that in such cases medicine is powerless."[3]

The Council on Ethical and Judicial Affairs of the American Medical Association simply affirms Hippocratic dogma in stating: "When efforts to resuscitate a patient are judged by the treating physician to be futile, even if previously requested by the patient, CPR may be withheld."[4] Although the predominance of medical opinion continues to be that physicians are not and should not be required to provide futile treatment, defining futility may be a more difficult and critical task. It has been implied that medical futility should apply when there is an absence of at least a modicum of medical benefit or, in the setting of cardiac arrest, when the patient predictably has near

Clinical Ethics in Anesthesiology: A Case-Based Textbook, ed. Gail A. Van Norman, Stephen Jackson, Stanley H. Rosenbaum and Susan K. Palmer. Published by Cambridge University Press. © Cambridge University Press 2011.

0% survival after CPR. For patients with diseases such as metastatic cancer, acute stroke, sepsis, or multilobar pneumonia, CPR should probably not be offered in the event of a cardiac arrest. Schneiderman *et al.* suggested that, in terms of probability, futile therapy be defined as a chance of success being less than 1 in 100.[5] Although isolated cases of long-term survival in these instances may exist, if these occurrences are so rare as to be unexplainable and therefore have little predictive value, then this definition of futility would still apply.

In discussing futility, it is imperative to differentiate "physiologic" or "quantitative" definitions of futility – based on scientific data that suggest that CPR will not be effective – from more value-laden or "qualitative" definitions of futility, in which physicians may impart their own beliefs on what they perceive as the patient's preference, and suggest in this context that CPR is not worth attempting.

Within the framework of "physiologic" futility, a DNR order should be written and CPR should be withheld when an arrest occurs. Patients and/or their families should be informed of this decision, although to suggest that a choice exists could imply that there may be a potential benefit from CPR, inadvertently sending a mixed message. Respect for patient autonomy does not mean that patients have a right to demand nonbeneficial and potentially harmful treatment. Physicians who agree to such demands act purely on behalf of the patient's psychological welfare rather than on the patient's rights. Brody reiterates "that there are some questions of professional ethics that physicians are entitled to decide among themselves unilaterally. Regarding those matters, the society is entitled to decree that the profession of medicine will not be practiced in that way … But the society is not entitled to dictate to the profession the contents of professional integrity."[6] In protecting the integrity of the medical profession, however, public trust must not be compromised. DNR policies founded on the premise of cost containment tend to be value laden and, if implemented, are likely to foster a paternalistic approach to patient care, as well as to erode patient confidence that physicians are acting with their best interests in mind.

Guidelines for establishing standards of medical futility have been suggested in an effort to create an open dialogue with society, in general, and the medical community. These guidelines include (1) acknowledging that the word futility is widely used and (2) defining futility as a treatment that fails to achieve the goals of medicine. Social and medical acceptance of futility as it pertains to CPR can then hopefully be attained by using this definition in formal outcome studies.

DNR orders may be written based on physician assessment of futility, or based on patient request. The majority of patients who request DNR orders do so not because they wish to die, but rather as a reflection of how they perceive their quality of life before or after the resuscitation. Diminished quality of life has been defined as diminished capacity to resume work and/or impaired cognitive function specifically as it applies to awareness of one's environment. It has been shown that, in patients who survive critical illnesses, quality of life is worse if the patient requires CPR. Physical or mental impairment, chronic disability, or persistent vegetative states are additional reasons patients or their surrogates may request a DNR order. Patients also express desires for DNR orders when they believe that CPR will merely prolong the dying process. Irrespective of the reasons behind the decision, the individual patient's values are more relevant than those of the physician in determining resuscitation status when quality of life is the issue in question.

Physician insecurity in applying a DNR order has sometimes led to the ethically and medically inappropriate practice of the "slow-code" or "show code." Additionally, a DNR order should not be misinterpreted as an order to withhold or withdraw other vital therapies. Indeed, the misconception of this order to mean "do-not-round" has led to the suggestion that the order be renamed no-CPR, or do-not-attempt resuscitation, to convey the idea that even if CPR were to be initiated, the likelihood of success would be extremely low. A DNR order does not preclude the use of other life support therapies including, in selected instances, surgery or intensive care. Most recently a call for renaming these orders to "allow natural death" (AND) has been suggested in order to eschew the negative connotation of do-not-resuscitate.[7] The problem with this term is that it may inappropriately lead to the withholding of all other forms of therapy exclusive of CPR.

Our patient is justified in requesting a DNR order in advance of ECT as he perceives his life to be insufferable should he require prolonged mechanical ventilatory support. An argument for a physician-initiated

DNR or AND order based on medical futility does not apply because of a lack of scientific evidence citing survivability if this type of patient suffers a respiratory or cardiac arrest.

Combinations of both medical and social factors have led to the more frequent application of the DNR order both in a pre-hospital and in-hospital setting. An aging population with end-stage malignancies, stroke syndromes, multiple organ failure, and Alzheimer's dementia contributes to the growing use of the DNR order. They are also major social factors related to the enactment of patient's Self-Determination Act of 1990,[8] which mandated that all hospitals receiving Medicare reimbursements provide patients with information that would aid in their decisions regarding end-of-life issues such as a DNR order. As DNR orders continue to be written, it is inevitable that new ethical dilemmas will arise. Such dilemmas are increasingly common in the pre-hospital and pre-surgical settings.

Pre-hospital DNR orders

Pre-hospital DNR policies have emerged recently and serve three primary purposes: (1) to provide continued respect for patient autonomy following hospital discharge, (2) to prevent futile resuscitation efforts in the field, and (3) to protect the well-being of emergency medical service (EMS) personnel. Patients who maintain a DNR order following discharge from the hospital should have this order honored in a pre-hospital setting should an arrest occur at home or at a chronic care facility.

Attempts to clarify whether a patient has a pre-existing DNR order based on quality of life in an out-of-hospital setting may be difficult and time consuming. Therefore recommendations have been made to identify such patients preemptively, and include a DNR identification bracelet or "no-code" tattoo, or a central, computerized file system allowing EMS personnel to access and verify resuscitation status at the scene. In the event that the patient's wishes are unclear, full resuscitative measures often are instituted by medical rescue technicians irrespective of the probability of successful resuscitation. Emergency department physicians and ethicists have thus considered the need for a pre-hospital DNR policy based on medical futility. As of 1991 when the US Federal Patient Self-Determination Act was mandated, Montana was the only US state to have a policy that provided civil and criminal immunity for EMS technicians who terminated resuscitative efforts in good faith in the field. At that time, other states restricted the use of pre-hospital DNR orders to only hospice programs, patients being transferred between institutions or terminally ill patients. Difficulty was felt to arise in establishing the validity of an advance directive or the competency of a conscious patient who refused such therapies as endotracheal intubation or intravenous vasopressors.

As of 2002, however, 42 US states had enacted out-of-hospital DNR protocols based on scientifically validated studies assessing the futility of CPR in the field. Futility in a pre-hospital setting needs to be determined completely on a physiologic basis (as was previously discussed), and without value-laden quality of life judgments. Outcome data in these multiple, large studies indicate a near 0% survival if there is no return of spontaneous circulation in the field, especially in the setting of blunt trauma.[9] Although studies of these types seem to validate the definition of physiologic futility as it relates to CPR in the field, application of "termination of resuscitation rules" based solely on futility are not absolute. Significant variability regarding the timing of termination of resuscitative efforts and the pronouncement of death has been noted despite having defined rules, especially in large cities where many different base hospitals provide on-line medical control of EMS personnel during out-of-hospital cardiac arrest.

Finally, concern regarding the health of both EMS personnel and innocent bystanders during high-speed ambulance transports, the increase of risks of HIV and hepatitis B exposure during resuscitation, economic constraints in terms of use of limited resources (especially in small communities), and costs of futile resuscitation have all been offered as additional reasons to establish pre-hospital DNR policies. Although fear of medical liability, in concert with the public's expectations that EMS personnel will initiate and continue CPR, may have limited the use of pre-hospital DNR orders in the past, federal and/or widespread state adoption of such preset rules of out-of hospital termination of basic and advanced cardiac life support appear imminent.

Pre-anesthesia DNR orders

Patients with preexisting DNR orders often require anesthesia for surgical procedures necessitated by the need to improve quality of life. Common surgical procedures that are often performed as a means of palliation or comfort of care in patients with DNR orders include the following:

- Tracheostomy
- Indwelling central line access
- Feeding gastrostomy/jejunostomy
- Emergency surgery (hemorrhage, bowel obstruction, peritonitis).

In addition, it is not uncommon for patients with DNR orders to require an anesthetic for nonsurgical procedures such as electroconvulsive therapy as described for our patient. Given that the practice of anesthesiology is inseparable from the process of intraoperative resuscitation, an ethical dilemma may occur when a patient with a DNR order presents for surgery. In this setting automatic resuscitation may violate patient autonomy and give rise to a situation directly prohibited by the DNR order, whereas automatic withholding of life-support may mean ignoring a reversible complication, thus violating the spirit of patient's wishes.

Although arguments have been made in favor of maintaining the DNR order at the time of surgery, the majority of medical and ethical opinion favors a policy that has been best termed "required reconsideration."

In keeping with the philosophy of Mills, the anesthesiologist should stress to the patient that to have the greatest likelihood of surgical success, simple intraoperative interventions and/or resuscitation may be necessary. These may include pharmacologic reversal of residual anesthetic agents (e.g., naloxone for the respiratory depressant effects of opiates, or flumazenil for similar effects of benzodiazepines), antiarrhythmic therapy for iatrogenically induced arrhythmias (e.g., ventricular tachycardia secondary to either an accidental intravascular injection of a local anesthetic or direct myocardial irritation from a central venous catheter placement), or correction of hypoxemia due to accidental esophageal or unilateral bronchial intubation. The contention that these mishaps are more likely to result in an intraoperative arrest in a patient with a preexisting DNR order has not been substantiated. Indeed patients should understand that survival following resuscitation, specifically CPR, has been shown to be considerably improved if the arrest occurs in an operating room versus the general hospital ward. With these

"exhortations," it is hoped that most patients or their surrogates would opt to have the surgery performed with the DNR order temporarily suspended. Patients should be reassured that resuscitation measures would be employed only if necessary, and any form of life support would be discontinued if no longer required or no longer beneficial in reversing the patient's underlying condition. This approach also allows distinguishing between, and treatment of those arrests that are readily reversible and those in which resuscitation is physiologically futile.

Within the context of this "informed consent" discussion, the patient or surrogate is entitled to certain options as they relate to the pre-anesthesia DNR order. The patient may: agree to undergo the surgery with the DNR order temporarily suspended; undergo surgery but may stipulate that only specific resuscitative measures be used (e.g., vasopressors but no CPR or mask ventilation but no endotracheal intubation); refuse surgery unless the DNR order is maintained throughout the procedure, thus accepting the risk of potentially reversible causes of death. If the patient demands the last option, both surgeon (or in our patient's case, psychiatrist) and anesthesiologist must decide if it is proper to proceed without the ability to institute life-support measures should a complication occur. Although physicians are not obligated on moral or legal grounds to operate under these constraints, they do have a duty to try to secure other physicians to care for the patient, so as to avoid potential charges of patient abandonment.

The American Society of Anesthesiologists[10] and the American College of Surgeons[11] have drafted guidelines for the management of the patient with a presurgical DNR order. Although both societies have adopted a policy of "required reconsideration," neither offers recommendations for either postoperative resumption of the DNR order or discontinuation of life support should intraoperative CPR be necessary. Recommendations for weaning or terminating life support in this setting have been proposed by Franklin and Rothenberg.[12] Should resuscitation be required in the operating room, necessitating life support either in the form of mechanical ventilation, inotropic agents or vasopressors, then postoperatively, the patient should be transferred to an appropriate care area such as the intensive care unit, and an attempt to wean the patient from support should commence. This type of management should probably not take place in a post-anesthesia care unit where the discussion and enactment of possible termination of life support may be distressing to other recovering patients. Weaning should ideally be achieved within a reasonably short period (i.e., 24 hours) should the etiology of the arrest be iatrogenic or unrelated to the patient's underlying disease. If successful, the DNR order may be reinstated and the patient transferred to an appropriate care area.

Should the weaning process fail, then provisions for terminating life support should be considered. Prior preoperative discussions in this regard are essential so that patients and their families may be assuaged of their fears of being left on life support systems indefinitely. Appropriate medical consultation to ensure that the patient's condition is irreversible and to support the decision to withdraw support is encouraged. Constant communication with the patient and/or surrogates and documentation of these discussions in the medical record is also mandatory.

The actual termination of life support should be done in accordance with well-established guidelines and be conducted with the sole purpose of minimizing patient suffering.

Case resolution

Our patient agreed to undergo ECT and suspend his DNR order during the time surrounding his treatment and the immediate recovery period with the stipulation that should he require endotracheal intubation and mechanical ventilation, these supportive modalities would be discontinued in an expeditious fashion (24 hours). Appropriate sedative/analgesic therapies would be instituted if tracheal extubation would likely lead to respiratory and subsequent circulatory arrest, assuring comfort at the end-of-life and in keeping with the principle of the "double effect". The patient was able to successfully complete a series of eight treatments and was discharged from the hospital with a DNR to be maintained at his chronic care facility.

Key points

- DNR orders may be written if CPR would be physiologically futile, or at the request of patients who feel that CPR would result in poorer quality of life.
- Pre-hospital DNR orders to prevent futile or unwanted CPR in the field are becoming

increasingly common and are likely to be widely inacted.

- DNR orders in the setting of anesthesia and surgery should undergo "required consideration" in which the risks and benefits of resuscitation in the OR are reviewed and patient desires determined.
- When a patient desires that a DNR order be maintained during anesthesia and surgery, providers who feel they cannot proceed nevertheless have an obligation to try to secure alternative physicians who are willing to respect the DNR order.
- Plans should be formulated for postoperative resumption of the DNR order, if suspended, or for discontinuation of life support after intraoperative CPR if appropriate.

References

1* Mills, J.S. (1978) *On Liberty*. Indianapolis, IN; Hackett Publishing, p. 75.

2 Schloendorff v Society of NY Hospital, 105 N.E. 92, 1914.

3* Chadwick J, Mann WN (eds). *The Medical Works of Hippocrates*. (1950). Boston, MA: Blackwell Scientific.

4* Council on Ethical and Judicial Affairs, American Medical Association (1991). Guidelines for the appropriate use of do-not-resuscitate orders. *JAMA*, **265**, 1868–71.

5* Schneiderman, L.J., Jecker, N.S., and Jonsen, A.R. (1990). Medical futility: Its meaning and ethical complications. *Ann Intern Med*, **112**:949–53.

6* Brody, H. (1994). The physician's role in determining futility. *J Am Geriatr Soc*, **42**, 875–8.

7* Venneman, S.S., Narnor-Harris, P., Perish, M., and Hamilton, M. (2008). "Allow natural death" versus "do not resuscitate": three words that can change a life. *J Med Ethic*, **34**, 2–6.

8 Omnibus Budget Reconciliation Act of 1990, Public Law 101–508, Section 4751.

9* Vayrynen, T., Kuisma, M., Maatta, T., *et al.* (2007). Medical futility in asystolic out-of-hospital cardiac arrest. *Acta Anaesthesiol Scand*, **52**, 81–6.

10* Committee on Ethics, American Society of Anesthesiologists: Ethical guidelines for the anesthesia care of patients with do not resuscitate orders or other directives that limit treatment. American Society of Anesthesiologist Directory Members, Park Ridge, IL, ASA, 1994, pp. 746–7.

11 Committee on Ethics. (1994). American College of Surgeons: Statement on advance directives by patients: Do not resuscitate in the operating room. *Am Coll Surg Bull*, **79**, 29.

12* Franklin, C.M. and Rothenberg, D.M. (1992). Do-not-resuscitate orders in the presurgical patient. *J Clin Anesth*, **4**, 181–4.

Further reading

Bishop, J.P, Brothers, K.B., Perry, J.E. and Ahmad, A. (2010). Reviving the conversation around CPR/DNR. *Am J Bioeth*, **10**(1), 61–7.

Consent and refusal

3

Informed refusal – the Jehovah's Witness patient

James M. West

The Case

A 41-year-old female with hepatitis C cirrhosis complicated by hepato-pulmonary syndrome is listed for liver transplant. She has high priority status due to the severity of her pulmonary disease, which is usually reversible with liver transplant. Pertinent lab results are: hemoglobin 12, INR 1.1, bilirubin 1.0, creatinine 1.0 and platelet count 75 000. Her situation is further complicated by the fact that she is one of Jehovah's Witnesses and will not accept blood transfusions.

Should this patient be a candidate for a liver transplant, given the relatively common need for blood transfusion during the operation? What are the anesthesiologists' obligations to the patient, to themselves and even to other patients on the transplant recipient list? Is the decision to follow through with this case different from any other major surgeries, such as coronary artery bypass surgery or liver resection?

Jehovah's Witnesses

Jehovah's Witnesses (JWs) began as a Bible study group formed in 1870 by C.T. Russell in Allegheny, PA. They believe that God's name is Jehovah, which is an English translation of the name that appears in Hebrew texts. They also believe in the literal interpretation of the bible, except in cases in which it is obvious that it is allegorical. JWs believe that only one government is owed allegiance – God's Kingdom. They do not salute flags, serve in the military, or vote in political elections. They also believe we are living in the "last days" of the present system.[1]

Like many religions, JW beliefs and teachings have evolved as society has evolved. In 1945 there was a ban placed on blood transfusions based on three quotes from scripture:[2]

Genesis 9:3 - Every moving thing that liveth shall be meat for you; even as the green herb have I given you all things. But flesh with the life thereof, which is the blood thereof, shall ye not eat.

Leviticus 17:10–16 - … I will set my face against the soul that eateth any manner of blood, and will cut him off from among his people. … no soul of you shall eat blood, neither shall any stranger that sojourneth among you eat blood. … Ye shall eat the blood of no manner of flesh; for the life of all flesh is the blood thereof; whosoever eateth it shall be cut off.

Acts 15:28–29 - … that ye abstain from things sacrificed to idols, and from blood, and from things strangled, and from fornication; from which if ye keep yourselves, it shall be well with you. Fare ye well.

A 1951 article in *Watchtower*, a publication of the JW governing body, explained the ban:

" … when sugar solutions are given intravenously, it is called intravenous feeding. … the transfusion is feeding the patient blood and …(the patient) is **eating it (blood)** through his veins." [Bold type added]

Over the years, adaptation has been required to keep up with advances in medicine. Guidelines have been developed to help members deal with renal dialysis, cardiopulmonary bypass, blood harvesting including cell saver, acute normovolemic hemodilution, and autologous blood donation as well as organ transplant. See Table 3.1 for a timeline of significant events in the Jehovah's Witness faith.

Ethical principles

Ethical dilemmas can be examined in the context of the four basic principles of medical ethics defined by Beauchamp and Childress: (1) respect for autonomy – a norm of respecting the decision-making capacities of autonomous persons, (2) beneficence – a group of norms for balancing benefits against risks, (3) nonmaleficence - a norm of avoiding harm, and (4) justice – a group of norms for distributing benefits, risks, and costs fairly.[3] In the US, the principle of respect for patient autonomy is usually the most heavily weighted of the four, while in many European countries, the

Clinical Ethics in Anesthesiology: A Case-Based Textbook, ed. Gail A. Van Norman, Stephen Jackson, Stanley H. Rosenbaum and Susan K. Palmer. Published by Cambridge University Press. © Cambridge University Press 2011.

Table 3.1. Events in the history of the Jehovah's Witness church and transfusion

1870	Study group formed
1879	First Issue of Watchtower published
1901	Discovery of ABO blood groups
1914	First blood bank transfusion
1931	Changed name to Jehovah's Witnesses
1945	Ban placed on transfusions
2008	7.1 million members worldwide and 1.1 million members in US

principle of beneficence may weigh more heavily than respecting individual autonomy.

Adults with appropriate decision-making capacity express their autonomy through the informed consent process. Physicians demonstrate respect for the autonomy of competent patients by accepting their informed decisions, whether or not they consent to medical treatment. It seems self-evident that without respect for informed refusal, the concept of informed consent is invalidated: "consent" would then merely be acquiescence of the patient to the physician's recommendations. Adults are therefore even allowed to make what doctors may sometimes consider unwise or foolish decisions. The physician does not have to agree with the patient, but neither can a physician be compelled to give inappropriate, bizarre, or substandard care. (For more on informed consent, please see Chapter 1.)

In order to give informed consent, a patient must have appropriate decision-making capacity, be able to understand the nature of the procedure, the risks, benefits and alternatives including that of doing nothing, and the probable outcomes of both acceptance and refusal of the proposed procedure. In addition the decision must be made free of coercion. Coercion is present if the patient feels threatened, bullied or subjected to irresistible pressure to make a decision he or she would otherwise not make.

Legal precedents

Although legal decisions are not always synonymous with "ethical" ones, a review of some legal precedents regarding JWs and how they have changed provides some insights into how medical ethics has shifted in the US from a paternalistic and/or beneficence-based emphasis, to one of respect for autonomy.

In 1964, two US courts compelled transfusion for adult patients. In Georgetown College v. Jones[4] the court of appeals ruled that the "patient's religion merely

prevented her from consenting to a transfusion, not from receiving one" and a transfusion was ordered. In Raleigh Fitkin Memorial Hospital v. Anderson, a pregnant Jehovah's Witness was not permitted to refuse a necessary transfusion.[5]

Over the last 40 years, US courts have rejected these cases and consistently upheld the rights of adult Jehovah's Witnesses to refuse blood even when a transfusion would be life saving – and even when others, such as dependent children, may be indirectly affected. On the other hand, when the patient is a minor child and hospitals have sought court orders to give blood believed to be absolutely necessary to preserve life, such orders have usually been granted. Exceptions have sometimes been made when an older teenager is committed to his/her religion and seems to fully understand the scope and consequences of his/her decision. Legal precedents in many European countries have paralleled those in the US.[6]

Specific issues to consider in this case

Key questions arise in most cases involving Jehovah's Witnesses and others who refuse certain types of treatment on religious or other grounds.

Does the patient have appropriate decision-making capacity?

All patients over the age of majority are assumed to have adequate decision-making capacity unless proven otherwise. Anesthesiologists can usually tell whether patients have decision-making capacity, which is generally present if the patient understands the nature of his/her illness/condition, the nature of the proposed procedure and its inherent risks and benefits and alternatives, and the consequences of refusing treatment. In doubtful cases, evaluation by a psychiatrist may be helpful.

Have all appropriate risks, benefits and alternatives been explained?

There are other important issues in this case that need to be addressed, aside from the usual explanation of anesthesia and surgical risks. These include assuring that the patient understands that there are some blood cells in solid organs; explaining the specifics of blood conservation techniques; and clarifying the risks of not accepting blood in the face of massive hemorrhage.

In nonemergent cases such as these, there is also often time to plan. Patients should be encouraged to discuss their options not only with the surgical team, but also with the local hospital liaisons from their church (who can be a resource for physicians as well). Preoperative treatments with erythropoietin, iron supplements, or other methods to improve baseline hematocrit should be discussed. Consideration should also be given to intraoperative use of DDAVP and any other measures that will minimize blood loss during the procedure.

Can a surrogate decision-maker refuse transfusion for an incompetent patient?

All JWs are encouraged to carry a durable power of attorney that explains in detail what their beliefs are concerning blood and blood products (see Fig. 3.1). If this is not available and it cannot be verified that the patient is a practicing JW, then physicians generally err on the side of transfusion. Consultation with hospital legal affairs or an organization's ethics committee may be helpful if the appropriate action remains unclear.

Can a surrogate decision-maker change a plan made by a previously competent patient?

A surrogate decision-maker's task is to make decisions for the patient when the patient cannot make them for himself. Ideally, surrogates are not supposed to express their own wishes, but are supposed to make the same decision that a patient would make if he/she were able to do so. Once the patient's decisions are known, whether physicians agree or not, those decisions should stand unless new information becomes available that brings the previous decision into question. This can be particularly difficult if the patient has refused a treatment that the physician thinks is life saving, and the physician knows, believes, or even hopes that the surrogate would capitulate and allow the prohibited treatment. That is when physicians discover if they truly believe in patient autonomy. (For more on surrogate decision-making, see Chapter 4.)

Is the patient making a decision that is free of coercion?

Patients should be free of coercion from healthcare providers and feel safe that regardless of their personal choices their doctors will not abandon them. Additionally, providers must also strive to ensure that the choices a patient makes are *truly* his/her own. It is not unusual for members of the JW church community, as well as family members, to flock to the bedside of a JW patient, both to support their loved one and also to protect him/her from receiving blood.

Sometimes the decisions JW patients express in the presence of family and church members are different from those they later express in private. In the author's experience, this is extremely rare. However, it is important that at some point prior to surgery and anesthesia, patients have an opportunity to express their transfusion preferences to the anesthesiologist in private.[7] This might be done in a preoperative holding area after the family and/or church members have been sent to the waiting room. The intent should *not* be to talk the patient into receiving blood, which would be itself coercive, but to insure that his/her true wishes are known and followed. If the patient does recant, it is then important to determine what, if anything can/should be told to family members about whether blood products were given. Principles of patient confidentiality demand that specifics of treatment such as this only be discussed with the patient unless there is an agreement with them to do otherwise.

Which blood products will and will not be acceptable?

It is not a given that a patient professing to be a JW will not accept any blood products. In one study, for example, up to 10% of pregnant JW patients indicated they would accept blood in an emergency.[8] Nevertheless, in general, few if any baptized Jehovah's Witnesses will accept whole blood, packed red blood cells, plasma, platelet concentrates, or white blood cell transfusions.[9] Stored autologous blood is also not acceptable because it is out of contact with the body for an extended period. Fractionated products such as albumin, cryoprecipitate, cryo-poor plasma, and individual factors are left to the "discretion of the practicing Christian," as are organ and bone marrow transplantation.

Other "gray areas" include, but are not limited to, cell saver, acute normovolemic hemodilution (ANH), cardiopulmonary bypass, and renal dialysis. In these situations, *The Watchtower* has stated that if the blood is kept in continuous circuit with the body and not stored for any length of time, then accepting its transfusion is a personal decision.

Cardiopulmonary bypass and dialysis would almost always involve a continuous circuit. Cell saver and ANH do not necessarily involve a continuous circuit, but one can be created by flushing the cell saver bag and tubing with crystalloid and connecting the circuit to the patient's IV prior to blood collection. If, after collecting blood for ANH, the line to the

(a)

Health Care Proxy
(New York Public Health Law §§ 2980-2994)

1. I, _____ (print or type full name),
fill out this document to set forth my treatment instructions and to appoint a health-care agent in case
of my incapacity.

2. I am one of Jehovah's Witnesses, and I direct that **NO TRANSFUSIONS of whole blood, red cells, white cells,
platelets, or plasma** be given me under any circumstances, even if health-care providers believe that such
are necessary to preserve my life. I refuse to predonate and store my blood for later infusion.

3. **Regarding minor fractions of blood:** [initial those that apply]

    (a) _____ I REFUSE ALL   (b) _____ I REFUSE ALL EXCEPT: _____
    _____

    (c) _____ I may be willing to accept some minor blood fractions, but the details will have to be dis-
    cussed with me if I am conscious or with my health-care agent in case of my incapacity.

4. **Regarding medical procedures involving the use of my own blood,** except diagnostic procedures, such as blood
samples for testing: [initial those that apply]

    (a) _____ I REFUSE ALL   (b) _____ I REFUSE ALL EXCEPT: _____
    _____

    (c) _____ I may be willing to accept certain medical procedures involving my blood, but the details will
    have to be discussed with me if I am conscious or with my health-care agent in case of my incapacity.

5. **Regarding end-of-life matters:** [initial <u>one</u> of the two choices]

    (a) _____ I do not want my life to be prolonged if, to a reasonable degree of medical certainty, my situ-
    ation is hopeless.

    (b) _____ I want my life to be prolonged as long as possible within the limits of generally accepted med-
    ical standards, even if this means that I might be kept alive on machines for years.

6. **Regarding other health-care instructions** (such as current medications, allergies, and medical problems):

    _____
    _____
    _____
    _____
    _____

7. I give no one (including my agent) any authority to disregard or override my instructions set forth herein. Family members, relatives, or friends may disagree with me, but any such disagreement does not diminish the strength or substance of my refusal of blood or other instructions.

8. Apart from the matters covered above, I appoint the person named below as my agent to make healthcare decisions for me. I give my agent full power and authority to consent to or to refuse treatment

Page 1 of 2

Figure 3.1 Sample form for Jehovah's Witness Patients Refusing Blood Transfusions. www.watchtower.org

(b)

(including artificial nutrition and hydration) on my behalf, to consult with my doctors and receive copies of my medical records, and to take legal action to ensure that my wishes are honored. If my first appointed agent is unavailable, unable, or unwilling to serve, I appoint an alternate agent below to serve with the same power and authority.

9. _____   _____
   Signature   ·   Date

   _____
   Address

10. STATEMENT OF WITNESSES: [Note: If the person who signed this document above resides in a mental hygiene facility, you should ask a staff member at the facility to explain any special witnessing requirements.]

   The person who signed this document or directed another to sign it did so willingly in my presence. He or she appears to be of sound mind and free from duress, fraud, or undue influence. I am 18 years of age or older. **Also, I am <u>not</u> the person appointed as agent or alternate agent by this document.**

   _____   _____
   Signature of witness   Signature of witness

   _____   _____
   Address   Address

HEALTH-CARE AGENT*

Name: _____

Address: _____

_____

Telephone(s): _____

_____

ALTERNATE HEALTH-CARE AGENT*

Name: _____

Address: _____

_____

Telephone(s): _____

_____

dpa-E   Uny   11/04   Page 2 of 2

* Note: You may appoint any adult to be your agent. However, your agent may <u>not</u> be (1) your attending physician; (2) anyone who is already an agent for ten or more people unless that person is your spouse, child, parent, brother, sister, or grandparent; or (3) an operator, administrator, or employee of a health-care facility in which you are a resident or patient, or to which you have applied for admission at the time you sign this document unless that person is related to you by blood, marriage, or adoption.

Health Care Proxy
(signed document inside)

NO BLOOD

Figure 3.1 (Cont.)

Table 3.2. Blood product guidelines for Jehovah's Witness patients

Type of blood product or procedure	Accept/refuse/personal decision (PD)	Specific concerns
Whole blood	Refuse	
PRBCs	Refuse	
Plasma	Refuse	
Platelets	Refuse	
White cells	Refuse	
Cryoprecipitate	PD	
Cryo-poor plasma	PD	
Fractionated factors	PD	
Albumin	PD	
Erythropoetin	PD	Most erythropoietin is albumin coated and is a PD. Darbepoetin contains no albumin
Recombinant Factor VII	Accept	Not made from blood, though some may still object
Cell saver	PD	If kept in continuous circuit
Acute normovolemic hemodilution	PD	If kept in continuous circuit
Cardiopulmonary or veno-venous bypass	PD	Continuous circuit rule
Renal dialysis	PD	Continuous circuit rule
Stored autologous blood	Refuse	Not in continuous circuit
Organ and bone marrow transplant	PD	

collection bags remains connected to the patient then it, too, is considered to be a continuous circuit. (See Table 3.2)

What are the capabilities of the surgical team?

When large surgical procedures are planned that may involved significant hemorrhage, it is important to assess whether the surgical and anesthesia team have the skills, experience, and resources necessary to perform this procedure on a patient who has limited their ability to care for him/her by refusing blood. The principle of nonmaleficence, doing no harm, might suggest refusing to do the surgery if the team does not have sufficient experience, modifying the surgical plan, or referring the patient to another center with more experience in "bloodless" surgery techniques. There are centers in the US, for example, that have created a niche in caring for high-risk Jehovah's Witness patients. They can be found by contacting the official Jehovah's Witness website.[10] Consultation with, or referral to, such centers may be useful.

Is it appropriate to undertake liver transplantation or other major surgery in a JW patient?

In many routine surgical and anesthesia cases, distributive justice (fair allocation of scarce resources) is not a large consideration in the decision-making process. However, except in the case of a living related donor, solid organ transplantation involves use of a very limited resource. Even centers that specialize in organ transplants in Jehovah's Witnesses have strict criteria for selecting the proper candidates for organ transplantation. If there is relative certainty that the preoperative status of the patient will mandate the use of blood products during the transplantation, then a Jehovah's Witness patient should not be a candidate if they would refuse such transfusions. On the other hand, many potential candidates for liver transplant are not in severe failure but are at the top of the recipient list due to other complicating factors such as hepato-pulmonary syndrome, hepatocellular carcinoma, or hepato-renal syndrome. Many of these patients have normal coagulation and hemoglobins and have a reasonable chance of receiving a liver transplantation without transfusion, whether they are one of Jehovah's Witnesses or not. Such patients may be appropriate candidates for organ transplantation.

What are the anesthesiologist's rights and obligations?

Many anesthesia providers feel that refusal of standard care in the operating room, such as blood transfusions, places them in an untenable position in which a seemingly irrational patient choice prevents them from fulfilling their professional obligations to provide life-saving therapy. The American Society of Anesthesiologists has developed guidelines for the anesthesia care of patients with do-not-resuscitate orders or other directives that limit treatment[11] that specify the following:

> When an anesthesiologist finds the patient's or surgeon's limitations of intervention decisions to be irreconcilable with one's own moral views, then the anesthesiologist should withdraw in a nonjudgmental fashion, providing an alternative for care in a timely fashion.
>
> [if such] alternatives are not feasible within the time frame necessary to prevent further morbidity or suffering, then in accordance with the American Medical Association's Principles of Medical Ethics, care should proceed with reasonable adherence to the patient's directives, being mindful of the patient's goals and values.

In nonemergent situations, anesthesiologists have the right to excuse themselves from a patient's care, as long as they are willing to refer the patient to another provider. This referral could even be to another medical center that has developed expertise in caring for Jehovah's Witness patients, and may be desirable in certain situations even if the anesthesiologist would personally be willing to care for the patient.

If the situation is a life-or-death emergency with no time to make a referral, then the anesthesiologist is obligated to care for the patient, trying as much as possible to adhere to the patient's wishes.

These guidelines are similar to the Guidelines on Clinical Management of Jehovah's Witnesses published by the National Health Service in Great Britain in 2005.[12] European countries vary somewhat in the depth of obligation a physician has to honor a patient's wishes to not be transfused. In France, for example, an autonomous patient's wishes are generally respected, but the law gives leeway to physicians acting in the course of an emergency. In Germany, transfusion even to save a life would be in direct conflict with constitutional guarantees of autonomy – although it is uncertain how this would play out in court if challenged.

Case resolution

In this case, the patient had been advanced on the recipient list due to her hepato-pulmonary syndrome, the only cure for which was a liver transplant. In addition, her pulmonary status was worsening and it was felt that she soon would not be a candidate at all. Though the transplant team did not have extensive experience in transplanting Jehovah's Witnesses, the most experienced surgeon did have a track record of operating on patients such as this with minimal blood loss and minimal use of blood products. The lead anesthesiologist had extensive experience with Jehovah's Witnesses in other major surgeries such as cardiac surgery. Both of these individuals committed to being involved in this case, whether on call or not, at the time a liver became available for this patient.

The patient agreed to acute normovolemic hemodilution and cell saver as long as a continuous circuit was maintained. She also agreed to albumin and recombinant factor VII if necessary. At the time of surgery three units of blood was drawn off and left in circuit with the patient. The surgery went smoothly and the patient received the three units of blood and two units of cell saver after the new liver had been revascularized. DDAVP was also administered. She tolerated the surgery and was discharged ten days later, having had a slightly extended postoperative ICU stay due to her pulmonary status.

Key points

- Due to strongly held beliefs, most practicing Jehovah's Witness patients will refuse transfusion of blood and many blood products.
- Respect for patient autonomy is the primary ethical principle applied in the United States, while the principle of beneficence is more strongly held in many other countries.
- Respect for autonomy supports the concept that adult, competent patients have the right to refuse blood transfusions, as well as any other therapy.
- Commitment to principles of beneficence and nonmaleficence require anesthesiologists to offer the best care available within the constraints of the patient's wishes – this includes appropriate preoperative planning for adjunctive therapies, and even referring

JW patients to other providers if they are more experienced, and likely to accomplish procedures with less blood loss.

- Many other Western countries follow laws and practices similar to that of the United States – the wishes of competent patients to forgo transfusions are generally respected, although individual countries may differ in whether and how strongly they penalize doctors who choose to transfuse rather than lose a patient's life in the operating room.

References

1* Jehovah's Witnesses – Who are they? What do they believe? (2006). Watch Tower Bible and Tract Society of Pennsylvania. http://www.watchtower.org/e/jt/index.htm.

2 *New Revised Standard Bible*.

3* Beauchamp T.L. and Childress, J.F. (2001). *Principles of Biomedical Ethics*, 4th edn. Oxford, UK: Oxford University Press, p. 12.

4 Georgetown College v Jones. 118 U.S. App. D.C. 80 (1964).

5 Raleigh Fitkin–Paul Morgan Memorial Hospital v. Anderson, 42 N.J. 421 (1964).

6 Re T (Adult: Refusal of Medical Treatment). Great Britain Court of Appeal, Civil Division. All Engl Law Rep 1992; 30[1992]4:649–70.

de Cruz, P. Comparative Health Care Law. Page 295. Cavendish Publishing Ltd, London UK. 2001.

Loriau, J., Manaoulli, C., Montpellier, D., *et al.* (2004). Surgery and transfusion in Jahovah's witness patient. Medical legal review. *Ann Chir*, **129**(5), 263–8.

* Honig, J.F., Lilie, H, Merten, H.A., and Braun, U. (1992). The refusal to consent to blood transfusion. Legal and medical aspects using Jehovah's Witnesses as an example. *Anaesthesist*, **41**(7), 396–8.

7* Muramoto, O. (2000). Medical confidentiality and the protection of Jehovah's Witnesses; autonomous refusal of blood. *J Med Ethics*, **26**(5), 381–6.

8* Gyamfi, C. and Berkowitz, R.L. (2004). Responses by pregnant Jehovah's Witnesses on health care proxies. *Obstet Gynecol*, **104**(3), 541–4.

9* Jehovah's Witnesses – religious and ethical position on medical therapy, child care, and related matters. (2001) Watch Tower Bible and Tract Society of Pennsylvania

10 www.watchtower.org

11* Ethical Guidelines for the Anesthesia Care of Patients with Do-Not-Resuscitate Orders or Other Directives that Limit Treatment. American Society of Anesthesiologists. Park Ridge, Il. Approved by HOD, October 2008. http://www.asahq.org/publicationsAndServices/standards/09.pdf.

12* Guidelines on Clinical Management of Jehovah's Witnesses. January 2005. Maidstone and Tunbridge Wells NHS Trust. London, UK.

Consent and refusal

Surrogate decision-making

Elizabeth K. Vig, Allen Gustin, and Kelly Fryer-Edwards

The Case – Part 1

Ethel Smith, an 80 year-old widowed woman, is admitted for elective total hip replacement. She has a history of well-controlled diabetes and hypertension, but is otherwise healthy. Her functional status has declined because of hip pain. Preoperatively, she is cognitively intact. Her surgery proceeds uneventfully; however, she develops postoperative delirium in the recovery room. Her medical team decides that she should be transferred to an intensive care unit for support and monitoring. They schedule a meeting with her three children to discuss her condition. During this meeting, her family states that she never designated any family member to act as her decision-maker.

Who is the legal decision-maker?

As long as Mrs. Smith has decision-making capacity, she can make her own medical decisions. Surrogates do not become legal decision makers until a patient loses decision-making capacity. Many places (including 44 of the United States) have laws identifying a hierarchy of legal surrogates. Different states vary in who is included in the hierarchy, but the order is often as follows: Court appointed guardian, Durable Power of Attorney for Healthcare (DPOA), spouse, adult children, parents, and adult siblings. Five states include attending physicians in this hierarchy. In Mississippi, the "owner, operator, or employee of a residential long term care institution" is included in the hierarchy. In Texas, a "member of the clergy" is included.

If there are multiple people within a category, such as Mrs. Smith's three children, in the US they all have equal legal standing as decision-makers. The legal decision-maker is not automatically the oldest, smartest, or most involved child. When there is not agreement between the surrogates within a category, some states require consensus, while others only require a majority opinion.

Many European countries have autonomy-based models of decision-making for competent patients, and hierarchies for surrogate decision-making for incapacitated patients that are similar to that in the US. A recent review of laws of eight European countries (Belgium, Denmark, England, France, Germany, the Netherlands, Spain and Switzerland) showed that all recognize the autonomy of competent patients to make medical decisions. All except France recognize the legally binding power of written advance directives. Decisional powers of family members, close friends, and family doctors vary from country to country. Similarities and differences are summarized in Table 4.1.[1]

A **Durable Power of Attorney for Healthcare** is a legal document in which individuals can designate one or more individuals whom they want to make decisions on their behalf if they lose decision-making capacity. There are some exceptions to this, such as some documents from the State of California that allow the DPOA to make decisions even if the patient retains decision-making capacity.

Patients usually want their families to make decisions for them if they lose the ability to make their own decisions. In one study, older patients explained that the reason they chose a given surrogate decision maker was because that person was the person they felt closest to (33%), the person who understood them the best (26%) and the person who was geographically the closest (17%).[2]

A **living will** is a type of **advance directive** in which an individual expresses his/her preferences for care in future health states. Most of these documents are not very specific, but can be used by the family and the patient's healthcare team in order to guide decisions when the patient can no longer express preferences.

Clinical Ethics in Anesthesiology: A Case-Based Textbook, ed. Gail A. Van Norman, Stephen Jackson, Stanley H. Rosenbaum and Susan K. Palmer. Published by Cambridge University Press. © Cambridge University Press 2011.

Table 4.1. Surrogacy in medical decisions for incapacitated patients in eight European countries, 2009

	Patient has AD	Patient has No AD but has a designated Surrogate	Patient has No AD and no designated Surrogate
Belgium	AD has decisional power	Surrogate has decisional power but must show it is consistent with pt wishes	Family member has decisional power: order is spouse; child; parent; sibling
Denmark	AD has decisional power only for end-of-life	Surrogate has decisional power	Family member or close friend has decisional power
England	AD has decisional power Treatment refusal must be expressed unequivocally for the physician to comply	Surrogate has decisional power Only a power of attorney can refuse life-sustaining treatment	Family member has consultative role Physicians have decisional power
France	AD has consultative role	Surrogate has consultative role	Family member has consultative role
Germany	AD has decisional power but Surrogate may challenge	Surrogate has decisional power Court approval is required to refuse life-sustaining treatment or there is disagreement with the physician	Family member and family doctor have consultative roles
The Netherlands	AD has decisional power	Surrogate has decisional power	Family member has consultative role Family order is spouse; parents, children, siblings
Spain	AD has decisional power; there is a National Directory of ADs	Surrogate has decisional power	Family member or close friend have decisional power
Switzerland	AD has decisional power If not sufficiently specific, AD has a consultative role	Surrogate has decisional power	Family member or close friend has decisional power The order is spouse; decendents; parents; siblings

AD: Advance Directive

When is a surrogate decision-maker needed?

Patients who are at risk of losing decision-making capacity include hospitalized patients, patients with some types of psychiatric illness (such as depression and schizophrenia) and cognitive impairment (such as dementia, delirium, and strokes), residents of nursing homes or assisted living facilities, and patients who are approaching the end of life. However, merely being in one of these categories does not automatically indicate that an individual is incapable of making his/her own decisions. An evaluation of a patient's decision-making capacity (discussed later in this chapter) can determine whether a patient can make a specific decision. Patients with decision-making capacity sometimes voluntarily defer decision-making to loved ones. This is an ethically and legally acceptable action. The literature has identified that patients from certain ethnic and immigrant groups and older patients are more apt to delegate decision-making.

What are the limits of surrogate decision-making?

Regional differences exist with regard to the decisions that surrogates are allowed to make. In California, surrogates cannot make decisions about whether or not a patient receives electro-convulsive therapy. In North Dakota, surrogates cannot make decisions about sterilization or abortion. In New York State, surrogates cannot make decisions about stopping artificial nutrition and hydration unless there is "clear and convincing evidence" of a patient's preferences.[3] States are variable regarding the descriptions of the abilities of surrogate decision makers; these specifications can be found in the state codes and laws, often searchable online. Clinicians also can contact the risk manager of their facility to obtain guidance on the specifics of each state's surrogate decision-maker statutes.

The Case – Part 2

Mrs. Smith's children understand the need for transfer of her care to an intensive care unit and initially agree to continue medical care with the goal of getting her back to her pre-operative state. Four days later, she is still in the intensive care unit with delirium. She is unable to participate in her own care, and she develops aspiration pneumonitis. At this time, she is supported with supplemental oxygen, however the family is told that she may need to be intubated. The orthopedic surgeon also notes purulent drainage from the wound and feels the need to re-explore the wound in the operating room. The patient's family begins to disagree about what to do. They do not agree on whether she would want to be reintubated.

How should surrogates make decisions?

As determined by law, surrogate decision-makers can make their decisions on two bases: substituted judgment or best interests. The preferred is the **substituted judgment** standard, in which the surrogate makes the decision s/he believes the patient would have made. If the surrogate does not have enough familiarity with the patient's care preferences, s/he then makes a decision using the **best interests** standard, that is, making the decision that is in the patient's best interests. Both of these standards are intended to be used based on the surrogate's knowledge and understanding of the patient's interests, values, and preferences.

How do surrogates make decisions?

Although surrogates are expected to make decisions based on substituted judgment or best interests, there is evidence in the literature that surrogates factor their own beliefs and preferences into the medical decisions they make for loved ones. One study of experienced surrogate decision makers found that surrogates make decisions in different ways.[4] Most surrogates relied, in part, on the substituted judgment standard and made decisions based on their knowledge of their loved one's preferences or thresholds of "living versus existing;" and a small percentage (10%) of the surrogates relied on written documents, such as the patient's living will. Another small group (18%), deferred decision-making to someone more experienced, such as a clinician family member. The third group based decisions on a sense of shared values with their loved one, which they believed obviated the need to formally discuss care preferences with their loved one. The final group was made up of 28% of surrogates who made decisions based on their own personal values and/or preferences, not necessarily those of their loved one.

There is not clear consensus amongst ethics experts as to whether it is ethically permissible for family members to incorporate their personal values and preferences into decisions they make for their loved ones. Some ethics experts have espoused the principle of **relational autonomy** which recognizes that the patient is not the only stakeholder in a medical decision.[5]

In favor of relational autonomy is evidence that patients are concerned about burdening loved ones and surrogates will often be the ones most affected by decisions made for incapacitated patients.[6] For example, if Mrs. Smith's children decide that she would not want to be reintubated and she dies as a result of this decision, they then have to live with the emotional and psychological implications of this decision. On the other hand, if they decide that she would want to be reintubated and hospital care continued, she might have a prolonged hospital course and recovery period that might have financial implications for her children. While no one would condone making these decisions on the basis of personal gain or loss, relational autonomy asks surrogates and clinicians to consider a broad interpretation of what decision is best.

The Case – Part 3

After much discussion, Mrs. Smith's older son convinces her two daughters that she would want life-sustaining treatment continued. He argues that she opted for the hip replacement to improve her quality of life and that she was not ready to die. Her daughters assert that she would not want prolonged mechanical ventilation, and would not want to be dependent on others indefinitely, but eventually agree to a time-limited trial of continued care in the intensive care unit.

What if the surrogate isn't making decisions that appear to be what the patient would have wanted?

When a surrogate's decision seems to diverge from a patient's known preferences, medical teams may find it challenging to decipher whether the decision stems from family beliefs/needs or from more dubious motives. In most cases, deviations from patient's preferences result from surrogates' authentic love for the patient, not malice. For example, family members may opt for more aggressive care for a terminally ill loved one than the patient would have wanted because they have not yet come to terms with their loved one's grim prognosis. However, some family members may have ulterior motives behind their decisions. Asking family members to explain the reasons for their decisions may help. Ethics and palliative care consultants can also help evaluate these difficult situations.

If there is clear evidence of a patient's preferences, such as in a living will, which the surrogate isn't honoring, and the medical team doesn't believe that the surrogate's reasons for disregarding the patient's preferences are acceptable, then the medical team may consider taking the case to court. At least three cases have involved discordance between the patient's preferences in their living will and the opinions of the patient's legal decision-maker (the cases of Dorothy Livadas in New York in 2008, Hanford Pinette in Florida in 2004, and Doris Smith in Louisiana in 2004). In all cases, the living will trumped the legal decision-maker. Prior to taking a potential case to court, the medical team and/or ethics consultants should consider whether the patient would have allowed the surrogate leeway in implementing his/her preferences and whether taking the case to court might have serious adverse effects on the surrogate(s) and/or patient's family.

How accurate are surrogate estimates of patient preferences?

Numerous studies have investigated the accuracy of surrogates' estimates of their loved ones' preferences.[7]

In these studies, patients fill out a questionnaire identifying their care preferences in numerous health states, and their preferred surrogate decision-makers estimate their care preferences in these same states. Surrogates' accuracy in estimating patient preferences is then calculated. A review of these studies found that surrogates correctly estimated their loved ones' preferences 68% of the time. Of note, clinicians are less accurate than family members in estimating patient preferences.

The Case – Part 4

After 9 days, Mrs. Smith remains unable to recognize her children, appears delirious, and is still intubated in the intensive care unit. Mrs. Smith's son remarks to the ICU nurse, "I realize that there's not much we can do but wait, and I hate to see her suffer, but I think we need to keep things going for now because I need to have something that I can live with."

What are the burdens of decision-making on surrogates?

Patients recognize how their illness, caregiving needs, and need for decision-making may impose stress on their loved ones. In previous research, many different types of patients have expressed concern about burdening their loved ones with their illness and needs. In order to lessen the burden on loved ones, many patients allow their loved ones some degree of **leeway** in how strictly to follow their preferences. For example, a patient may prefer not to remain on a ventilator for an extended period of time, but also may recognize that his/her surrogate decision-maker may need time to get comfortable with making the decision to withdraw care. Patients may recognize this and agree to remain on the ventilator temporarily.

Additionally, it is stressful both to have a loved one who is seriously ill and to make life or death decisions for that loved one. The literature on the after-effects of caregiving and surrogate decision-making is becoming more extensive. In studies from France[8] and the US[9], families who made decisions for a loved one in an intensive care unit were found to have anxiety, depression, and even symptoms of PTSD up to six months after their loved one was discharged from that unit.

There are some data from the perspective of surrogate decision-makers on what clinicians could have done to make decision-making easier for them. In one study, surrogates reported that decision-making was easier when clinicians were available to answer their questions, gave them frank information about chances of recovery and prognosis, made treatment recommendations, and treated them with respect.[10] When too many clinicians were involved, decision-making was harder for surrogates. When the medical team can frame their recommendations in terms of the patient's known values and preferences, such a recommendation can be a strong guide and support for the surrogate. That is, the team can help shift the burden of owning the decision from the surrogate to the patient (e.g., just enacting his/her wishes for him/her) or to the disease state (e.g., there is little more we can offer that will help her).

The Case – Part 5

After 2 weeks, Mrs. Smith's aspiration pneumonitis and her delirium show signs of improvement. She is still intubated, but her confusion begins to wane. She now recognizes her children. She has periods where she is quite lucid and other periods where she is still quite confused. She probably would benefit from a tracheostomy in the operating room, but her clinicians don't know if they should ask Mrs. Smith or her family to make this decision.

How do we determine if a patient can make his/her own medical decisions?

The team needs to assess Mrs. Smith's decision-making capacity. Unlike **competence**, which is determined in a court of law, **decision-making capacity** is determined by a clinician. Psychiatrists and psychologists aren't the only clinicians who can evaluate decision-making capacity – any physician can determine whether a patient has decisional capacity.

Decision-making capacity is made up of four decision-making abilities: understanding, appreciating, reasoning, and choosing. Though she may be intermittently delirious, Mrs. Smith may still be capable of making some decisions, especially when her mental status is clearest. For example, Mrs. Smith may be able to designate one of her children as her Durable Power of Attorney for Healthcare, but at the same time, she may not be able to make more complex decisions such as whether or not to undergo an additional surgical procedure.

When assessing whether Mrs. Smith can make the decision about a tracheostomy, her medical team would want to talk to her when she is most alert and lucid. They first would want to assess her **understanding** of her condition and the decision at hand. The team should review her condition, the need for a tracheostomy, and the risks, benefits, and alternatives to the procedure. They might ask Mrs. Smith to repeat this information back in her own words – by writing, or indicating her preference on a tablet or computer screen, for example. Next, her **appreciation** should be assessed. Does she realize that the decision will affect her body? For example, if she is in denial about how sick she has been and her continued need for mechanical ventilation at night, she might not appreciate why a tracheostomy is needed. The team next would want to ask Mrs. Smith to indicate her treatment **choice** and the **reasons** for that choice. Her reasons should be consistent with her beliefs and values. Her choice should follow this reasoning and be stable over time. If she changes her mind when she is more confused, but then reverts to her previous choice when less confused, the choice voiced when she is less confused should be honored.

After assessing a patient's decision-making abilities, the clinician uses his/her judgment to determine if the patient has decision-making capacity. Patients do not need to have all four abilities present to have decisional capacity. The clinician determines how much of each ability needs to be present for capacity to be present, and may vary the requirements depending on the decision at hand. In other words, when assessing a patient's decision-making capacity, the evaluation will be more stringent if the consequences of the decision are more serious and irreversible, such as the decision to withdraw life-sustaining treatment.

Key points

- It may be possible to prevent confusion about the appropriate surrogate by asking all hospitalized and preoperative patients with decision-making capacity to identify their preferred surrogate decision maker(s) early in their hospital stay.
- Most patients are concerned about burdening loved ones and allow their surrogates some leeway in interpreting and implementing their care preferences.
- Surrogates estimate loved one's preferences with moderate accuracy. When they choose treatment plans that seem to be contrary to a patient's preferences, it is more often because of love than malice. Ethics and palliative

care consultants can help evaluate apparent discrepancies.

- Disagreement between surrogates about the "best" plan of care happens often. Although surrogates are expected to interpret a patient's preferences, they may have trouble putting their own preferences aside. Clinicians may need to investigate the reasons for each surrogate's opinion when there is disagreement and try to refocus the discussion from each party's interest to a general discussion of the patient's life and values.

- Decision-making capacity is assessed by evaluating patients' abilities to (1) understand information about their condition and treatment options; (2) appreciate that the decision at hand will affect them; (3) explain their reasoning; and (4) arrive at a choice consistent with their values and beliefs or a discussion of the patient's life and values.

References

1* Lautrette, A., Peigne, V., Watts, J., *et al.* (2008). Surrogate decision makers for incompetent ICU patients: a European perspective. *Curr Opin Crit Care*, **14**(6), 714–19.

2 Cohen-Mansfield, J., Rabinovich, B.A., Lipson, S., *et al.* (1991). The decision to execute a durable power of attorney for health care and preferences regarding the utilization of life-sustaining treatments in nursing home residents. *Arch Intern Med*, **151**(2), 289–94.

3 In re Westchester County Medical Center, 72 NY 2d 517 (1988)

4* Vig, E.K., Taylor, J.S., Starks, H., *et al.* (2006). Beyond substituted judgment: how surrogates navigate end-of-life decision-making. *J Am Geriatr Soc*, **54**(11), 1688–93.

5* Verkerk, M.A. (2001). The care perspective and autonomy. *Med Health Care Philos*, **4**(3) 289–94.

6* Stewart, A.L., Teno, J., Patrick, D.L., and Lynn, J. (1999). The concept of quality of life of dying persons in the context of health care. *J Pain Symptom Managem*, **17**(2), 93–108.

7* Shalowitz, D.I., Garrett-Mayer, E., and Wendler, D. (2006). The accuracy of surrogate decision makers: a systematic review. *Arch Intern Med*, **166**(5), 493–7.

8* Azoulay, E., Pochard, F., Kentish-Barnes, N., *et al.* (2005). Risk of post-traumatic stress symptoms in family members of intensive care unit patients. *Am J Respir Crit Care Med*, **171**(9), 987–94.

9* Anderson, W.G., Arnold, R.M., Angus, D.C., and Bryce, C.L. (2008). Posttraumatic stress and complicated grief in family members of patients in the intensive care unit. *J Gen Intern Med*, **23**(11), 1871–6.

10* Vig, E.K., Starks, H., Taylor, J.S., *et al.* (2007). Surviving surrogate decision-making: what helps and hampers the experience of making medical decisions for others. *J Gen Intern Med*, **22**(9), 1274–9.

Further reading

Beauchamp, T.L. and Childress, J.F. (1994). *Principles of Biomedical Ethics*. 4th edn. Oxford, UK: Oxford University Press.

Buchanan, A.E. and Brock, D.W. (1990). *Deciding for Others: The Ethics of Surrogate Decision Making*. Cambridge, UK: Cambridge University Press.

Grisso, T. and Appelbaum, P. S. (1998). *Assessing Competence to Consent to Treatment. A Guide for Physicians and Other Health Care Professionals*. New York: Oxford University Press.

DISCOVERY LIBRARY
LEVEL 5 SWCC
DERRIFORD HOSPITAL
DERRIFORD ROAD
PLYMOUTH
PL6 8DH

Informed consent and the pediatric patient

David Clendenin and David B. Waisel

The Case

During the preanesthetic discussion for resection of pulmonary metastases of osteosarcoma, the anesthesiologist advises the 14-year-old boy and his parents that a thoracic epidural catheter would be the best way to manage post-thoracotomy pain. The anesthesiologist initiates a discussion commensurate to the adolescent's age, experiences and cognitive ability. The patient immediately refuses the thoracic epidural stating, "I don't want a needle in my back while I'm awake." Despite reassurance by the anesthesiologist and parents of adequate sedation and analgesia, the patient still refuses. The parents, frustrated, scared and wanting the best for their child still ask the anesthesiologist to insert the epidural.

The child's role in medical decision-making

The American Academy of Pediatrics Committee on Bioethics 1995 recommended integration of children into the informed consent process[1] (Table 5.1), and this has been reaffirmed both nationally and internationally.[2] Indeed, the ASA has incorporated the principle of pediatric assent into its *Guidelines for the Ethical Practice of Anesthesiology* (Section I.2):

> Anesthesiologists respect the right of every patient to self-determination [and] should include patients, including minors, in medical decision-making that is appropriate to their developmental capacity and the medical issues involved.[3]

Anesthesiologists should choose to involve children in medical decision-making with the ethical objective of enhancing the child's self-determination, while keeping the child engaged in their care.

Anesthesiologists can use the patient's age as a first approximation of a patient's cognitive and emotional development. Children under the age of 7 generally do not have decision-making capacity. Children between ages 7 and 14 years are considered

unlikely to have complete decision-making capacity but are able to voice preferences about increasingly complex questions. Children older than 14 are considered to have decision-making capacity unless proven otherwise.

This chapter will discuss the issues raised by incorporating the ethical concept of pediatric patient assent into the traditional process of parental (surrogate) informed consent.

Competency and decision-making capacity

In discussing pediatric decision-making, it is important to distinguish between competency and decision-making capacity. In the US, *competency* is a legal status determined by the judicial system and is not determined by clinicians, although the judicial system relies on clinical specialists such as psychiatrists when determining competency. By law, except under specific circumstances, children are not legally competent to authorize medical care for themselves.

Distinct from competency, *decision-making capacity* is the ability to make specific decisions at specific times.[a] Clinicians determine decision-making capacity. Children exhibit ranges of decision-making capacity, depending on age, risks and benefits of the decision, emotional and cognitive maturity, and temporary (e.g., sedation) and permanent limitations on cognitive function.

Developmental progression of pediatric assent

For children younger than 7 years old, anesthesiologists should focus on obtaining parental[b] *informed permission* or "assent." (Table 5.1) "Informed permission"

Clinical Ethics in Anesthesiology: A Case-Based Textbook, ed. Gail A. Van Norman, Stephen Jackson, Stanley H. Rosenbaum and Susan K. Palmer. Published by Cambridge University Press. © Cambridge University Press 2011.

Table 5.1. Elements of consent and assent as defined by the American Academy of Pediatrics Committee on Bioethics

Consent

(1) Adequate provision of information including the nature of the ailment or condition, the nature of the proposed diagnostic steps or treatment and the probability of their success; the existence and nature of the risks involved; and the existence, potential benefits, and risks of recommended alternative treatments (including the choice of no treatment)

(2) Assessment of the patient's understanding of the above information

(3) Assessment, if only tacit, of the capacity of the patient or surrogate to make the necessary decisions

(4) Assurance, insofar as it is possible, that the patient has the freedom to choose among the medial alternatives without coercion or manipulation

Assent

(1) Helping the patient achieve a developmentally appropriate awareness of the nature of his or her condition

(2) Telling the patient what he or she can expect with tests and treatment

(3) Making a clinical assessment of the patient's understanding of the situation and the factors influencing how he or she is responding (including whether there is inappropriate pressure to accept testing or therapy)

(4) Soliciting an expression of the patient's willingness to accept the proposed care

is used instead of informed "consent" because "consent" implies that the patient is providing the legal consent. The implication of "informed permission" is that, although clinicians nearly always honor parental decision-making, parental decision-making does have boundaries. Physicians honor parental decision-making because they assume that parents desire the best for their children, parents have to live with the consequences of that decision, and parental values and goals often approximate their child's future values and goals.

Boundaries of parental decision-making are informed by the "best interests" standard, which requires that parents and clinicians choose their decisions from within a range of reasonable options. This standard does not require clinicians to dogmatically insist on what they think is best for the child. However, if the parents are making a decision that is unacceptably outside the boundaries of reasonable decision-making options, then clinicians are expected to intervene in an escalating manner as necessary to protect the child.[4] For example, if the child in the introductory case were 9 years old, then it is acceptable, if perhaps suboptimal, for the parents to choose intravenous pain management instead of epidural analgesia. If, however, the parents wanted to forgo all pain management out of fear of exacerbating a known family risk of narcotic addiction, then that decision would be an unacceptable treatment option and would require intervention by the anesthesiologist.

As children increase in age from 7 to 14 years, they are beginning to seek independence and are progressively capable of assimilating, analyzing, and using complex information. As a result, anesthesiologists should begin seeking both age-appropriate assent and parental informed permission from these children. Age-appropriate assent varies by age and the complexity of the decision, with particular focus on the potential risks of the decision. It ranges from involving a 7-year-old in determining whether to use preoperative premedication, to discussing preoperative intravenous placement with a 10-year-old, to seeking assent from a 12-year-old for placement of a peripheral nerve block. More important than the specifics is that anesthesiologists make an effort to integrated children into the decision-making process based on their maturity. As these children approach adolescence, they become increasingly able to understand parental and physician motives. For example, a 13-year-old child fearful of an awake intubation may recognize the importance of a sound medical decision and assent to the process. Anesthesiologists who involve children in decisions related to their care frequently cite patient autonomy, education and the protection of a child's rights as the focus of the involvement.

Adolescents older than age 14 prioritize independence and have fully developed abstract thought and complex reasoning. Anesthesiologists must engage these adolescents in decision-making.

However, fully developed cognitive abilities do not necessarily translate into good decision-making skills. Adolescents do not fully develop impulse control and consideration for long-term consequences until their early twenties. For this reason, decisions of significant risk and consequences (such as refusal of potentially life-saving transfusion therapy in the child of a Jehovah's Witness) must undergo greater scrutiny and require significant evidence of decision-making capacity. Evidence of decision making capacity includes internally coherent reasoning, appreciation of cause and effect, appreciation of the range of outcomes and the effects that the different possibilities would have on loved ones, and the ability to imagine what circumstances would have to be different for them to choose an alternate path. Determining the extent of risk includes considering the amount of potential harm to the child by the intervention or its absence, the likelihood of occurrence for each of the likely outcomes, and the overall risk-to-benefit ratio.

Engaging children in decision-making

The American Academy of Pediatrics emphasizes that "no one should solicit a patient's views without intending to weigh them seriously."[1] *Pro forma* and insincere engagement of children is easily recognized and brings harms to current and future patient-doctor relationships. A common mistake is well-intentioned vagueness in explaining options to children, leading the child to choose untenable options.

In non-emergent care, anesthesiologists should honor a child's refusal of care. Some suggest the ability to refuse elective procedures begins around the age of 10, although in practice is seems to be older, perhaps around age 12.[5] Clinicians should explore the child's refusal in the hopes of addressing specific concern. Short delays, a change of location, changing into street clothes, or using pediatric mental health professionals often help address most refusals. Given the harm of ignoring a child's preferences, clinicians should disregard pressures to proceed forthwith from operating room administrators, physicians or parents. Strategies such as using the operating room for other cases may help ameliorate these production pressures. To minimize the harm of *pro forma* solicitation of a child's opinion, children should never be offered illegitimate choices. Moreover, they should be directly informed when they will undergo procedures despite their objections.

Anesthesiologists can minimize the harm of limiting a child's decision-making authority by overtly honoring their authority about more negotiable decisions. For example, while a 12-year-old girl may not be permitted to choose whether to have an anterior cruciate ligament reconstruction because of potential long-term harm, it would be reasonable to permit a healthy adolescent to choose between a peripheral nerve block or intravenous narcotics to provide postoperative analgesia. The anesthesiologist still should explain to the patient that a nerve block may provide superior pain management, but should respect the patient's wishes should she choose the alternative. This approach helps balance the sometimes unaligned goals of self-determination and safe and quality care for the adolescent.

Medical decisions: who ultimately chooses?

Disagreements about the appropriate clinical plan occur in any combination within the patient–parent–clinician triad. As with all disagreements about patient care plans, clinicians should focus on continued communication and transparent exchanges among the parties. Divining misunderstandings may resolve disagreements. Unfortunately, clinicians tend to avoid patients and family members that are complicated or are considered to be "difficult." Avoidance appears to be the easier option, but in the long term, it entrenches opinions and exacerbates discord.

When the preferences of the parent and patient diverge, clinicians should attempt to define the reason for the disagreement. Parental and adolescent disagreement often is rooted in the dynamic of the adolescent establishing independence from the parent. Clarifying the merits of the options, offering an objective opinion based on stated values, and improving intra-family communication can help resolve these challenging problems.

When differences persist within the patient–parent–clinician triad, clinicians may want to consult multidisciplinary conflict resolution experts such as social workers, ethics consultants, and chaplains. The enhanced communication that often results from third party consultation may increase decision-makers' appreciation of the shared interest in the child's well-being. Improved communication may also enable clinicians to recognize previously unappreciated fears or misunderstandings. Legal counsel may be necessary in the rare instances of impasse. Even when legal intervention is necessary, clinicians should continue to seek common ground and a functional patient–parent–clinician relationship.

Case resolution

In the situation of the 14-year-old with pulmonary metastases of osteosarcoma, the parents and the patient disagree about whether to have a thoracic epidural catheter placed. This patient's fear of an epidural needle does not obviate the risks of inserting a thoracic epidural placement in an anesthetized patient. Exploration of his refusal reveals that his fear is based on "ward gossip' that getting an epidural really hurts, despite what the anesthesiologist says. Such gossip is formidable. Extensive conversations emphasizing the differences among patients and their situations and the promise to stop if the procedure became too uncomfortable do not ameliorate his concerns.

Four options present themselves: (1) insert the thoracic epidural catheter after inducing anesthesia; (2) insert the thoracic epidural catheter after heavily sedating the patient, either surreptitiously or after informing the patient he did not have a choice about the epidural; (3) insert a lumbar epidural catheter after inducing anesthesia, although a lumbar epidural may be less effective; or (4) use intravenous postoperative pain management.

The decision rests heavily on the relative benefits of placing a thoracic epidural. If he would strongly benefit from the attributes of a functional thoracic epidural (such as pain control enhancing pulmonary hygiene in a patient with pulmonary disease or minimizing intravenous narcotics in a patient at risk for apnea), then with appropriate parental informed permission (consent), it may make sense to risk inserting the epidural catheter after inducing anesthesia or to inform him that his preference is being overridden in his best interest. Lying to the patient might be devastating in a child who will continue to undergo extensive therapy. On the other hand, if the clinically significant benefits of using a thoracic epidural for postoperative analgesic are minimal, then the benefits of not inserting a thoracic epidural catheter outweigh the risks of inserting the thoracic epidural catheter in an anesthetized, surreptitiously sedated, or coerced patient. In the example case, it is ethically proper to explain to the parents why it is more important to honor their child's requests than to insert a thoracic epidural catheter.

Requests for non-disclosure to children

Parental non-disclosure requests range from "do not tell him he is having surgery" to "details will only scare him" to "she doesn't know the diagnosis and we want to keep it that way." Thoughtful consideration of parental nondisclosure requests should serve solely the goal of patient benefit. Although dishonesty jeopardizes the physician–patient relationship, frightening children for the sake of a principle is often unwise. A pragmatic approach is to disclose issues that the child will find out in the imminent future and is within the domain of anesthesiology, but to defer disclosure about issues that would be better served by discussions with other experts. For the most part, children should be told in age-appropriate terms that they are having surgery and anesthesia, but it would be inappropriate for the anesthesiologist to insist that the child be told that he has been diagnosed with cancer. Anesthesiologists who believe that information is being inappropriately withheld from the patient should approach the primary physicians to discuss their ethical concerns.

Emancipated minors and mature minors status

Emancipated minors can legally give informed consent for their medical decisions. Emancipated minor status is determined by state statuted, and varies from state to state, but commonly included determinants are pregnancy, marriage, military service, or being self-supporting. *Mature minor status* differs from emancipated minor status. Mature minor status is awarded by a judge and permits minors to be an autonomous decision-maker for specific decisions (such as refusing transfusion therapy for the perioperative period). These minors tend to be near the age of consent and are more likely to be granted mature minor status in decisions of lesser risk.

Emergency care

Consistent with the idea that nearly all people want emergency therapy to preserve life and functional status, emergency treatment should be initiated in children even if their parents are unavailable to provide consent.[6] This unambiguous presumed consent wilts when unaccompanied adolescents refuse emergency care or when adolescents and parents differ in their preferences. Honoring an adolescent's preferences in an emergency medical situation depends on the adolescent's rationale and the extent of potential harm. If there is considerable risk in honoring the adolescent's desires and the adolescent cannot exhibit substantial decision-making capacity, then it is appropriate to supersede the adolescent's preferences and use the "best interests" standard. Indeed, in emergencies, it is rare for an adolescent to demonstrate sufficient decision-making capacity to convince other decision-makers to override standard medical practices.

Confidentiality

Physicians are obligated to protect patient information from unauthorized disclosure. Breeches of confidentiality often cause adolescents to eschew future medical care.[7] Clinicians should only consider breeching confidentially if they believe that maintaining confidentiality exposes the patient to serious risk. If the risk of non-disclosure is not significant, then clinicians may wish to encourage adolescents to confide in their parents, but clinicians should respect decisions not to confide. Emancipated and mature minors have a right to complete confidentiality.

Given the principles of confidentiality, it is nearly always ethically appropriate to inform only the adolescent of a positive pregnancy test. Similarly, most states have statutes that limit disclosure of a positive pregnancy test *only* to the adolescent.[8] When an adolescent has a positive preoperative pregnancy test, the anesthesiologist should seek consultation with experts such as pediatricians, gynecologists and social workers as to how best to proceed. Informing parents or other family members may expose the minor to other serious risks, in part because family incest is not an uncommon etiology. If the adolescent, anesthesiologist, and surgeon were to postpone surgery, and the adolescent chooses not to tell her parents of the pregnancy, then the physicians must be careful not to inadvertently breech confidentiality when informing the parents about postponing surgery. (For more on pregnancy testing, see Chapter 14)

Key points

- Pediatric patients should be integrated into the process of informed consent.
- Competency is a legal term while decision-making capacity is the ability to make a specific decision at a specific time.
- Children exhibit ranges of decision-making capacity, and there is a developmental progression of the capacity of a child to assent.
- Insincere engagement of children is harmful.
- It is important to resolve disagreements among the pediatric patient–parent–physician triad about the appropriate clinical plan.
- Response to requests for nondisclosure by parents must weigh the goal of the "best interests" of the patient.
- Emancipated minor and mature minor status pose distinct ethical and practical issues.
- Confidentiality must be honored, and failure to do so may be harmful to the patient.

Notes

[a] Editor's note: in the UK, the terms "competency" and "capacity" are reversed from the US. "Competency" generally refers to functional ability, and "capacity" to legal status.

[b] The term "parental" will be used in this chapter to refer to the adult decision-maker(s) and should be considered inclusive of all other adult surrogate decision-makers.

References

1* Committee on Bioethics, American Academy of Pediatrics. (1995). Informed consent, parental permission, and assent in pediatric practice. *Pediatrics*, **95**, 314–17.

2* De Lourdes Levy, M., Larcher, V., and Kurz, R. (2003). Informed consent/assent in children. Statement of the Ethics Working Group of the Confederation of European Specialists in Paediatrics (CESP). *Eur J Pediatr*, **162**, 629–33.

3 Guidelines for the Ethical Practice of Anesthesiology (2003). American Society of Anesthesiologists. Park Ridge, IL. (last amended 2008) http://www.asahq.org/publicationsAndServices/standards/10.pdf.

4* Edwards, S. D. (2008). The Ashley treatment: a step too far, or not far enough? *J Med Ethics*, **34**, 341–3.

5* Diekema, D.S. Boldt v. Boldt: a pediatric ethics perspective. (2009). *J Clin Ethics*, **20**, 251–7.

6   Committee on Pediatric Emergency Medicine. (2003). Consent for emergency medical services for children and adolescents. *Pediatrics*, **111**, 703–6.

7*   Council on Scientific Affairs, American Medical Association. (1993). Confidential health services for adolescents. *JAMA*, **269**, 1420–4.

8*   American Academy of Pediatrics. Committee on Adolescence. (1998). Counseling the adolescent about pregnancy options. *Pediatrics*, **101**, 938–40.

Further reading

Committee on Adolescence, American Academy of Pediatrics. (1996). The adolescent's right to confidential care when considering abortion. *Pediatrics*, **97**, 746–51.

Hagger, L.E. (2004). The Human Rights Act 1998 and medical treatment: time for re-examination. *Arch Dis Child*, **89**, 460–3.

6

Do not resuscitate decisions in pediatric patients

Kelly N. Michelson and Joel E. Frader

The Case

A 4-year-old boy with metastatic neuroblastoma undergoes stem cell transplantation following intensive chemotherapy and radiation. 17 days post-transplant, with the success of anti-cancer treatment and stem cell rescue unclear, he develops an acute bowel obstruction. His parents feel that, after many months of therapy, especially over the last few weeks, their son should not have to endure "heroic" treatment. They do not want him to have cardiopulmonary resuscitation (CPR) and the oncologists have agreed to a "do not resuscitate" (DNR) order, given the boy's overall poor prognosis. The parents would like him to have palliative surgery to relieve the bowel obstruction. The anesthesiologists and surgeons request suspension of the DNR order for the surgery. The parents do not understand why it is acceptable to forgo resuscitation on the oncology unit, but not in the operating room.

Attempts to resuscitate a person from an apparently "lifeless" state date back to at least biblical times:

> When Elisha came into the house, he saw the child lying dead on his bed. So he went in and closed the door on the two of them, and prayed to the Lord. Then he got up on the bed and lay upon the child, putting his mouth upon his mouth, his eyes upon his eyes, and his hands upon his hands; and while he lay bent over him, the flesh of the child became warm.(2 Kings 4:32–34)[1]

In 1878, Boehm described closed chest cardiac massage in cats, the basis for current CPR. The first successful resuscitation in humans using CPR, reported in 1960, involved five patients who experienced in-hospital cardiac arrests.[2]

The use of CPR spread and in 1966 the National Academy of Sciences' National Research Council recommended all health care providers obtain CPR training. CPR became a nearly ubiquitous final procedure for all hospitalized patients experiencing cardiopulmonary arrest, regardless of circumstances. Later, healthcare providers questioned the indiscriminate use of CPR, particularly with terminally ill patients for whom resuscitations seemed to provide no benefit and who might experience suffering related to CPR. In some circumstances, professionals began to decide, albeit arbitrarily and without input from patients or their loved ones, who should or should not have CPR. Language such as "show code," "Hollywood code," or "slow code" emerged to describe sham resuscitations when healthcare providers chose not to make serious efforts to revive patients.

In 1974, the American Medical Association (AMA) described CPR as a procedure meant to prevent sudden, unexpected death that has no valid use in patients with terminal, irreversible illnesses. They stated, "Resuscitation in these circumstances may represent a positive violation of an individual's right to die with dignity," and proposed that actual orders be written in the patient's chart when a physician determines that CPR is not indicated.[3] In response, hospitals developed specific DNR order policies.

Arguments about the patients' right to self-determination ensued. Some felt practitioners should assume that all patients prefer resuscitation unless they or their valid surrogates have clearly stated otherwise. Others argued for only offering CPR when "medically indicated." A 1983 report of the President's Commission for the Study of Ethical Problems in Medicine and Biomedical and Behavioral established a standard whereby consent for CPR was presumed unless specifically withdrawn following discussion between the patient or surrogate and the involved physicians.[4]

Terminology

The original term, DNR, persists at many institutions. Some institutions use "DNAR" ("do not attempt

---

Clinical Ethics in Anesthesiology: A Case-Based Textbook, ed. Gail A. Van Norman, Stephen Jackson, Stanley H. Rosenbaum and Susan K. Palmer. Published by Cambridge University Press. © Cambridge University Press 2011.

resuscitation"), arguing it better recognizes that CPR often does not succeed. Recently, some have advocated using "AND" (allow natural death) noting that it focuses attention on improving the dying process, rather than on withdrawing therapies.

Simple DNR orders do not convey information about a patient's goals for care and views about life-prolonging technology. Resuscitation goals do not always fit into a "yes" or "no" response. Patients may prefer to make specific decisions about multiple therapies, including intubation, vasoactive medication, defibrillation, chest compression, antibiotics, and laboratory testing. A patient might want intubation in the event of respiratory decompensation, for example, but prefer not to undergo chest compression or defibrillation for cardiac arrest. Which interventions make sense depends on patient/surrogate goals and the specifics of the clinical situation.

DNR orders in adults vs. children

In the US competent adults have the legal right to refuse unwanted medical therapies, provided they understand the consequences of refusal. A competent adult can refuse therapies based on: (1) religious or moral views, (2) views about what constitutes a good quality of life, or (3) a determination that a particular therapy is inappropriate for medical or other reasons. Often adults lack decision-making capacity at the time when a decision is required. Anticipating such a possibility, some adults have written or oral instructions, known as "advance directives," that communicate their wishes should they lose decisional capacity. Alternatively, adults may identify a decision-maker and confer on them a "durable power of attorney for healthcare decisions" for situations when the patient cannot make or communicate their own decisions about care. The law generally expects alternative decision-makers to choose based on what the patient would have wanted. This is called substituted judgment.

Pediatric patients often lack the capacity to make medical decisions, either because of their neuro-developmental status or their medical conditions. Principles of law and ethics rely on parents to make medical decisions on behalf of their children, based on the best interest of the child.[5] The best interest standard requires that the decision-maker determine the net benefit for the patient of each option, and the appropriate course of action is the one with the greatest overall patient benefit. Older children or adolescents have some capacity to make, or assist in making medical decisions. The American Academy of Pediatrics recommends that the pediatric patients contribute to decisions to the extent of their ability.[6] (More in-depth discussions of pediatric informed consent and the rights of minors can be found in Chapter 5)

DNR in the OR

The Federal Patient Self-Determination Act of 1990 requires hospitals and healthcare organizations to advise patients during every admission of their right to create advance directives and to inquire if the patient has completed one. The law refocused attention on limits of resuscitation and intensive care. Professionals noticed that many advance directives provided inadequate clarity and specificity for clinical decision-making. Ambiguities included whether limits on resuscitation applied in the operating room. Even at end-of-life, surgical interventions may be undertaken to ease continuing care (e.g. placement of tracheostomy or gastrostomy tubes or ports for IV medications), or to surgically palliate acute problems (e.g., relief of pain from a pathologic fracture or nerve root interruption to prevent pain transmission).

Many surgeons and anesthesiologists argue that providing general anesthesia is similar to providing continuous resuscitation. During surgery patients are under continuous close observation that differs fundamentally from care outside the OR. Most patients dying on hospital units die from causes directly related to their underlying conditions, such as cancer, congestive heart failure, and degenerative neurological disease. By contrast, in the OR cardiopulmonary collapse can occur as a direct result of anesthesia or surgical manipulation (e.g. hemorrhage). Moreover, resuscitative efforts under the well-monitored and expectant conditions of the OR have higher success in returning patients to their baseline functioning than do resuscitations outside the OR. Finally, some argue that the OR provides a poor environment for end-of-life care. OR personnel typically do not deal with terminal situations and the OR has no readily available space to accommodate grieving families and clergy.[7]

In the early 1990s, institutional policies honoring patients' or surrogates' DNR wishes, as reflected in physicians' orders, typically permitted automatic suspension of DNR orders for surgical procedures and during the immediate post-operative period. Such policies did not sufficiently reflect respect for patients' autonomy. Over time, there has been more general acknowledgment of the rights of patients and their valid surrogates to authorize or reject available treatments, particularly at emotionally and religiously sensitive periods, such as the end of life.[8] A shift occurred from paternalistic physician-centered decisions, to shared decision-making between patients or surrogates, and healthcare professionals. Mirroring guidelines from the American Society of Anesthesiologists, the American College of Surgeons, and the Association of OR Nurses, some hospitals have adopted "required reconsideration," whereby a review of existing directives limiting treatments occurs before a procedure is undertaken. Discussion of perioperative DNR orders should involve the patient or surrogates, the anesthesiologist, the surgeon, and other professionals involved in the patient's care.[9] It should include the following points:

(1) Careful review of the goals of the procedure(s);
(2) Discussion of the meaning of the treatment limits and how proscriptions on interventions might compromise or complicate the anesthetic and/or the operation;
(3) Discussion of the likelihood of successful reversal of any anesthesia- or surgery-related complication;
(4) Agreement on what, if any, limits on resuscitation will remain during the procedure;
(5) Establishment of time boundaries for reinstituting the DNR orders if they are suspended;
(6) Assurance that suspension of treatment limitations will not inhibit sound decision-making – including a decision to withdraw life support – should the patient's evolving condition alter the expected clinical course.

The anesthesiologist and/or surgeon should provide clear and comprehensive documentation of the agreement in the medical record and ensure that all those involved with the proposed surgery understand and accept the agreement.

Is the cause of cardiac arrest relevant?

Reluctance of OR personnel to accept DNR orders rests to a great extent on the notion that actions by surgeons or anesthesiologists which cause or appear to cause life-threatening events (e.g. hypotension,

hypoxemia, hemorrhage, arrhythmia, etc.) differ fundamentally from events that may happen elsewhere. The assumption is that iatrogenic death, or near death, deserves a different response from other events. This claim has some merit in that instability in the OR is often easily reversed with a small likelihood of major adverse effects. But it does not explain why one would not have a similar responsibility to attempt to reverse all potentially fatal events that could be "blamed" on medical interventions. For example, a patient may experience cardiac arrest as a result of severe sepsis, a known complication in immunocompromised patients who have received anti-neoplastic agents. Few would insist on reversing DNR orders for every event whose etiology could possibly be traced to a medical intervention. A patient, parent, or other surrogate might well ask why acceptance of death in one circumstance (on the nursing unit) should not apply in the OR, especially in a setting where the patient is mercifully unconscious and will likely not suffer. The temporal and causal relationship between anesthetic delivery or surgery and death may well affect how physicians and surgeons feel about what happens, but does not necessarily make an important moral or psychological difference to the patient or loved-one who accepts the inevitability of the patient's death.

This points to potential conflicts in the goals of care for patients and loved-ones, versus those of the professionals. All parties need to clarify these goals and develop practical guides that all parties can accept. In many cases, everyone will agree on preserving life if temporary instability develops in the OR, so that remaining expected weeks or months pass with greater comfort or even function. In others, patients or surrogates may feel that some measures, such as chest compressions, electroshock, or even mechanical ventilation beyond the surgical suite or recovery room imply a level of personal invasion or indignity which is unacceptable, given the patient's overall condition and prognosis. In those cases, there are few ethical arguments that support the idea that the preference of anesthesiologists or surgeons for life extension should simply override the feelings and beliefs of patients and family members.

Case resolution

The fact that the bowel obstruction occurs so soon after transplantation makes this case especially problematic, because there is likely little reliable information

41

regarding prognosis. Decision making with such uncertainty makes physicians uncomfortable. The oncologists may well favor "aggressive" treatment, hoping the patient will remain free of neuroblastoma and have marrow recovery. The surgeons and anesthesiologists, also hoping for a good medical outcome, may view relief of bowel obstruction as relatively simple and limits on trying to sustain the boy's life as wrongheaded.

The child's parents see this picture quite differently. Their son has already endured the rigors of initial cancer surgery and chemotherapy that failed to eliminate the disease. He has also experienced considerable discomfort and distress related to "conditioning" prior to the stem cell transplant, felt the difficulties of post-transplant, pre-engraftment treatment, and faces a very uncertain outcome. Bowel obstruction represents "one more blow" and while they accept an attempt at surgical correction, they feel "heroic" attempts to revive him from a cardiac arrest in the OR would only impose additional burdens on their son and on them.

Extensive conversations between professionals and parents may or may not overcome their concerns about cardio-pulmonary arrest and CPR. They may accept a time-limited reversal of a standing DNR order. Or they may persist in their view that CPR and mechanical ventilation beyond the OR represent unacceptable invasiveness, given the boy's overall prognosis. Should they refuse to accept a temporary suspension of the DNR order, few ethical theories could justify ignoring their wishes.

A somewhat thornier ethical issue concerns whether professionals have an obligation to proceed with surgery if they voice "conscientious objection" to providing care without authorization to resuscitate. In the absence of finding substitute physicians who could willingly respect the parents' wishes, simply refusing to give the anesthetic may be regarded as "abandoning" the patient and/or exerting coercive power over the patient/surrogates. Such willful expressions of power over patients raise questions about what it means to accept the mantle of "professional" as one who puts the interests of patients ahead of self-regarding considerations. (For more on physician conscientious objection see Chapter 43.)

Key points

- DNR orders developed in response to the realization that CPR is not appropriate for all patients, particularly those with terminal illness and otherwise dismal prognosis.
- The patient's/surrogates' goals should determine the appropriateness of resuscitative interventions in and outside of the OR.
- Pediatric patients may or may not have the capacity to participate in medical decision-making, depending on age and medical condition. They should be involved in decision-making to the degree they are capable. In general, parents function as surrogate decision-makers, acting in the overall "best interest" of the child.
- Automatic suspension of DNR orders in the setting of anesthesia and surgery does not sufficiently recognize patients' rights to self-determination.
- DNR orders in pediatric patients undergoing anesthesia and surgery, as in adults, should undergo "required reconsideration" in which the involved parties review treatment limitations in light of their benefits and risks, and agree upon and document changes in orders, if any.
- When patients or their surrogate decision-makers, such as parents, do not wish to suspend DNR orders in the setting of surgery, few ethical arguments support ignoring their wishes.

References

1   *The Holy Bible. The New Revised Standard Version.* (1989). New York: Oxford University Press.

2   Kouenhoven, W.B., Jude, J.R, and Knickerbocker, G.G. (1960). Closed-chest cardiac massage. *JAMA*, **173**, 1064–7.

3* Standards for cardiopulmonary resuscitation (CPR) and emergency cardiac care (ECC). (1974). *JAMA*, **227**(7), Suppl:837–68.

4* Burns, J.P., Edwards, J., Johnson, J., *et al.* (2003). Do-not-resuscitate order after 25 years. *Crit Care Med*, **31**(5), 1543–50.

5* American Academy of Pediatrics Committee on Bioethics. (1994). Guidelines on foregoing life-sustaining medical treatment. *Pediatrics*, **93**(3), 532–6.

6* Committee on Bioethics, American Academy of Pediatrics. (1995). Informed consent, parental permission, and assent in pediatric practice. *Pediatrics*, **95**(2), 314–17.

7* Ewanchuk, M. and Brindley, P.G. (2006). Perioperative do-not-resuscitate orders – doing 'nothing' when 'something' can be done. *Crit Care*, **10**(4), 219.

8* Waisel, D.B., Burns, J.P., Johnson, J.A., *et al.* (2002). Guidelines for perioperative do-not-resuscitate policies. *J Clin Anesth*, **14**(6), 467–73.

9* Fallat, M.E. and Deshpande, J.K. (2004). Do-not-resuscitate orders for pediatric patients who require anesthesia and surgery. *Pediatrics*, **114**(6),1686–92.

7

Consent in laboring patients

Joanna M. Davies

Case 1

Sarah is a 32-year-old, gravida 1, para 0 in active labor at 4 cm cervical dilatation. She is experiencing considerable pain and requests an epidural for analgesia. However, as the anesthesiologist arrives, the patient's husband, Tom, is telling the nurse that, prior to labor, his wife specifically told him that she did not want an epidural for pain, even if she begged for one, and he should not let her change her mind. This information is also written in her birth plan. Sarah is now screaming with each contraction and, despite receiving a total of 150 mcg of intravenous fentanyl, is adamant that she wants an epidural "now."

Principle-based medical ethics focuses on the four concepts of autonomy, beneficence, nonmaleficence and justice. Over time, there has been movement from the beneficence driven paternalism of "doctor knows best" towards increasing patient autonomy. Authentic patient autonomy requires that the patients make their own decisions after they have received all of the relevant information pertinent to their situation and are therefore fully informed. Informed consent requires several elements: (1) capacity of the patient to make a decision, (2) freedom or voluntariness of the patient in decision-making, (3) disclosure of adequate information to the patient, (4) understanding of that information by the patient, and (5) consent by the patient to the procedure. Ensuring that these elements have been addressed and obtaining consent for procedures in laboring patients can be extremely challenging.

Can informed consent be obtained during the pain of labor?

There are conflicting views on whether informed consent is even possible during active labor. Black and Cyna, analyzed responses from 291 anesthesiologists surveyed about the risks they discussed with laboring patients, and whether it was possible to gain fully informed consent from them.[1] Seventy percent considered active labor a barrier to the ability of a woman to give consent. However, a Society of Obstetric Anesthesia and Perinatology Anesthesiologists (SOAP) survey, published the same year (2006), found that 68% of 448 anesthesiologists thought that women in active labor are able to give informed consent.[2] Scott has gone so far as to say "the only time when consent to an epidural to relieve the pain of labor is truly informed is in labor itself … when the person concerned knows what the pain is like."[3]

Several studies of the patient's perspective of informed consent during labor show that the pain of labor does not appear to interfere with the patient's ability to hear and comprehend the information relevant to consent.[4] Furthermore, a woman's ability to understand epidural risks does not correlate with level of labor pain, anxiety, duration of pain, opioid medication, previous epidural experience or the desire for an epidural.[5] In fact, the ability to recall the risks has been found to be similar in both laboring and nonlaboring, nonobstetric patients.[6] Ideally, written or visual information about labor analgesia should be provided or at least available during prenatal visits to the obstetrician's office in the antenatal period or during early labor allowing time for consideration of the available options and any questions.

Is Sarah's consent impeded by the fentanyl she has received? In general the answer is poorly addressed in the literature. There are no US legal precedents regarding this issue and most institutions have inconsistent policies. Anesthesiologists can and do routinely make judgments about a patient's capacity for informed consent based on the elements described above. There is normally no need to contact a psychiatrist or obtain legal advice. Sarah must have the mental capacity to comprehend and participate in the consent process and analgesia may allow her to do this. Withholding

Clinical Ethics in Anesthesiology: A Case-Based Textbook, ed. Gail A. Van Norman, Stephen Jackson, Stanley H. Rosenbaum and Susan K. Palmer. Published by Cambridge University Press. © Cambridge University Press 2011.

appropriate analgesia, particularly if there is a delay in the anesthesiologist obtaining consent, may in itself put the anesthesiologist in an unsupportable ethical position.

Ulysses directives

At this stage in her care, the literature supports that Sarah, despite being in severe pain and having received fentanyl, should be able to provide fully informed consent for epidural placement. However, an additional ethical dilemma has developed. Sarah's husband, Tom, is insistent that Sarah does not really want an epidural and produces a written birthing plan which includes a statement that Sarah does not want to be permitted to deviate from this plan or her wishes concerning an epidural. Such a document is known as a "Ulysses directive" and brings into conflict the anesthesiologist's beneficent desire to provide Sarah with analgesia, and the wish to respect Sarah's autonomous decision to have a "natural" delivery.

However, autonomous decision-making brings with it the privilege for a woman to change her mind, especially if she has never experienced the pain of childbirth before. One might argue that Sarah's directive be considered invalid because it was made at a time when the she was not fully informed. Antenatally, she may have been determined not to have an epidural. However, she may not have received appropriate information regarding the risks and benefits of epidurals, nor had she experienced labor pain previously. Information and valid experience are critical prerequisites for autonomous decision-making. While Scott considers it unethical "to withhold pain relief from a greatly distressed woman … solely because of a statement written in her birth plan..", Thornton and Moore have argued that this "… does not respect her long-term preferences", and hence her autonomy."[7] Other authors have even postulated that the duty of beneficence (in this case to relieve pain) may allow an intervention to proceed in the absence of informed consent until evidence of patient refusal is forthcoming.[8] In this instance there is no unequivocal ethical ground upon which to stand and it has been suggested that the anesthesiologist be guided by the circumstances.[9]

Sarah is a primiparous woman at 4 cm cervical dilatation and is likely to be in labor for many more hours. Placing an epidural for analgesia is certainly an ethically defensible decision in this case. Interestingly, frequently it is the legal ramifications rather than the ethical debate that cause anesthesiologists the most concern. As a woman with capacity, Sarah can legally overrule her birth plan at any point. However, there is a risk after delivery, when the pain is long gone, that Sarah might feel she somehow "failed" during the birthing process by agreeing to have an epidural and see the anesthesiologist as an accomplice in this failure. This could result in an accusation of assault, or unconsented touching of the patient.

The anesthesiologist should be encouraged to see the patient and her family postpartum. At that time the anesthesiologist can discuss the events and reassure the patient that her decision was the correct one for the circumstances in which she found herself. It may help to inform the patient that relief of pain and stress during labor has benefits for the fetus and the course of labor. It is also wise to document the decision-making process that occurred. An example chart note might read:

> After an appropriate consent process, the patient has decided to withdraw her previous refusal of epidural analgesia for labor. I will proceed based on her currently stated request for epidural analgesia.

In this particular case the ethical tension was resolved when the anesthesiologist conducted a patient and lengthy discussion with both Tom and Sarah. They agreed that they may not have appreciated how painful the labor would be, that an epidural would allow Sarah to enjoy the birth more, and that perhaps they had been naïve in her inexperience to completely refuse to consider all of her analgesic options.

How much information is enough?

How much information is too much and how long a discussion is too long during the throws of active labor? The amount of information given to Sarah regarding the risks and benefits of an epidural needs to be balanced against her level of pain and urgency to proceed. If possible, discussions should be held between contractions when the woman can focus on what she is being told. It is prudent to have this conversation with the patient's support person present. Tom, in this case, will be able to ask questions and witness that the information has been provided. Every anesthesiologist has their own routine when providing information to a patient during the consent process. Brooks and Sullivan have aided the practitioner by developing a list of recommended issues that should be discussed with the patient.[10] This list includes:

(1) benefits of the epidural to the mother, i.e., excellent pain relief;
(2) potential beneficial effects of an epidural on the baby and labor;
(3) risks of epidurals, such as epidural failure, side effects, and rare but serious risks;
(4) information relevant to the individual patient, e.g., the effect of an epidural on preexisting medical conditions she may already have, e.g., chronic back pain or neurological disease;
(5) alternatives for analgesia and any further information requested by the patient.

Which risks should be disclosed?

As is frequently the case, Sarah does not wish to hear a lot of details about the procedure and urges the anesthesiologist to "just get on with it." While being flexible in the approach to providing information under these conditions, it is imperative that the anesthesiologist cover the risks of the procedure. There is no universal standard of care when disclosing risks associated with an epidural to obtain informed consent, although different rules have been proposed. Several studies have found that the majority of women want to hear all the risks associated with regional anesthesia, particularly those that occur commonly but are less severe, and those which are rare but could be serious or life-threatening.[11]

Should informed consent be written or verbal?

There is no consensus about whether it is better to have patients sign consents or, simply verbally consent: both are ethically and legally acceptable in many states. Documentation of this discussion can include either a separate anesthesia consent form signed by the patient or a detailed note in the patient's chart verifying verbal consent.

Is informed consent during labor a liability issue?

Knapp examined three legal cases that addressed the issue of adequacy of informed consent during labor.

In every instance the cases were found in favor of the defending anesthesiologist because the courts felt there was not only evidence of "reasonable" information having been provided to the patients but also, the patients had not objected to, and in fact, had actively cooperated with the procedure.[12]

Case 2: Refusal to consent to treatment

Fatima is a non-English speaking, 19-year-old, gravida 2, para 1, Somalian Muslim married to 40-year-old Mohammed. It is 3:00 am. Because of the hour there is no formal Somali interpreter available so Mohammed has been providing interpretation. Fatima has been in labor for more than 20 hours with slow progress. She is at 9 cm cervical dilatation and the fetus is showing signs of distress with severe variable heart rate decelerations into the 60s. The obstetricians want to perform an urgent cesarean section but Mohammed is refusing, despite being told that the baby could die if surgery is delayed. In spite of his refusal for surgery Fatima continues to say that she wants her baby to be delivered safely. There is concern that Mohammed is not giving his wife the correct information or providing the practitioners with an adequate representation of Fatima's wishes.

Frequently, such dilemmas are resolved by further discussion regarding the risks and benefits of the Cesarean section, understanding the fears of surgery that the patient brings to the table, and gentle persuasion as to the best course of action to gain the consent of the husband to proceed. However, that is not always the result. There are several ethical issues that must be considered in this situation. The first is that of "maternal–fetal conflict," also discussed in Chapter 8, under "CDMR from the Fetus's Perspective."

Maternal–fetal conflict

This case demonstrates how two fundamental ethical principles, autonomy and beneficence, can come into conflict. A competent pregnant woman such as Fatima, has the autonomous right to refuse medical intervention, even if that decision may adversely affect her fetus. This can be distressing to the obstetrician who is advising a cesarean section in accordance with the ethical principle of beneficence to ensure the best outcome for both Fatima and her baby.

Some physicians may feel that the obvious solution in this case would be to obtain a court order to perform the cesarean section and save Fatima's baby. It has long been debated as to whether the fetus should be considered as a patient, with its own rights, separate from the mother. This stance does consider the fact that the fetus is dependent on the mother for its existence. While delivery of the fetus may respect the right to life of the fetus, it compromises Fatima's right to autonomy.

There has been much discussion in the literature regarding forced medical intervention and its possible justification in certain situations. The American College of Obstetricians and Gynecologists (ACOG) has provided clear guidance on this, stating that in cases of maternal refusal of treatment for the sake of the fetus, "court-ordered intervention against the wishes of a pregnant woman is rarely, if ever acceptable."[13] The American Medical Association (AMA) considers forced intervention to be counter-productive, stating that "women may withhold information from the physician … Or they may reject medical or prenatal care altogether."[14] A compounding issue is whether the obstetrician's prognosis regarding the fetal outcome without intervention is correct. There have been cases where the woman has refused emergency cesarean section on religious grounds, only to deliver a healthy baby vaginally.[15] When court orders have been sought in the US, different states and judges have come to different judgments in these difficult cases. The risk to the primary patient, the mother, may often decide these cases. Specifically, there is a foreseeable risk for a mother with a complete placenta previa, not just a threat to her undelivered fetus.

Cultural and religious beliefs

Some cultures and religions place constraints on medical care. Physicians must have respect for different belief systems and work with laboring patients to achieve the best outcome for both mother and baby.

In Western culture, Fatima's autonomy regarding her medical care is paramount and we would expect her to decide whether she is willing to consent to a Cesarean section only after receiving all the pertinent information. According to the Islamic faith, Mohammed has the right to make decisions for his wife. This is seen as a positive, caring aspect of their marriage. Personal autonomy is not considered important. Even if Fatima is asked her decision,

there is no guarantee that she has not been influenced by others. In this case, while respecting the cultural and religious basis upon which Mohammed is operating – and thereby potentially manipulating Fatima's care – we also want Fatima to understand the situation, so that she could at least discuss it with her husband.

There some is concern that critical information is not being conveyed accurately to Fatima. Muslim women are allowed to voice their opinion but, like anyone, they need all the facts before making their decision. The absence of an interpreter is a problem. One solution is to use a telephone interpreter service, to which many hospitals subscribe. Such services provide access to most languages at any time of day. This service was unfortunately not available on that particular night. Interpreter help in urgent situations can also be sought from hospital employees, religious community members, or relatives of the patients who might be reachable by phone.

Ultimately, Mohammed and Fatima stood by their decision, despite prolonged discussions with the obstetricians. Fatima's baby was still-born several hours later. Although distressed by their loss, they were comforted by their belief that this was Allah's will. The obstetricians were devastated.

Could this case have been managed differently? Ethically, the obstetricians behaved correctly by respecting Mohammed's autonomous decision to refuse a cesarean section for Fatima. There will always be concerns that Fatima was not given all the facts about the fetal condition and may have been able to persuade her husband to allow a Cesarean delivery.

Ethical considerations are of primary importance in cases such as these, but there are also legal issues that need to be considered and managed. Whenever a patient refuses medical care, the American College of Obstetricians and Gyencologists suggest that following information should be documented:[16]

(1) The patient's refusal to consent to a medical treatment, surgical procedure, or diagnostic test

(2) Confirmation that the need for this treatment, procedure, or test has been explained

(3) The reasons stated by the patient for refusal of treatment

(4) Confirmation that the consequences of the refusal, including possible jeopardy to health or life, have been described to the patient.

Key points

- Although many anesthesiologists believe that laboring women may not be able to give informed consent, most studies indicate that laboring women are similarly capable to nonlaboring patients of hearing and remembering the risks involved and consenting to treatment.

- The informed consent process in laboring patients has requirements to disclose risks, benefits, and alternatives to anesthesia care that are similar to that in nonlaboring patients.

- Ulysses directives – advance directives that include irrevocable instructions – are sometimes included in birth plans, but are ethically problematic in laboring women who retain personal autonomy during labor. Women have the right to change plans and may do so in light of valid new experience. It is questionable whether such directives are ethically or legally binding in most cases. Deviation from Ulysses directives requires appropriate discussion and documentation.

- Every labor carries the risk of maternal–fetal conflicts. ACOG and AMA guidelines discourage forced intervention in all but rare cases, and recognize that respect for maternal autonomy is usually the dominant ethical principle to follow.

- Cultural and religious beliefs may complicate care of the laboring patient and require consideration in managing ethical conflicts.

- When a laboring woman refuses critical intervention, all efforts should be made to inform her of the risks and benefits of refusal of treatment, including the use of interpreter services if needed to a conduct careful and complete discussion.

References

1 Black, J. and Cyna, A.M. (2006). Issues of consent for regional analgesia in labour: a survey of obstetric anaesthetists. *Anaesth Intens Care*, **34**, 254–60.

2 Saunders, T.A., Stein, D.J. and Dilger, J.P. (2006). Informed consent for labor epidurals: a survey of Society for Obstetric Anesthesia and Perinatology anesthesiologists from the United States. *IJOA*, **15**, 98–103.

3* Scott, W.E. (1996). Ethics in obstetric anaesthesia. *Anaesthesia*, **51**, 717–18.

4* Pattee, C., Ballantyne, M. and Milne, B. (1997). Epidural analgesia for labour and delivery: informed consent issues. *Can J Anaesth*, **44**, 918–23.

5* Jackson, A., Henry, R., Avery, N., *et al.* (2000). Informed consent for labour epidurals: what labouring women want to know. *Can J Anaesth*, **47**, 1068–73.

6* Affleck, P.J., Waisel, D.B., Cusick, J.M., *et al.* (1998). Recall of risks following labor epidural analgesia. *J Clin Anesth*, **10**, 141–4.

7* Brooks, H. and Sullivan, W.J. (2002). The importance of patient autonomy at birth. *IJOA*, **11**, 196–203.

8* Hoehner, P.J. (2003). Ethical aspects of informed consent in obstetric anesthesia – new challenges and solutions. *J Clin Anesth*, **15**, 587–600.

9 Brooks, H. and Sullivan, W.J. (2002). The importance of patient autonomy at birth. *IJOA*, **11**, 196–203.

10 Brooks, H. and Sullivan, W.J. (2002). The importance of patient autonomy at birth. *IJOA*, **11**, 196–203.

11 Jackson, A., Henry, R., Avery, N., *et al.* (2000). Informed consent for labour epidurals: what labouring women want to know. *Can J Anaesth*, **47**, 1068–73.

12* Knapp, R.M. (1990). Legal view of informed consent for anesthesia during labor. *Anesthesiology*, **72**, 211.

13* Patient choice in the maternal–fetal relationship. In *Ethics in Obstetrics and Gynecology*. 2nd edn. (2004). Washington, DC: American College of Obstetricians and Gynecologists, pp. 34–6.

14 Hoehner, P.J. (2003). Ethical aspects of informed consent in obstetric anesthesia – new challenges and solutions. *J Clin Anesth*, **15**, 587–600.

15* Weiniger, C.F., Elchalal, U., Sprung, C.L., *et al.* (2006). Holy consent – a dilemma for medical staff when maternal consent is withheld for emergency caesarean section. *IJOA*, **15**, 145–8.

16* Informed refusal. In *Ethics in Obstetrics and Gynecology*. 2nd edn. Washington, DC: American College of Obstetricians and Gynecologists, pp. 105–6.

Further reading

Beauchamp, T.L. and Childress, J.F. (2001). *Principles of Biomedical Ethics*, 5th edn. Oxford, UK: Oxford University Press Inc.

Walton, S. (2003). Birth plans and fallacy of the Ulysses directive, *I5OA*, **12**, 138–45.

Maternal–fetal conflicts: Cesarean delivery on maternal request

Ruth Landau and Steve Yentis

The Case

Jane and Jim, successful lawyers in their mid-forties, are expecting their first child. Immediately after they learned that their 4th in-vitro fertilization attempt was successful, they decided to request a Cesarean delivery. At 36 weeks, Jane and Jim confirm again their desire to have a 'maternal request' Cesarean section and ask for the Cesarean delivery to be performed the following week at 37 weeks' gestation to accommodate Jim's busy agenda. In addition, Jane is adamant she wants to have a general anesthetic due to her fear of experiencing any kind of discomfort or pain during the Cesarean section.

Until recently, debate around the indications for and choice of Cesarean section have focused on rights of women to *refuse* a Cesarean section when urgent delivery is medically indicated. In terms of the "principlism" (four principles) approach to ethical analysis, this debate has highlighted the balance between the obligations of the obstetrician to both the mother and fetus and obligations of the mother to the fetus, based on *beneficence* and *non-maleficence*, and the duty to respect the mother's *autonomy*. Legally, many courts recognize an absolute right of women with capacity to refuse medical treatment even when that decision may result in their death or the death of their baby. Doctors have duties to respect a woman's autonomy and obligations to inform fully, counsel honestly, and avoid coercion.

Recently, a new phenomenon has emerged in which patients *demand* a cesarean section. More women are switching their birth plan from a "natural childbirth/no epidural" perspective towards a more "controlled", medicalized or surgical childbirth. What ethical implications does this growing phenomenon have for clinicians?

Cesarean section upon maternal request

Cesarean section rates are rising in developed countries. Reasons include a decline in vaginal births after previous Cesarean delivery, a decline in vaginal breech deliveries, and a reluctance among many obstetricians to "risk" a vaginal delivery when labor is not straightforward. The number of Cesarean deliveries at maternal request (CDMR) – i.e., in the absence of any medical or obstetrical indications – has been increasing, accounting for 48–18% of all Cesarean deliveries.[1] An independent panel of the National Institute of Child Health and Human Development and the Office of Medical Applications of Research of the National Institutes of Health (NIH) reviewed CDMR in 2006[2] and drew the following conclusions.

(1) The incidence of cesarean delivery without medical or obstetrical indications is increasing in the US, one component of which is CDMR.

(2) There is insufficient evidence to fully evaluate the benefits and risks of CDMR compared to planned vaginal delivery. More research is needed.

(3) Until evidence becomes available, the decision to perform CDMR should be individualized and consistent with ethical principles.

(4) The risks of placenta previa and accreta rise with each Cesarean delivery, and CDMR is not recommended for women desiring several children.

(5) CDMR should not be performed before 39 weeks' gestation or without verification of lung maturity because of the significant danger of neonatal respiratory complications.

(6) Unavailability of effective labor pain options should not influence the decision to perform CDMR.

Ethical considerations for CDMR go beyond the principles of respect for autonomy and beneficence/non-maleficence. They include issues of resource allocation and the impact of CDMR on healthcare

Clinical Ethics in Anesthesiology: A Case-Based Textbook, ed. Gail A. Van Norman, Stephen Jackson, Stanley H. Rosenbaum and Susan K. Palmer. Published by Cambridge University Press. © Cambridge University Press 2011.

costs (i.e., the principle of justice) as well as idealistic and philosophical reflections on future societal implications if Cesarean deliveries become the norm.

CDMR from the mother's perspective

Common reasons reported by women requesting a cesarean delivery are fear of labor pain and stress; uncertainty of outcome; fear of emergency intervention such as forceps; fear of fetal distress during labor; fear of future sexual dysfunction, stress incontinence or pelvic prolapse; and convenience. Ultimately, women may invoke a right to have their autonomy respected, and to participate in all decisions related to their healthcare; in other words, if an informed woman wants a cesarean delivery, she should have the right to request a cesarean delivery regardless of any medical risk that her decision may inflict on her or her baby.

Respect for patient autonomy requires that a patient be fully informed about the benefits and the risks of a recommended treatment, and then has the right either to consent to the treatment or refuse it. But broadening this principle to create an obligation to respect a patient *request* for treatment that is *not recommended* and might even be harmful stretches the concept of patient autonomy to a point that many ethicists and lawyers believe goes beyond what is reasonably acceptable within the usual doctor–patient relationship. In the UK, non-obstetrical patient treatment requests have been tested in the courts, which have confirmed that doctors are not legally or ethically obliged to provide treatment requested by a patient if they consider it not in his/her best interests.[3]

With CDMR, the situation is further complicated by the involvement of a third party – the fetus. A woman may desire CDMR to avoid a complicated vaginal delivery that may be harmful not only to herself but also to her baby. Furthermore, the risk of a primigravidae requiring an urgent unplanned cesarean delivery during labor are significant – approximately 10%–20%. Cesarean section following a prolonged trial of labor involves higher maternal morbidity than a scheduled Cesarean, due to increased risk of uterine atony and hemorrhage. For the baby, a scheduled Cesarean delivery may reduce risks, such as reduced availability of neonatal resuscitative measures, associated with a possible "out of office hours" delivery. Indeed, concern for the baby is one of the most common motivations cited by women requesting CDMR.[4]

Autonomy of decision-making implies that the benefits and risks are known, disclosed and discussed. In the case of CDMR, this may not be entirely possible. Evidence on the risks and benefits of CDMR in low risk pregnant women has never been entirely assessed, leading the NIH to call for more randomized clinical trials.

CDMR from the fetus's perspective

The concept of "fetal rights" contributes to a notion that the pregnant woman and her fetus are potential adversaries. Much of the debate around "fetal rights" has been in the context of abortion, an area of great political, ethical, and legal controversy. The fetus is in an intermediate ethical, and legal position. Lacking capacity, it cannot have autonomy. Furthermore, the fetus is dependent for its well-being on the choices made by the mother. In UK and Canadian common law "the fetus does not have legal rights until it is born alive and with complete delivery from the body of the pregnant woman."[5] If a competent woman refuses medical advice, her decision must be respected even if the doctor believes that her fetus will suffer as a result. According to the ACOG Committee on Ethics[6]:

> Pregnant women's autonomous decisions should be respected. Concerns about the impact of maternal decisions on fetal well-being should be discussed in the context of medical evidence and understood within the context of each woman's broad social network, cultural beliefs, and values. In the absence of extraordinary circumstances, circumstances that, in fact, the Committee on Ethics cannot currently imagine, judicial authority should not be used to implement treatment regimens aimed at protecting the fetus, for such actions violate the pregnant woman's autonomy.

Regarding CDMR, the fetus's best interests are usually considered in terms of the risks of prematurity and trauma if delivered by elective cesarean section, weighed against the risks of injury arising from difficult delivery, emergency intervention, or post-maturity.

In the case of Jane and Jim, CDMR is particularly controversial because they request it at 37 weeks' gestation. Compelling evidence concludes that neonatal outcomes are improved if Cesarean delivery is delayed until 39 weeks.[7] The risks should clearly be presented to Jane and Jim as well as the option to perform fetal lung tests prior to scheduling the surgery.

CDMR from the doctor's perspective

Do doctors have the choice whether or not to perform a CDMR?

Principles of beneficence and nonmaleficence are particularly challenging with CDMR, since they must balance benefits and harms for both mother and baby in a situation where (1) there is a lack of reliable authoritative data, (2) physicians' own personal views may vary widely, and (3) there is heated political as well as medical debate.

The most compelling arguments against performing an elective Cesarean section relate to complications. To reduce fetal morbidity, CDMR should at least not be performed before fetal lung maturation has been established, and therefore should not be scheduled before 39 weeks' gestation. Data regarding *maternal* morbidity are generally based on nonscheduled procedures in women with medical and obstetrical conditions that both increase risks and may require general rather than regional anesthesia. Data for maternal morbidity following scheduled procedures are few. In addition, maternal risks are known to increase with successive Cesarean sections. From a nonmaleficence perspective, therefore, CDMR risks to future pregnancies must be thoroughly examined and discussed.

Should obstetricians ever be compelled to provide a Cesarean delivery they do not believe to be medically necessary? Most doctors believe that *professional autonomy* protects them from providing such therapy, and ensures their "clinical freedom." There are cases (e.g., abortion) in which doctors are excused from obligations to provide treatment to which they have a moral or religious objection. Obstetricians might argue it is against their moral integrity to perform a nonindicated surgical procedure such as a CDMR. However, as reinforced in the UK by the *Burke* ruling,[8] a much stronger argument may be one based on risks and benefits and the interests of the patient(s), rather than one based on physicians' personal morals. In the UK, National Institute for Health and Clinical Excellence (NICE) guidelines suggest that doctors have the right to "decline a request for a caesarean section in the absence of an identifiable reason."[9]

What do obstetricians believe?

Surveys show disagreement among obstetricians regarding CDMR, and that a significant proportion of obstetricians would either choose CDMR for themselves or their partners and/or would comply with women's requests. Their reasons include fears of complications of vaginal delivery, desires to avoid medicolegal consequences if such complications develop after refusing to perform CDMR, and desires to respect women's autonomy. In a survey involving eight European countries and over 1500 obstetricians, wide differences in culture and case law appeared to account for variation in compliance with a woman's request for CDMR, which ranged from 15% (Spain) to 79% (UK).[10] A survey of ACOG members found that of 699 respondents, just over half believed that women had the right to CDMR and a similar proportion had complied with such a request.[11]

CDMR from a public health perspective

In a world of finite resources, we might question the ethics (*distributive justice*) of promoting CDMR as a standard of care to endorse women's autonomy when millions of citizens do not have access to even basic health coverage. If healthcare resources are diverted to increased Cesarean deliveries, theoretically such resources will not be available to others. Should individual women therefore bear financial responsibility for their CDMR just as they do for other "non-medically" indicated procedures such as cosmetic surgery? Limiting CDMR to women able to afford the extra cost of surgery, however, creates another inequality in healthcare access. How would this model take into account the percentage of women who ended up with an urgent, complicated, and costly unplanned Cesarean delivery after a failed trial of labor and delivery?

Finally, how do we anticipate the true cost of CDMR when most studies assessing such costs compare vaginal deliveries with all cesarean sections, including those with sicker women and/or babies? Taken to an extreme, if all women who wanted CDMR obtained it, the need for labor and delivery rooms, and the incidence of lengthy failed labors, urgent instrumental or cesarean deliveries would significantly decline, potentially being replaced by a less costly obstetrical practice. Although cesarean section without labor would seem to be more expensive than uncomplicated vaginal delivery, studies attempting to compare such costs are often methodologically flawed, involve few randomized trials, are plagued by inadequate power, and often omit important considerations including costs accruing to patients.

Other societal issues not directly related to costs include the medicalization of childbirth and a paradoxical transfer of power from women to the medical profession if CDMR becomes the norm.

CDMR from the anesthesiologist's perspective

The anesthesiologist probably would not have been directly involved in the patient's and obstetrician's decisions regarding mode of delivery. However, one of the reasons cited by women choosing CDMR is fear of pain during labor and delivery, and adequate information and access to optimal labor analgesia may be crucial in shaping this discussion. Anesthesiologists are obliged to inform women that early neuraxial analgesia is safe and available. For women who fear loss of control, access to low-dose neuraxial labor analgesics with patient-controlled epidural analgesia (PCEA) may be one way to "avoid" a CDMR. Pain during and after Cesarean section is a major concern for women, and these issues also need to be addressed.

At minimum, the following information regarding general anesthesia should be discussed with Jane and Jim:

Maternal risks of general anesthesia

Anesthesia-related maternal mortality, though low, has been associated with difficult airway management and aspiration during induction of anesthesia and recovery.[12] However, these risks are clearly increased when patients are obese and surgery is unplanned and urgent, mitigating this concern when it is applied to elective surgery.

Risk of pain after Cesarean delivery

A woman who requests a general anesthetic to avoid all pain and discomfort during Cesarean section should be informed that the gold standard for post-Cesarean analgesia, neuraxial opioids, cannot be administered. The clear association of severe acute post-delivery pain, post-partum depression, and chronic pain must also be disclosed.

Risk of awareness during general anesthesia

Although the risk of awareness is low, this potentially traumatic and devastating outcome must be disclosed to women who are seeking the utmost comfort and stress-free experience when choosing a CDMR under general anesthesia.

Fetal risks of general anesthesia

A recent study in a cohort of very preterm infants comparing neonatal mortality after epidural, spinal and general anesthesia for cesarean reported no increased risk after general anesthesia when controlling for gestational age.[13] However, a large population-based study reported higher neonatal risks with general anesthesia even in scheduled cesarean sections.[14] Women therefore need to be informed that the risk for neonatal resuscitation and intubation are potentially higher after general anesthesia than after regional anesthesia.

Long-term effects of general anesthesia on the developing brain have been of growing concern,[15] but further studies are necessary before firm conclusions can be drawn regarding the adverse effect of short perinatal exposure to general anesthetics.

Alternative regional anesthesia

In order to make an informed choice the risks of alternatives, including regional anesthesia must also be discussed, including hypotension, inadequate anesthesia requiring conversion to general anesthesia, severe headache, nerve damage, epidural abscess or meningitis, epidural hematoma, and severe injury including paralysis. Benefits such as being awake to bond with the baby, and the opportunity for postoperative neuraxial analgesia should also be presented.

Can the anesthesiologist refuse to participate in CDMR?

Examples of refusal by physicians to provide anesthesia when it conflicts with their personal beliefs include abortions and care of Jehovah's Witnesses undergoing scheduled surgery. The NICE guidelines give doctors the right to decline a request for a Cesarean section in the absence of an identifiable reason. However, Camman argues that unlike terminations of pregnancies or refusal of blood transfusion by Jehovah's witnesses, elective Cesarean sections do not have a religious or moral component, since Cesarean section is an accepted medical intervention that does not intentionally result in harm or loss of life.[16] Refusal to provide anesthesia based on beneficence and nonmaleficence arguments are therefore stronger than those based on moral objection, although Gass, in a counter to Camman, has argued that there are moral grounds for refusal to participate in CDMR based on the utilitarian need to maximize societal benefit.[17]

Conscientious objections could be applied to any treatment where the doctor might have personal beliefs that conflict with the patient's. But rights of physicians to invoke conscientious objection is limited by the (usually) overriding duties to provide patient care. In the UK, the General Medical Council has stated the following[18]:

> You must make the care of your patient your first concern.
>
> You must treat your patients with respect, whatever their life choices and beliefs.
>
> You must not unfairly discriminate against patients by allowing your personal views to affect adversely your professional relationship with them or the treatment you provide or arrange.
>
> If carrying out a particular procedure or giving advice about it conflicts with your religious or moral beliefs, and this conflict might affect the treatment or advice you provide, you must explain this to the patient and tell them they have the right to see another doctor. You must be satisfied that the patient has sufficient information to enable them to exercise that right. If it is not practical for a patient to arrange to see another doctor, you must ensure that arrangements are made for another suitably qualified colleague to take over your role. You must not express to your patients your personal beliefs, including political, religious or moral beliefs, in ways that exploit their vulnerability or that are likely to cause them distress.

(For more on physician conscientious objection, see Chapter 43.)

With regards to the choice of anesthetic, there is no difference between CDMR and any other Cesarean section. It is generally accepted that regional anesthesia is safer and better than general anesthesia. However, there may be cases, such as when the parturient's anxiety and fear are so great – even if irrational – that her interests are best served by undergoing a general anesthetic.

The authors would personally be agreeable to Jane and Jim's request to perform a Cesarean section as soon as fetal lung maturity has been established (or at 39 weeks), preferably under regional anesthesia. When the desires of a pregnant woman are in conflict with usual medical indications for treatment or with the best interests of the baby, the following key points should be kept in mind:

Key points

- The principle of respect for patient autonomy supports a pregnant woman's rights to refuse recommended medical treatments, even if such refusal may be detrimental to her or to her fetus. Physicians generally are ethically obliged to honor these rights.
- The obligations of physicians to accede to requests for *nonrecommended treatments* are less straight forward.
- Principles of beneficence and nonmaleficence require that consideration be given to the maternal benefits against the maternal harms, as well as benefits and harms for the fetus.
- When patients request unnecessary interventions, additional ethical considerations include issues of distributive justice (does CDMR divert healthcare resources away from more basic needs to fulfill the wishes of a few privileged persons, or does it have the potential to reduce health care costs overall by avoiding the costs of complications of more traditional care?).
- Some patient care situations allow physicians to withdraw out of conscientious objection based in personal religious or moral beliefs, but refusing to provide requested and accepted (albeit unnecessary) therapies are better supported by arguments using principles of beneficence and nonmaleficence.
- When a physician objects to providing medical services that are acceptable within the standard of care, they have obligations to transfer the care of such patients to a suitably qualified colleague who can provide such care.

References

1. ACOG Committee Opinion No. 394, December 2007. Cesarean delivery on maternal request. *Obstet Gynecol* **110**, 1501.

2. NIH State-of-the-Science Conference Statement on cesarean delivery on maternal request. NIH (2006). *Consens State Sci Statements*, **23**, 1–29.

3. R (Burke) v General Medical Council and Disability Rights Commission (interested party) & The Official Solicitor (Intervener) [2004]. EWHC 1879

4. Wiklund, I., Edman, G., and Andolf, E. (2007). Cesarean section on maternal request: reasons for the request, self-estimated health, expectations, experience of birth and signs of depression among first-time mothers. *Acta Obstet Gynecol Scand*, **86**, 451–6.

5. Flagler, E., Baylis, F., and Rogers, S. (1997). Bioethics for clinicians: 12. Ethical dilemmas that arise in the

care of pregnant women: rethinking :maternal-fetal conflicts. *CMAJ*, **156**, 1729–32.

6* ACOG Committee Opinion N. 321. Maternal decision making, ethics, and the law. November 2005. American College of Obstetrics and Gynecology. Washington DC.

7 Tita, A.T., Landon, M.B., Spong, C.Y., *et al.* (2009) *N Engl J Med*, **360**, 111–20.

8 R (Burke) v General Medical Council and Disability Rights Commission (interested party) & The Official Solicitor (Intervener) [2004]. EWHC 1879

9 (NHS) NIfCE: Caesarean section. www.nice.org.uk/CG013NICEguideline 2004.

10 Habiba, M., Kaminski, M., Da Fre, M., *et al.* (2006). Caesarean section on request: a comparison of obstetricians' attitudes in eight European countries. *BJOG*, **113**, 647–56.

11 Bettes, B.A., Coleman, V.H., Zinber, S., *et al.* (2007). Cesarean delivery on maternal request: obstetrician-gynecologists' knowledge, perception, and practice patterns. *Obstet Gynecol*, **109**, 57–66.

12 American Society of Anesthesiologists' Practice Guidelines for Obstetric Anesthesia: update 2006. American Society of Anesthesiologists. Park Ridge, Il. http://www.asahq.org.

13 Laudenbach, V. Mercier, F.J., Roze, J.C., *et al.* (2009). Anaesthesia mode for caesarean section and mortality in very preterm infants: an epidemiologic study in the EPIPAGE cohort. *Int J Obstet Anesth*, **18**, 142–9.

14 Algert, C. S., Bowen, J.R., Giles, W.B., *et al.* (2009). Regional block versus general anaesthesia for caesarean section and neonatal outcomes: a population-based study. *BMC Med*, **7**: 20.

15 Loepke, A.W. and Soriano, S.G. (2008). An assessment of the effects of general anesthetics on developing brain structure and neurocognitive function. *Anesth Analg*, **106**, 1681–707.

16* Camann, W. (2006). It is the right of every anaesthetist to refuse to participate in a maternal-request caesarean section. *Int J Obstet Anesth*, **15**, 35–7.

17* Gass, C.W. (2006). It is the right of every anaesthetist to refuse to participate in a maternal-request caesarean section. *Int J Obstet Anesth*, **15**, 33–5.

18 General Medical Council. (2008). Consent: patients and doctors making decisions together www.gmc-uk.org/guidance.

Further reading

ACOG Committee Opinion No. 385. (2007). The limits on conscientious refusal in reproductive medicine. American College of Obstetrics and Gynecology. Washington DC.

Bergeron, V. (2007) The ethics of cesarean section on maternal request: a feminist critique of the American College of Obstetricians and Gynecologists' position on patient-choice surgery. *Bioethics*, **21**, 478–87.

Hawkins, J.L. (2007). American Society of Anesthesiologists' Practice Guidelines for Obstetric Anesthesia: update 2006. *Int J Obstet Anesth*, **16**, 103–5.

Kukla, R., Kuppermann, M., Little, M., *et al.* (2009). Finding autonomy in birth. *Bioethics*, **23**, 1–8.

Maclean, A.R. Caesarean Sections, Competence and the Illusion of Autonomy (St George's Healthcare NHS Trust v S; R v Collins and others, ex parte S [1998] 3 All ER 673, [1998]). *Web Journal of Current Legal Issues* 1999.

Minkoff, H. and Paltrow, L.M. (2004). Melissa Rowland and the rights of pregnant women. *Obstet Gynecol*, **104**, 1234–6.

Nilstun, T., Habiba, M., Lingman, G., *et al.* (2008). Cesarean delivery on maternal request: can the ethical problem be solved by the principlist approach? *BMC Med Ethics*, **9**, 11.

Samanta, A. and Samanta, J. (2005). End of life decisions. *BMJ*, **331**, 1284–5.

Weiniger, C.F. (2007). Cesarean delivery on maternal request: implications for anesthesia providers. *Int J Obstet Anesth*, **16**, 186–7.

Consent for anesthesia for procedures with special societal implications: psychosurgery and electroconvulsive therapy

Sadek Beloucif

The Case

A 20-year-old patient suffers from severe psychiatric disorders (agitation, hetero-aggressivity, threatened self-mutilation) for which he had been hospitalized almost continuously for 7 years. His condition is refractory to the usual psychiatric medication, and psychosurgery may reduce his potential for violence and make him less dangerous to himself and to others. The health care team thus hopes the intervention will provide more humane treatment than the prison-like incarceration to which he is currently subjected. However, given the history and grim connotation of lobotomy as well as its irreversibilty, it raises major issues of appropriate consultation and informed consent more than for any other treatment. These concerns continue to be at the forefront of ethical considerations in psychosurgical techniques and other functional psychiatric interventions, such as electroconvulsive therapy (ECT).

Historical perspective

Psychosurgery has a controversial history, in which medical, moral, social, and political considerations intermingle. First described in 1936, and defined as a surgical ablation or destruction of nerve transmission pathways with the aim of modifying behavior, the conventional "lobotomy" of the 1940s and 1950s flourished. There was a strong desire to relieve overpopulation in asylums and hospitals, and lobotomy came to be seen as a means for calming down and even discharging an appreciable proportion of committed patients,[1] or of at least of making caring for them easier. Little attention was paid to patient selection and consent. The unrestrained application of lobotomy makes it difficult to this day to gain an objective evaluation of its true efficacy.

Almost immediately after its introduction, lobotomy was noted to have severe collateral effects on the patient's personality and their emotional experience of the world. Caregivers described them as listless, dull, apathetic, without drive or initiative, passive, preoccupied and dependent. A horror among the public developed that the operation actually excised free will.

In 1948, Norbert Wiener remarked,

> Prefrontal lobotomy … has been recently been having a certain vogue, probably not unconnected with the fact that it makes the custodial care of many patients easier. Let me remark in passing that killing them makes their custodial care still easier.[2]

In 1950, physicians in the Soviet Union banned lobotomy, concluding that it was "contrary to the principles of humanity," and that it "turned an insane person into an idiot."[3] Notorious outcomes involving lobotomy, both in real life (e.g. Rosemary Kennedy and Rose Williams, sister of Tennessee Williams), as well as in fiction (e.g. Ken Kesey's *One Flew Over the Cuckoo's Nest*) perpetuated a horror of psychosurgical techniques.

After neuroleptics and chlorpromazine were discovered in the 1950s, psychosurgery declined rapidly, although it continued to be used in cases viewed as otherwise refractory to treatment. Following spirited social controversy in the US, a Federal commission was convened in 1977, which discredited growing public allegations claiming that psychosurgery was used to control minorities, restrict individual rights, and that its undesirable effects were nonethical. The Chairman of National Committee for the Protection of Human Subjects of Biomedical and Behavioral Research, even went so far as to declare:

> We have looked at the data and they did not support our prejudices. I, for one, did not expect to come out in favor of psychosurgery. But we saw that some very sick people had been helped by it … The operation should not be banned.[4]

Clinical Ethics in Anesthesiology: A Case-Based Textbook, ed. Gail A. Van Norman, Stephen Jackson, Stanley H. Rosenbaum and Susan K. Palmer. Published by Cambridge University Press. © Cambridge University Press 2011.

Nevertheless, lobotomy was subsequently prohibited in a number of states in the US and in other countries such as Germany or Japan. Psychosurgery continues to be performed, but is strictly regulated and controlled in the US, Finland, Sweden, the UK, Spain, India, Belgium, and the Netherlands[1].

Psychosurgery techniques

Conventional lobotomy

Prefrontal leucotomy – or "standard" prefrontal lobotomy – and transorbital leucotomy destroyed parts of the frontal lobes or their connections to the limbic system. Significant "frontal lobe" syndrome was a common complication, characterized by permanent apathy or euphoria, inconsistency, puerility, boorishness, impaired judgment, and chaotic behavior. Harmful side effects included epileptic seizures or aggressiveness.

Functional neurosurgery

Earlier techniques have since been abandoned in favor of much more limited – although still destructive – procedures. Grouped under the heading of "psychosurgery," these procedures based on a "functional" neurosurgical approach are:

(1) anterior capsulotomy – interrupting fronto-thalamic connections in the internal capsule
(2) cingulotomy – partial destruction of the cingulate gyrus, altering certain connections within the limbic system
(3) subcaudate tractotomy – acting on the lower portion of the frontal cortex to destroy the fibres which connect it to the hypothalamus and the head of the caudate nucleus and
(4) bilimbic leucotomy – combining cingulotomy and subcaudate tractotomy.

Results are generally considered effective, although this is on the basis of small case series due to the paucity of acceptable indications. The severe cognitive behavioral disorders experienced by early lobotomy patients are no longer observed. More recently, the administration of highly focused gamma radiation ("gamma-knife") has produced clinical results similar to functional neurosurgical techniques, while being minimally invasive.

Cerebral stimulation techniques

New hopes are arising for new, nondestructive techniques based on stereotaxic neurostimulation. Initially used to treat severe Parkinson's disease, they appear to be comparatively free of complications, as there is no permanent cerebral damage. They achieve psycho-modulation, even the equivalent of a reversible anterior capsulotomy, by inducing radiofrquency stimulation to the brain in specific locations of the cerebral parenchyma via implanted electrodes. Although very different from surgery mutilating the cerebral parenchyma, these stimulation techniques will probably always remain less psychologically and socially acceptable than, for instance, cardiac electrical pacing. However, because the patient is free to interrupt the neurostimulation, the voluntariness of the patient's submission to treatment is preserved. In fact, these new treatments share many points in common with behavioral modification induced by pharmaceutical treatment.

Ethical issues

The present indications for psychosurgery, although exceptional, have not entirely disappeared. In 2001, a prominent specialist stated:

> "However, despite the plethora of pharmacological agents that are available today, there remains a small but significant proportion of patients who suffer horribly from severe, disabling, intractable psychiatric illness. It is in these patients that surgery might still be appropriate if intervention is safe, reasonably effective, and without significant morbidity."[5]

The main ethical issues connected to these interventions involve the scientific validity of the therapy and its evaluation, the validity of patient consent, and the possibility of conflict between the interests of the patient and those of society – particularly in the case of dangerous or violent individuals.

Accordingly, many questions remain to be answered. What are the indications? How are these techniques being evaluated and researched? What are the limits of informed consent? Are patients able to consent who have, in essence, lost a significant aspect of their freedom of judgment?

Current indications

A primary indication for psychosurgery is obsessive-compulsive disorder (OCD). Treatment-refractory OCD is both tormenting and disabling. About 70% of psychosurgical procedures are currently performed for OCD, with notable objective improvement. Patient consent is not usually an issue, since patients are frequently aware of their disability, competent, and eager to pursue treatment.

Other possible indications include severe depression refractory to extreme pharmacologic therapy and sismotherapy (ECT), selected affective disorders such as treatment-refractory schizophrenic psychosis, and selected cases of aggressiveness to self or others.

In practical terms, pre-surgical evaluation to enable medical selection of patients applies solely to patients suffering from OCD. Selection criteria that are considered are: (1) an established diagnosis for at least 5 years; (2) significant suffering evidenced by validated clinical and social function scores; (3) failure of the usual medications to control the disorder, either singly or in combination when administered for at least 5 years, or inability to continue medication due to intolerable side effects; (4) appropriate treatment of an associated co-morbid disorder, and (5) a poor prognosis for the disorder in question. In all cases, it is necessary to inform the patient of the risks, prefer less intrusive stereotaxic techniques, and obtain patient consent.

The relationship between therapy and research procedures

For all other indications, the scientific demand for research is dominant, in view of the uncertainties veiling both the pathology and its presumed treatment. Although a degree of tension emerges whenever potentially irreversible cerebral manipulation is considered, obviously the actual reversibility of new techniques can only be formally established through research. It therefore seems ethically improper to oppose research which aims to examine reversibility of the effects produced. According to a report of the French Bioethics Advisory Commission on the subject of consent[6]:

> The intricacy of the care and research relationship has become a major characteristic of "scientific medicine". This should be a subject of pride. When it engages in research, medicine questions its own principles, corrects its mistakes, and progresses. Good research is not sufficient in itself to ensure quality health care, but it does contribute.

Consent

The concept of consent has very different implications depending on whether the perspective is medical, legal, philosophical, or ethical; whether it only concerns the individual in question; or whether it is given for the benefit of a third party. Consent remains a crucial issue in psychiatry, more than for any other medical discipline, and particularly so when psychosurgery is one of the options.

In the case of severe obsessive psychoses and OCD patients are fully conscious of the torment they endure and are often the first to call for the intervention. In the presence of this desire, physicians need to recognize the anguish created by the pathology, and consider whether they should accede to such requests. Understanding and sensitivity to the reality and intensity of the patient's distress may bring the conviction that it non-ethical to deny such treatment to patients suffering from a disabling, chronic, and intractable disease. Furthermore, the risk of social, somatic and mental complications of non-treatment, including the risk of suicide cannot be discounted.

Consent may be easy to secure because some patients endure such suffering that they may be ready to accept, or for that matter demand, intrepid action. It is precisely this ease of securing consent that paradoxically raises ethical concerns. But an alternate, equally legitimate question is how long a patient can ethically be left to suffer medical therapeutic failure before offering the option of neurostimulation.

For patients suffering from aggressive delusional conditions (who may be dangerous for themselves or others), the question of consent is much more problematic. It is wishful thinking to imagine that the validity of consent ("free and informed") does not bear scrutiny in cases where judgment is severely impaired. Nevertheless, all efforts must be made to secure the patient's assent, even though this "consent" may be dubious in legal terms. Cerebral neurostimulation techniques may be appropriate in some particularly disabling treatment-refractory psychiatric pathologies. However, because neurostimulation for such patients is not established standard therapy and therefore is inextricably involved with research, a very specific concept of consent, validated by external appraisal, must be provided. For further discussion of consent for human subjects in research, see Chapter 27.

In situations where both therapy and research are involved, consent takes on a new dimension. A physician must inform his patient of the consequences of the expected therapeutic effects, and also of the value of the research activity. Although it is clear that consent may be defective for patients suffering from psychiatric disorders, every effort must nevertheless be made to obtain agreement prior to treatment. Even though a particular patient's "intervals of lucidity" may be very rare, assent should still be sought persistently to try to assure whenever possible that the patient has been able to understand, at least to some degree, the medical expectations and their consequences.

Confronted with a mentally disabled individual whose condition may risk violence to self or to others, society has a duty to protect the vulnerable, but while doing so, must also respect and protect the sick individual – who is also vulnerable. In the clinical setting as well as in biomedical research, pains should always be taken to do as much good and as little harm as possible, while respecting the freedom of decision of those one seeks to help. Even though duty calls for a constant effort to combine and reconcile these two principles, there often conflict between beneficence and autonomy. For example, the French Code of Ethics of the medical profession states:[7]

> Consent from the person under examination or care must always be sought .... when the patient is in a fit state to express his/her wishes, and rejects the investigation or treatment offered, the physician must respect that rejection, after having informed the patient of the consequences. If the patient is unable to express his/her wishes, the physician may not take action unless next of kin have been warned or informed, unless that is an impossibility or urgent action is required.

Therefore, the issue of "being or not being fit to express a wish" is the crux of the matter. Further detailed instruction in the Code of Ethics on this difficult matter is unambiguous:

> Consent from a mentally sick patient to treatment offered is most advisable and, if necessary, attempts to secure it may be insistent; however, in case of refusal, the physician and the family must, in certain cases, ignore the patient's wishes. When mental aberration is clearly established, or if the patient is dangerous, commitment by certification or voluntarily to a mental hospital or institution becomes necessary. The law dated June 27, 1990[8] on the commitment of the mentally ill, allows for the wishes of the patient to be ignored in certain cases, both as regards admission to a public hospital and administering treatment. When neurotic disorders or affective disturbances, even of a spectacular nature, do not alter the patient's personality nor prevent reasonable decision, no treatment may be applied without the patient's consent.

While the advisory and, in some cases, authoritative role of family members in providing consent for mentally disabled patients is recognized in Europe, such is not universally true elsewhere. In the US, where psychosurgical techniques and psychiatric interventions have been associated in public perception with manipulation or obliteration of free will, restrictions have been placed on consent for psychosurgical procedures

and ECT. In some of the US, such treatments can be obtained for decisionally incompetent patients only by court order.

In many cases, a casuistic approach, based on a case-by-case discussion, is needed. In fact, the Madrid Declaration of the World Psychiatric Association states:

> Ethical behavior is based on the psychiatrist's individual sense of responsibility towards the patient and their judgment in determining what is correct and appropriate conduct. External standards and influences such as professional codes of conduct, the study of ethics, or the rule of law by themselves will not guarantee the ethical practice of medicine.[9]

One solution might be the formation of a formal committee tasked with establishing decision-making procedures for the purpose of providing support and protection to such patients. In the presence of severe psychotic conditions, it may not be best to accept a surrogate consent between the attending physician, the expert, and the family or legal representative. Rather, a committee including non-medical personnel as well as individuals capable of evaluating both the handicaps and misery endured by the patient, the family, and the entourage, might attenuate the pain and anxiety of making such decisions.

For procedures that involve considerations of research and care, every protocol should be approved by a special committee, according to criteria which define: (1) conditions for approaching potential candidates; (2) criteria for patient selection such as severity, chronicity, gravity and failures of prior medical treatment; (3) validity of consent; and (4) mode of evaluation of results.

In view of new issues arising out of the emergence of experimental therapy, the committee's task would be to preserve the integrity of suffering human beings and safeguard respect for their autonomy, as well as to consider what alternative objective help can be given to them. On the subject of psychosurgery, a working group of the Steering Committee on Bioethics of the Council of Europe stated:

> where States continue to sanction the use of it, the consent of the patient should be an absolute prerequisite for its use. Furthermore, the decision to use psychosurgery should in every case be confirmed by a committee which is not exclusively composed of psychiatric experts.[10]

Electroconvulsive therapy

Electroconvulsive therapy (ECT) is a procedure performed under general anesthesia during which a seizure is induced by application of electricity through electrodes applied on the head. After its introduction in the 1940s, as with psychosurgery, excesses involving its use in the 1960s and 1970s led to sharp criticisms questioning its very necessity. As with psychosurgery, negative associations of its use in public perceptions, both real (e.g., Frances Farmer and Ernest Hemingway) and fictional (e.g., Robert Pirsig's *Zen and the Art of Motorcycle Maintenance*) perpetuate suspicion regarding ECT. It nevertheless remains widely used throughout the world. Current indications for ECT are severe psychiatric disorders (severe depressions, melancholia) with a tangible risk of suicide. It is also used in cases of documented resistance to medical therapies for severe depressions and in selected patients suffering from maniac-depressive psychosis or severe schizophrenic disorders.

General anesthesia including muscle relaxants is mandatory to prevent musculoskeletal complications of seizures. Preoperative clinical evaluation allows recognitions of classic contraindications such as certain arrhythmias, or intracranial hypertension complicating some neurological disorders. ECT might even, in selected patients, have less morbidity than certain antidepressants.

The main controversy surrounding ECT involves the fear of psychiatric pathologies and their therapies. An important symbolic question also raised by ECT is the issue of dignity, which is deeply embedded in the concept of free will. Accordingly, the aim of safeguarding the patient's freedom is central to the official declarations of psychiatric associations regarding patient rights. The World Health Organization recently condemned the abuses and violation of the human rights of people with mental disorders and Dr Jong-Wook Lee, former Director General of WHO urged:

> countries, international organizations, academia, the healthcare and legal sectors and others to take a hard look at the conditions of people with mental disorders and take action to promote and protect their rights.[11]

The question of how to best preserve the interests of the patient while having effecting human behavior, is key to this subject. The use of ECT should be performed in a non-passionate and dramatic way, and in cooperation with the patient. When obtaining consent, the clinician must believe that the treatment is performed in what he/she thinks is in the patient's best interests, yet always keep open the possibility of patient refusal.

Key points

- Special societal implications of psychosurgery and ECT lead us to reconsider the hierarchy of cardinal ethical principles.
- Because of the investigational nature of more recent, less invasive and potentially reversible techniques, research and patient care cannot always be disengaged from one another.
- When considering Autonomy, Beneficence, Non-Maleficence and Distributive Justice, the physician has a moral obligation to respect the common good, with a fair balance between beneficence and the autonomy of the patient.
- Psychosurgery raises fundamental questions, such as those linked to the definition of person and free will, concepts of dignity, integrity, and the validity of true consent.
- In the quest for authentic harmony in the relationships between the health care provider and the patient, tensions between means and ends should be recognized, as well as the understanding of contextual influences, such as economic, political, scientific, and social perceptions, that may alter the consent process.
- Ultimately, decisions regarding psychosurgical interventions and ECT must be made on a case-by-case basis, taking into account patient suffering and disability, and balancing these considerations with patient autonomy.
- Decisions regarding involuntary treatments may benefit from the input of established committees including non-medical personnel and representatives of the patient and their entourage.

References

1* Feldman, R.P. and Goodrich, J.T. (2001). Psychosurgery: a historical overview. *Neurosurgery*, **48**, 647–59.

2 Wiener, N. (1948). *Cybernetics*, The MIT Press.

3 Laurence, W.L. (1953). Lobotomy banned in soviet as cruel. *New York Times*, p. 13.

4 Cullinton, B.J. (1976). Psychosurgery; National Commission issues surprisingly favorable report – news and comment. *Science*, **194**, 299–301.

5 Cosgrove, G.R. (2001). *Neurosurgery*, **48**, 657–8.

6 CCNE, Opinion n° 58, Informed consent of and information provided to persons accepting care or research procedures. Text available at http://www.comite-ethique.fr.

7 Article 36 of the *Code de Déontologie*.

8 Law n° 90–527 June 27 1990 (J.O. June 30, 1990) ; art. L.326 – L.355 of the *code de la santé publique*.

9 Madrid Declaration of World Psychiatric Association, Approved by the General Assembly on August 25, 1996. Text available at http://www.wpanet.org/generalinfo/ethic1.html.

10 "White paper" on the protection of the human rights and dignity of people suffering from mental disorder, in particular those placed as involuntary patients in a psychiatric establishment. Council of Europe, January 3, 2000.

11 News Release WHO/68, 7 December 2005 : "End Human Rights violations against people with mental health disorders". Text available at http://whqlibdoc.who.int/press_release/2005/PR_68.pdf.

Further reading

Bell, E., Mathieu, G., and Racine, E. (2009). Preparing the ethical future of deep brain stimulation. *Surg Neurol*, **72**(6), 577–86.

Comité Consultatif National d'Éthique. CCNE, Opinion n° 71, Functional neurosurgery for severe psychiatric disorders. Text available at http://www.comite-ethique.fr.

Walter G, and McDonald A. (2004) About to have ECT? Fine, but don't watch it in the movies: the sorry portrayal of ECT in film. *Psychiatric Times*; **21**(7) http://www.psychiatrictimes.com/.

Ethical use of restraints

Joan G. Quaine and David B. Waisel

The Cases

Case 1

A muscular 25-year-old requires post-operative mechanical ventilation following laryngospasm-induced negative pressure pulmonary edema. The nurse applies restraints prior to lightening his sedation and calls the intensivist for an order, explaining that he is concerned that the patient will extubate himself as he wakes up.

Case 2

After a stroke, a 76-year-old man is intermittently communicative, occasionally aware of self and place. He is being physically restrained with wrist restraints to minimize the likelihood of dislodging his intravenous and arterial catheters. The wrist restraints occasionally agitate him for short periods. His non-medical daughter is extremely disturbed by the use of restraints and repeatedly requests their removal. His son, a physician, does not object.

Restraint therapy is instituted to prevent injuries to patients or others by restricting a patient's movement. If used improperly, restraint can cause accidental injury or even death. In order to reduce associated risks and protect a patient's health, safety and well-being, while concomitantly preserving a patient's dignity and rights, physicians are ethically obliged to limit the use of restraints to clinically and adequately justified situations.

What is medical restraint?

Intent, not mechanism, determines whether movement restriction is considered restraint. *Medically necessary restraints* are designed to avoid harms from unplanned interruption of therapy, such as self-extubation, removal of catheters, or interruptions to operative sites. *Behavioral restraints* are used to maintain safety for the patient and others. *Forensic restraints* are those used by law enforcement to constrain individuals. Medical care should not be hindered by forensic restraints. Medical immobilization to accomplish a procedure is *not* considered restraint therapy. Examples of medical immobilization including placing a baby in a papoose to perform a frenulectomy and holding down a toddler to perform a mask induction of anesthesia.

Restraint therapy should be used thoughtfully. Comprehensive, individualized assessments should be performed before and throughout restraint therapy. Clinicians should obtain informed consent from available decision-makers before instituting restraint therapy. If there are no available decision-makers, the decision to use restraints should be based solely on beneficence, the obligation to do good, or nonmaleficence, the obligation not to harm. It is assumed that appropriate use of restraint therapy is consistent with the desires of patients to receive safe and quality medical care. Restraints should not be used for clinician convenience, as a solution for insufficient staffing, or as a substitute for adequate medical care.

Common physical restraints include wrist, chest and waist restraints. Wrapping the hands in bandages is used to prevent patients from using fingers. Chemical restraint is the use of drugs to control behavior and limit movement. Medication is not considered a restraint when used to treat a clinical condition such as pain.

Principles

Restraint therapy should maintain the patient's dignity and comfort by using the least restrictive restraint possible (Table 10.1). Determining the least restrictive restraint involves determining both the extent of restraint needed to accomplish the goals and the specific benefits ostensibly obtained by restraint therapy.

To decrease the need for restraint therapy to treat agitation, clinicians should sooth patients through

Clinical Ethics in Anesthesiology: A Case-Based Textbook, ed. Gail A. Van Norman, Stephen Jackson, Stanley H. Rosenbaum and Susan K. Palmer. Published by Cambridge University Press. © Cambridge University Press 2011.

Table 10.1. Principles of restraint use

- Create the least restrictive but safest environment for patients.
- Restraints should only be considered after determining whether treatment of irritants or other problems would minimize the need for restraint therapy. Alternatives to restraints should be sought.
- Restraining therapies should only be used when the risk of harm from treatment interference outweighs the physical, psychological and ethical risks of restraint use.
- The rationale for restraints must be documented in the medical record.
- Orders for restraint therapy should be time-limited to encourage formal reassessment.
- Patients and significant others should receive education as to the need for, and nature of, the restraining therapies.
- Patients receiving neuromuscular blockade should receive adequate sedation and analgesia.
- The need for restraint therapy should be frequently reassessed and restraint therapy should be discontinued at the earliest possible time.

diversion, music, reorientation, enhanced comfort, and reduction of light and noise stimulation. At the same time, clinicians should treat potential medical sources of agitation such as hypoxemia, hypercarbia, electrolyte disorders, drug withdrawal and pain. Ventilation settings, endotracheal tube position and the fit of masks used for noninvasive ventilation should be optimized. Better methods of securing the endotracheal tube may also reduce the need to use restraint therapy.

Physicians should consider whether the benefits of restraint therapy are worth the harms. In certain situations, clinicians may consider removal of certain therapies, such as endotracheal tubes and extracorporeal membrane oxygenation lines in the very ill, to have potentially devastating consequences. Other times, however, maintenance of the therapy may be easily reinstituted, or the loss of the therapy may not be considered harmful. Between 63% and 89% of self-extubated patients do not require reintubation, suggesting that, for these patients, unplanned extubation was not harmful.[1]

Potential risks of restraint therapy include regurgitation and aspiration in the supine patient, skin breakdown, dehydration and accidental death. Straining against restraints may cause muscle injury and may increase agitation. It is unclear if restraints affect the extent of posttraumatic stress disorder that occurs in ICU patients.

Chemical restraints may be seen as kinder and less invasive than physical restraints and frequently are used without the requisite oversight and continual reassessment of physical restraints. However, use of chemical restraints in lieu of using other measures has individual and societal costs. Deep sedation used for restraint may increase intensive care unit stay, perhaps decreasing access to the limited resource of intensive care unit beds. Longer intensive care unit stays expose patients to more bacterial infection, muscle wasting, and critical illness polyneuropathy, among other problems.[2]

Lengthy withdrawal of sedation can be minimized by either conversion to physical restraints or use of multimodal therapy at the appropriate time. A 2004 editorial stated that in the UK, while "physical restraint of patients is considered unacceptable in the [UK] … the importance of the timely withdrawal of sedation cannot be overemphasized, and the judicious use of physical restraints may legitimately be built into an overall treatment plan …"[2]

Case discussion

We can apply these principles to both of the example cases. In the muscular 25-year-old man with negative pressure pulmonary edema, the desire for the restraints may be misguided. The nurse may worry that he will miss the onset of agitation because other nursing responsibilities keep him from the bedside, or that inadequate in-house coverage may mean that an unplanned extubation would have a devastating effect (note that unplanned extubation might well not be harmful). Unquestioned acceptance of the nurse's request for restraint therapy may lead to inappropriate therapy as well as a missed opportunity to highlight an institutional system-level problem. On the other hand, avoidance of restraint therapy may lead to the use of chemical restraints, which may increase the duration of mechanical ventilation and intensive care unit time. This complexity is best addressed by adopting well-considered protocols to help ensure appropriate use of restraint therapy in order to best achieve the desired goals.

The second case exhibits the effects of restraint therapy on the family. While restraints minimize the likelihood of catheter dislodgement (possibly necessitating replacement), they occasionally appear to agitate the patient. Wrapping the arterial line such that it could not be removed may be inconvenient for the nurses, who have to document the appearance of the arterial line site at specific intervals. The family's reaction to the restraints was perhaps indicative of the public's perception. The nonmedical adult daughter was horrified and campaigned daily for removal of the restraints. The physician-son recognized the benefits of the restraints, and was capable of assessing the appropriateness and possible consequences of restraint therapy. He may also have been inured to the use of restraints after years of working in intensive care units. Despite the son's explanation to his sister that there was no treatable cause of their father's agitation, that he appears to tolerate the restraints well, and that the loss of the arterial line would require painful reinsertion, the daughter continued to focus on the restrains. Following additional strokes, the patient had fluid and nutrition therapy withdrawn. Yet, several years after her father's death, the daughter's narrative of her father's death focused on the restraint therapy.

Key points

- Used appropriately, restraint therapy reduces patient risk and improves outcome.
- The general impression by oversight bodies is that physical restraint therapy is overused in the US, but may be underused in the UK and elsewhere.
- By considering the use of restraints as a therapy, clinicians will go through the natural process of seeking a thorough understanding of indications, risks, and benefits, and will likely use restraint therapy appropriately.

- The ethical principles of respect for patient self-determination (including informed consent obtained from surrogate decision-makers), beneficence and nonmaleficence should weigh heavily in the decision to employ restraint as a mode of treatment.

References

1* Maccioli, G.A., Dorman, T., Brown, B.R., *et al.* (2003). Clinical practice guidelines for the maintenance of patient physical safety in the intensive care unit: use of restraining therapies – American College of Critical Care Medicine Task Force 2001–2002. *Crit Care Med*, **31**, 2665–76.

2* Nirmalan, M., Dark, P.M., Nightingale, P., and Harris, J. (2004). Editorial IV: physical and pharmacological restraint of critically ill patients: clinical facts and ethical considerations. *Br J Anaesth*, **9**, 789–92.

Further reading

Council on Ethical and Judicial Affairs, American Medical Association. Opinion 8.17 Use of Restraints. Code of Medical Ethics.

http://www.ama-assn.org/ama/pub/physician-resources/medical-ethics/code-medical-ethics/opinion817.shtml.

Hine K. (2007). The use of physical restraint in critical care. *Nurs Crit Care*, **12**, 6–11.

The Joint Commission. (2010). Hospital Standards Manual: PC.03.02, 03.02,03.05. 3.

http://www.jointcommission.org/.

Kunken, F.R., McGee, E.M., and Stell, L.K. (2001). Strap him down. *Hastings Cent Rep*, **31**, 24; discussion -6.

Ofoegbu, B.N. and Playfor, S.D. (2005). The use of physical restraints on paediatric intensive care units. *Paediatr Anaesth*, **15**, 407–11.

Van Norman, G. and Palmer, S. (2001). The ethical boundaries of coercion and restraint of patients in clinical anesthesia practice. *Int Anesth Clin*, **39**(3), 131–43.

Zun, L.S. (2003). A prospective study of the complication rate of use of patient restraint in the emergency department. *J Emerg Med*, **24**, 119–24.

The use of ethics consultation regarding consent and refusal

Susan K. Palmer

The Case

A 63-year-old female unconscious patient involved in an MVA was brought urgently to the O.R for repair of bilateral femur fractures. The anesthesiologist administered a general endotracheal anesthetic for a 6-hour operation during which the patient received six units of packed red cells and other blood products. She was transferred to the intensive care unit (ICU) still intubated and ventilated. The following day the anesthesiologist visited the patient, who was now awake but still dependent on mechanical ventilation. She signaled that she wanted to write something given a pad and pencil. She wrote, "I am Christian Scientist, I want to go home NOW."

Mary Baker Eddy founded Christian Science in about 1866. Her textbook entitled *Science and Health with Key to the Scriptures* became the primary source for the Christian Science philosophy, which has unique beliefs concerning illness and healing. There are approximately 500 000 members of this group, found mostly in the US.

A foundational belief of the Christian Science church is that illness is an illusion and that an ill person can simply change their perception to alter or eliminate their illusory illness. All drugs, surgery, or other conventional medical treatments are unneeded and ultimately ineffective. Prayer is the only effective way to change the course of illness, by revealing the noncorporeal nature of all existence, including the nonphysical nature of the human body. A body that is spiritual is not in need of physical treatment.

Christian Science theology describes the corporeal world as a kind of shared illusion. In this sense, Christian Science bears a resemblance to the fundamental Buddhist idea that the world of the senses is illusory. Christian Scientists believe that immortality is actually and only achievable by the perfection of the spiritual mind. Disease is an imperfection of the spirit perceived as a physical problem.

Religious freedom and state interests

In the US there is a complex history of the relationship of the state to religious groups. Even though the framers of the Constitution were adamant that there should be a separation of church and state, such that the state could make no laws favoring any church, there have been times when religious groups were given special privileges or permission to indulge in what would otherwise be illegal conduct. Recently, religious groups and their followers are more commonly being held to the same standards as other members of society with their religious standing or preferences not allowed to excuse harmful conduct just because it conforms with religious preferences. For example, the tradition of churches providing "sanctuary" for people wanted by the civil authorities was abolished with the ecclesiastical courts in sixteenth-century England. But the idea that churches can still provide protection from civil prosecution for their own clergy and some church members lingers. Recent revelations that many Roman Catholic Churches in America and Europe failed to report the repeated criminal activities of its clergy are potent evidence that some churches still do not wholly submit to the authority of the state.

The Christian Scientist church and the state

Among the many aspects of her Christian Science philosophy, Mary Eddy was explicit in her direction that believers should be obedient to the authority of the law and of states, including state health laws. She was a progressive regarding the treatment of women and children, and was also a believer in civil liberties and individual freedom.

Clinical Ethics in Anesthesiology: A Case-Based Textbook, ed. Gail A. Van Norman, Stephen Jackson, Stanley H. Rosenbaum and Susan K. Palmer. Published by Cambridge University Press. © Cambridge University Press 2011.

However, the American tradition of "freedom of religious belief" is not identical with a right to freely practice religious behavior that may be harmful to others or to society. At times, Christian Scientists have come to public attention because a member or members have denied standard healthcare for their children. Rejection of vaccination for Christian Scientist children may lead not only to the suffering and complications of common childhood diseases for the unvaccinated children, but may also lead to the propagation of diseases like measles within the whole population, thus harming others. The state, however, has an enduring interest in the health of its children and its general population.

The majority of the US still has specific legislation that protects parents from charges of child abuse or neglect when they deny their children certain resources, including some medical care, for religious reasons. The 1972 case Yoder v. Wisconsin allowed Amish to be exempt from the duty to educate or to send their children to school.[1] The decision was justified on the basis that it was necessary for preservation of the Amish way of life. There are numerous examples of religion-based exceptions to public health requirements such as rules that children be vaccinated to attend public school.

However, there are no legislative protections for religious citizens accused of more serious crimes and felonious harms. In August, 1990 *the New York Times* reported on several cases of parents charged with felonies after deaths of their children occurred as a direct result of the parents' failure to seek medical care for them.[2] Although the majority of such cases resulted only in civil penalties such as fines or sentences requiring public service and promises to seek medical care for their remaining children, there are now some cases in which parents have been sentenced to prison time. A more recent example occurred in 2008 in Wisconsin wherein parents allowed their 11-year-old daughter to die of diabetes.[3] The child deteriorated while her parents and other couples treated her only with prayer. The father and mother were accused of reckless homicide and were sentenced to some prison time every year for 6 years and probation for 10 years.

In our case, the patient is an adult who appears to be decisionally competent and the complexities of dealing with minor or incompetent patients are (fortunately) not involved.

Case discussion

How should the anesthesiologist respond to this patient?

After reassuring the patient, the anesthesiologist decided to consult with several colleagues and hospital officials, with the following results:

(1) The attending orthopedic surgeon was called and suggested that his patient be sedated indefinitely so that she does not harm herself or disturb the surgical repairs.

(2) The Chief of Staff (COS), who was also a surgeon, agreed with the attending surgeon.

(3) The hospital Chief Executive Officer (CEO) decided to call the hospital system lawyers.

(4) Anesthesiology colleagues at the state university suggested calling the chair of their hospital ethics committee, and provided a name and phone number.

(5) An attempt was made to contact local elders/readers from the Church of Christ, Scientist, but there was no phone registered to the local church.

Can the advice of the orthopedic surgeon or the COS be justified by reference to ethical principles or ethical reasoning? Neither the orthopedic surgeon nor the COS suggested that their advice to chemically restrain the patient could be justified on any but practical grounds. Federal laws regarding physical and chemical restraint now require that the use of any restraint must be re-evaluated frequently. The patient was cooperative, so chemical restraint beyond appropriate analgesia was not needed.

The hospital CEO was advised by the hospital system lawyers that legally it would be safest to follow the patient's requests if she was considered to have medical decisional capacity. The lawyers were perplexed as to whether the patient had the ability to command the removal of her own ventilatory support if the physicians thought that death would ensue shortly.

When the anesthesiologist returned to the patient's bedside, she was conscious but dependent on ventilatory support. The anesthesiologist assured the patient that her requests were being seriously considered. He also indicated that her statement was tantamount to requesting euthanasia because she predictably would not survive extubation or cessation of intravenous support at that time. He explained that, when she was delivered to the hospital, treatment was started in the good faith assumption that she would want to survive her injuries. He told her that he could not in good conscience stop her medical support at this time, and certainly her metallic femoral implants could not be removed to satisfy her now stated wish not to receive medical care. He indicated to the patient that he was actively seeking advice about her situation and requests.

Advice from the Ethics Committee chair

During telephone consultation with the university Ethics Committee chair, she suggested a formal ethics consultation involving an in-person evaluation of the patient's situation by a member of the university's clinical ethics consultation team, who would travel to his hospital. Alternatively, the university clinical ethics consultation team could participate in a consultation by conferencing telephone. Finally, the Ethics Committee chair encouraged the anesthesiologist to lead an informal ethical consultation about the patient's situation.

A local ethics consultation process was initiated, with the invitation of all interested parties including the surgeon, the anesthesiologist, the hospital CEO, the patient and her choice of supportive relatives or advocates, and a representative from the patient's nurses. The patient's consent for the consultation was obtained and all the participants agreed that the consultation would be treated with the same respect and confidentiality afforded the rest of the patient's medical care. With the guidance of the university Ethics Committee chair, the anesthesiologist planned the consultation according to the following outline:

(1) What is the current medical situation?
(2) What are the legal considerations?
(3) What are the medical ethical considerations?
(4) What is included in the range of acceptable/ justifiable ethical and professional responses

What is the current medical situation?

All medical ethical consultations begin with explication of the patient's current medical condition and the range of recovery or therapeutic responses expected.

The patient's attending physician explained what the normal course of planned treatments would be. This patient was stable and expected to recover back to her baseline ambulatory condition. She had significant risks for continuing pain and for serious sequelae from her long bones fractures. Her ventilatory

insufficiency had not been definitively diagnosed. The differential list included fat emboli, pulmonary capillary leak syndrome, and transfusion reaction, all of which could have produced her current severe decrease in oxygenation and impairment of ventilation. However, the impairment was starting to resolve and she was expected to fully recover to her baseline ventilatory function. With standard medical care, she was expected to be able to be discharged from the ICU within 48 hours. She would normally need continued observation, wound care treatment for her incisions, and in-hospital physical therapy for return to ambulation.

What are the legal considerations?

The patient was on a ventilator, but able to communicate by writing. She was originally brought to the hospital for emergency care and treatment was undertaken without specific consent from the patient or any spokesperson. Now she was requesting that her medical treatment be stopped and that she be discharged from the hospital. She was on medications for analgesia and sedation while being weaned from mechanical ventilatory support. The orthopedic surgeon believed that the patient was incompetent because she failed to understand that the course of treatment he was prescribing should be followed. He believed that she may have had cerebral fat emboli as a basis for her apparent inability to understand her current medical difficulties. None of the other physicians or the nurses who had spoken to the patient and seen her consistent written responses believed that the patient was mentally impaired. Although a judge could be summoned to investigate and evaluate the patient's degree of legal competency, the majority of her health care providers already believed she was decisionally competent, but misguided by her religious beliefs.

What are the ethical considerations?

Respect for each patient's autonomy is a highly valued principle of the medical ethics of the patient–physician relationship. This is a particularly strong ethic in the in the United States. European principles emphasize autonomy, but may temper autonomy considerations with principles of beneficence ("doing good") and non-maleficence ("avoiding harm").

It is justifiable to continue standard medical care while doubts about the patient's understanding of her own medical situation are resolved. However, physicians are generally not free to define a patient as incompetent primarily because the patient disagrees with their physicians' recommendations. Capacity for medical decision-making is not identical with complete legal competence. A patient who is able to appreciate their medical condition, consider their alternative choices for treatment or refusal of treatment, and express a consistent choice with supporting reasons has decisional capacity. Physicians have a duty to place such a patient's interests above their own medical preferences.

What is included in the range of acceptable ethical and professional responses?

The integrity of the medical profession is a societal good which should not be easily ignored or thwarted by an individual patient. Physicians are obligated to treat all their patients with respect, but are also bound by the limits of professional integrity, which would not currently allow euthanasia in the US, even if the patient requests it. Even in countries where euthanasia is discussed, it is in the context of terminally ill patients or those with unrelievable suffering, neither of which applies to the patient in this case. The orthopedic surgeon was taken aback by the patient's request for cessation of orthopedic care and discharge from the hospital. His definition of his professional obligations to this patient included supervising her recovery from his surgery and starting her on the physical therapy required for her complete recovery. The anesthesiologist supervising her pulmonary care did not believe the patient would survive removal of her endotracheal tube at this time, and on that basis he could not accept the patient's requests for discharge.

The patient has a "right" to expect that her requests will be honored, but no one has an absolute right to command the actions of a physician when they conflict with the physician's deeply held personal beliefs or involve transgression of important elements of professional medical integrity. If/when the patient's request for discharge is not tantamount to a request for euthanasia, her request may have more power to change her physician's actions.

Possible courses of action in this case include the following:

(1) Do exactly what the patient requests.

(2) Do only what the orthopedic surgeon advises.

(3) Do what the patient requests as soon as it is compatible with important aspects of medical professionalism and the deeply held personal beliefs of the physicians and nurses who are caring for the patient (even if this requires that the care of the patient be transferred to other physicians and nurses).

(4) Compromise to the point that both the patient and the medical personnel get to do some of what they consider most important.

Case resolution

The patient and her advocate listened and participated thoughtfully in the ethics discussion. The patient recognized that it was not her right to command a physician, a nurse, or a hospital to do something that was clearly against their medical professional ethics. She agreed to request discharge from the hospital against medical advice (AMA) as soon as her physicians and nurses could in good conscience allow her release. The physicians and nurses were unhappy that they were unable to convince the patient to remain longer under their care as they recommended. Everyone agreed to the compromise that as soon as the patient's survival was more likely than not likely, she would be allowed to arrange for her own discharge from the hospital. The patient was released AMA but without malice or disrespect at a time much sooner than the surgeon's custom, but at a time when death was not likely to immediately result from cessation of hospital care.

Did they do the right thing?

Finding an ethically acceptable course of action is not the same as calculating a single correct answer to a simple mathematical problem. The multiplicity of ethically justifiable resolutions to a clinical scenario are often bewildering to scientifically trained physicians who would normally prefer to find a single most correct answer to any dilemma. In this case, they did the right thing by trying to balance the ethical principles of respect for the patient's autonomy with the important principle that medical professionals should avoid doing harm.

Ethical behavior can seldom be described as acting "perfectly" or in such a way as to provide a paradigm for all future actions by people in similar circumstances. Acting in a way that currently seemed thoughtfully ethical, but is later found to be less ethical than an alternative is not shameful. Difficult situations inspire thoughtful reconsideration of previous decisions and actions. Contemplating future situations so that future actions can be even more ethical is the response expected from medical professionals who are dedicated to serving their patients in ways that are consistent with each patient's consent and within the boundaries of acceptable professional behaviors. Respectful professional behavior will not only serve the patient at hand but it will also inspire respect for the medical profession by making future patients confident that their concerns will always be dealt with in a just manner.

Key points

- Religious freedom does not guarantee the free practice of religious behaviors if such behavior is harmful to others or to society. At times, conflicts between religious behavior and societal interests occur in the setting of medical care.
- Ethics consultation services can be useful when unusual or seemingly irresolvable conflicts between patient wishes and physician professional standards arise.
- An ethics consultation requires the participation of all interested parties, including the patient, patient's caregivers, family, and religious support if available, the physicians, and hospital representatives.
- Ethics consultation includes a process of outlining the medical situation, legal considerations, ethical concerns, a range of acceptable ethical and medical outcomes.
- Ethical issues may not lend themselves to a single correct answer; a number of solutions are usually possible, and none may ideally meet the desires of all parties.
- Difficult ethical problems should inspire thoughtful reconsideration of previous

actions with a goal of better understanding and preparing for future conflicts.
- Respectful physician behavior is key not only to caring for the present patient, but to assuring future patients that their concerns will be dealt with in a just manner.

References

1 Wisconsin v. Yoder, 406 US 205 (1972).
2* Margolick. D. (1990). In child deaths, a test for Christian Science. *The New York Times*, Aug 6. The New York Times.com http://www.nytimes.com/1990/08/06/us/in-child-deaths-a-test-for-christian-science.html?pagewanted=1.
3 Guzder, D. (2009) When parent call God instead of the doctor. *Time*. Feb 5. Time.com. http://www.time.com/time/nation/article/0,8599,1877352,00.html.

Further reading

Burton, R.A. (2008). *On Being Certain. Believing You are Right Even When You're Not*. New York: St. Martin's Griffin.

Code of Medical Ethics of the American Medical Association. (2006). Council on Ethical and Judicial Affairs, Current Opinions with annotations 2006–2007 edition. AMA, USA.

Etzioni, A. (1996). *The New Golden Rule: Community and Morality in a Democratic Society*. New York, NY: Basic Books.

Hamilton, M.A. (2005). *God vs. the Gavel. Religion and the Rule of Law*. New York: Cambridge University Press.

Luce, J.M. (2010). End-of-life decision-making in the intensive care unit. *Am J Respir Crit Care Med*, **Mar 1** [epub ahead of print]

Thaler, R.H. and Sunstein, C.R. (2008). *Nudge: Improving Decisions about Health, Wealth, and Happiness*. New York: Penguin Books.

Waisel, D.B. and Truog, R.D. (1997). How an anesthesiologist can use the ethics consultation service. *Anesthesiology*, **87**(5), 1231–8.

12

Consent and refusal

Consent and cultural conflicts: ethical issues in pediatric anesthesiologists' participation in female genital cutting

Maliha A. Darugar, Rebecca M. Harris, and Joel E. Frader

The Case

A healthy 5-year-old female patient is scheduled for "surgical correction of clitoral phimosis." The patient's Somali parents explain their custom of "circumcising" girls; a surgeon has agreed to perform the procedure. The anesthesiologist doubts the medical indications for the procedure. The parents assert the need to circumcise their daughter so she will be accepted in their community. They tell the anesthesiologist that if they cannot find a US physician to perform the procedure, they will go to Somalia where a village elder will do it, without benefit of anesthesia or aseptic conditions.

Female genital cutting (FGC) refers to procedures involving partial or total removal of external genitalia or other alteration of female genitals for nonmedical reasons. The World Health Organization (WHO) defines four types of FGC.[1] Type I (clitoridectomy) involves partial or total removal of the clitoris and/or the prepuce. Type II (excision) involves partial or total removal of the clitoris and the labia minora, with or without excision of the labia majora. Type III (infibulation) involves cutting and appositioning the labia minora and/or the labia majora to create a covering seal narrowing the vaginal orifice. Infibulation may or may not involve excision of the clitoris. Type IV involves all other procedures to the female genitalia for nonmedical purposes, including pricking, piercing, incising, scraping, or cauterization. Despite this categorization, significant overlap and ambiguity exist in the practice within and between the cultures that practice it. The procedure is most often performed between birth and 15 years of age, depending on tribal or regional custom. Adults occasionally undergo the procedure for the first time or request reinfibulation after childbirth.

Many different terms have been used to describe FGC, including female genital mutilation, female genital cutting/mutilation, and female circumcision, with continued debate about the best term. Some object to "circumcision" as suggesting an inaccurate parallel with male circumcision. The WHO adopted female genital mutilation as the term for this practice.[1] However, many researchers believe "mutilation" alienates the cultures practicing it, resulting in unproductive backlash. We use FGC as descriptive and as distinguished from male circumcision, while withholding judgment about the practice.

FGC is prevalent globally and not limited to any religious or ethnic group. Its highest prevalence occurs in western and eastern Africa where an estimated 90%–100% of females undergo some form of the practice in Egypt, Guinea, Mali, Somalia, and northern Sudan. Between 100 and 140 million girls and women have experienced FCG worldwide and three million girls may undergo the practice each year.[1] In an effort to preserve ethnic identity, immigrants from these countries have brought the practice to the West, including Europe and the US. Thus, first world physicians can no longer regard FGC as exotic and must confront requests for participation, especially where large concentrations of immigrants regard FGC as expected and routine.

FGC is deeply entrenched in cultures that practice it and persists despite large-scale international campaigns, including medical and health organizations condemning it. The WHO, the American Medical Association (AMA) and the International Federation of Gynecology and Obstetrics (FIGO) all oppose the practice and urge health professionals to abstain from participating. Ten international health and human rights organizations have created a consensus statement summarizing the international fight to end FGC.[2]

Commentators and analysts differ regarding the underlying influences promoting FGC. Many

Clinical Ethics in Anesthesiology: A Case-Based Textbook, ed. Gail A. Van Norman, Stephen Jackson, Stanley H. Rosenbaum and Susan K. Palmer. Published by Cambridge University Press. © Cambridge University Press 2011.

believe that patrilineal social, economic, and political values drive the practice of FGC. Some anthropologists think that women perpetuate the practice as a form of African cultural rebellion against encroaching Western societies. From the latter perspective, FGC has virtue, promoting female empowerment, strength, cleanliness, and purity. While some assert that FGC follows Islamic principles, the practice predates the beginning of Islam, is not practiced by the majority of Muslims, and is not universally endorsed by Islamic scholars and theologians. Some supporters believe FGC curbs sexual desire in women, preserving virginity prior to marriage.[3] Others consider FGC to enhance the appearance of female genitalia. Many women consider FGC part of a coming-of-age ritual inducting young girls as members of a community. In any case, women who reject the practice endure stigmatization and ostracism. Females without FGC are often considered unsuitable for marriage within their community, creating practical dilemmas, as marriage grounds economic and social stability. All of these factors contribute to perpetuating FGC.[3]

Community elders and birth attendants traditionally performed FGC. Campaigns from the West highlighting severe medical consequences of FGC performed under unhygienic conditions have backfired. Rather than halting the procedure, the efforts have shifted the practice to the medical sector. Women from cultures practicing FGC now ask physicians from many specialties, including obstetrics/gynecology, surgery, and family practice, to perform the procedure using sterile technique with analgesic agents to minimize pain and adverse medical outcomes.

Patients or other medical professionals may request the help of anesthesiologists for female genital surgeries. This may put an anesthesiologist in a difficult position, as s/he must consider the patients' wishes, the professional's relationships with and obligations to other members of the medical team, and the ethical implications of participating in a procedure with a cultural, rather than medical, justification.

Medical sequelae of FGC

Physicians must understand the potential medical sequelae of FGC to make reasoned decisions about whether or not to participate in the procedure. Both immediate and long-term medical complications arise from FGC. Most of the immediate adverse outcomes result from nonhygienic practices outside of medical settings by lay midwives or shamans. Some of the

long-term consequences occur regardless of the conditions under which the cutting occurred.

Immediate adverse outcomes of FGC include pain, post-operative infection, shock, tetanus, hemorrhage, and death. Long-term physical complications include urinary problems, dysmenorrhea, inflammation, keloids, introital and vaginal stenosis, painful vulvar masses, and fistulae. Long-term sexual dysfunction includes dyspareunia, loss of libido, inability to achieve orgasm, and partner dissatisfaction. Adult women may require defibulation procedures to allow for intercourse and childbirth. Subsequent obstetric complications include prolonged labor from mechanical obstruction, hemorrhage from perineal tears, and perinatal complications including fetal death. Studies suggest FGC can increase the risk of human immunodeficiency virus (HIV) infection from unsterilized instruments.[4]

No literature demonstrates specific health benefits of FGC, though no well-controlled, unbiased studies consistently show the physical harms of FGC. Existing studies do not adequately distinguish the adverse consequences associated with subtypes of FGC. A systemic review of the adverse consequences of FGC concluded that most studies had inadequate power or failed to show statistically significant increased risk of many complications, including urinary problems and infertility among women with FGC compared to uncut women. Data do not unequivocally demonstrate differences in frequency of intercourse, orgasm, and sexual desire in women who have undergone FGC compared to women who have not. Finally, the psychosocial and cultural value of the practice to women who practice it cannot be readily tallied.

Ethical issues

Whether an anesthesiologist should participate in FGC depends on his or her interpretation of ethical considerations. Primary among these is the weight to give cultural values, beliefs, and practices of a particular community, compared with claims of universal human rights, a concept known as cultural or moral relativity. Should Western concerns about gender equality, treatment of children as a protected vulnerable group, patient autonomy, avoiding paternalism, the need to stress nonmaleficence (prevention of harm), and the primacy of beneficence trump an ethnic or other community's belief that FGC preserves important and valid traditions?

Cultural/moral relativism

Cultural or moral relativism refers to the notion that moral or ethical norms must be understood in the context of particular circumstances rather than as universal moral standards. A cultural/moral relativist may argue that Westerners have no moral authority over those practicing FGC. The relativist would note widespread variation in what communities consider acceptable human activity, for example, polygamy vs. monogamy, proscriptions on vs. permissibility of pregnancy termination, allowing or prohibiting physical punishment for civil transgressions and so on, as well as a lack of a generally agreed upon system for resolving philosophical disputes. Others support a notion of universal, absolute human rights. From this perspective all humans have a right to live free of institutionalized suffering, meaning that policies or practices that systematically promote harms to a group of people are unethical. Further, minority and/or politically and economically marginalized persons deserve protection from injustice. Some see FGC as part of a long-practiced set of honored traditions that are common and widely accepted in Somalia. Others condemn FGC as unethical in the US as imposing physical and sexual harm on girls and women, perpetuating a social system that oppresses and disenfranchises females.

Human rights, children's rights and gender equality

Physicians must balance their duty to respect patient, or in the case of children, parental autonomy with their duty to respect and protect human rights. FGC challenges women's rights to gender equality and the WHO considers FGC a violation of women's rights. FGC also violates the rights of children in the view of many nongovernmental organizations such as Amnesty International and UNICEF, necessitating action to protect especially vulnerable young girls.

The United Nations *Declaration on the Elimination of Violence Against Women* classifies FGC as a type of violence against women, impinging on a woman's right to, "equality, security, liberty, integrity and dignity."[5] Proponents of FGC defend the custom as parallel to male circumcision. Some consider prohibition of FGC as a violation of equal rights in that it prevents women from participating in a custom in which men participate. However, women do not experience health benefits from FGC that parallel males benefits from circumcision (e.g., reducing HIV transmission); the adverse health effects of FGC have no similar set of poor outcomes for males who have penile circumcision. Furthermore, harms to women from FGC stem from more than the medical consequences of the procedure; any violation of rights is embedded in broad social structures supporting and perpetuating FGC, including male supremacy in education, political freedom, and economic opportunity. In this light, physician participation in FGC, while possibly reducing harm to the individual patient, legitimizes the practice as medically and socially acceptable, maintaining gender inequalities.

Medical decisions involving children have unique ethical considerations. The American Academy of Pediatrics Committee on Bioethics advises that children should be given age-appropriate information about medical decisions and the opportunity to provide assent for medical interventions.[6] Children also have a right to dissent to medical interventions when not urgently necessary to preserve the health or wellbeing of the child. FGC is a non-urgent procedure that has significant risks. The child will have to live with any complications or consequences of the procedure. Under such circumstances, the informed child should have the right to refuse the procedure and physicians should respect this right. When a young child does not have the capacity to make decisions about her medical care, the parents must make medical decisions according to the best interest of the child. In FGC, parents typically request the procedure on the grounds that FGC will preserves the girl's chances of obtaining a good marriage. Whether such social interests outweigh the medical and psychological harms of the practice comprises the ethical problem in FGC. Physicians have independent moral responsibilities toward their child patients and cannot rely solely on the views of parents. The risks and benefits (including the socio-cultural benefits) specifically for the child deserve careful consideration before physicians decide whether to participate in FGC.

Patient autonomy, conscientious objection, and paternalism

Patient autonomy is a fundamental principle of bioethics, underlying patients' rights to make informed and voluntary decisions about their medical care. It does not, however, mean that patients must receive any requested medical intervention. Two broad types of intervention that patients do not have an unequivocal right to receive from a given physician include: (a) interventions without medical indications and (b) interventions that violate the physician's ethics. In the former case, one often finds dispute about what constitutes a medical indication. For example, some individuals may feel, and courts have upheld, the right of a parent to request and receive mechanical ventilation for recurrent apnea in an infant with anencephaly despite medical claims that artificial respiration served no medical purpose. In the latter case, individual physicians may decline participation in pregnancy termination, removal of feeding tubes, or palliative sedation, though they may have obligations to explain legally available options and refer patients or families to other professionals willing and able to provide the requested service.

Of course, medical professionals routinely perform procedures without clear medical necessity, such as cosmetic surgery. Assuming an informed patient with adequate capacity to consent, FGC seems similar to elective female genital cosmetic surgery: no medical indication exists and each alters the shape of the genitals. Just as women request labiaplasty and vaginoplasty to alter their bodies to meet Western standards of beauty, women requesting FGC aim to meet cultural standards of beauty and gain social acceptance. The interventions may differ, however, with respect to the likelihood of negative consequences, such as diminished sexual pleasure, risk of fistula formation, and complications of pregnancy, labor, and delivery.

Highly contentious procedures like FGC can challenge physicians' values to the extent that they feel they cannot reconcile participation and must refrain from any involvement. Conscientious objection involves the refusal to participate in activities on religious, moral, or ethical grounds. Frader and Bosk argue that invoking conscientious objection for medical interventions acceptable to society and to the medical profession generally undermines patient autonomy, professional ethics, and trades on the imbalance of power in the patient-physician relationship.[7] They oppose opting out of any interaction with the patient or surrogate about an objected-to intervention and suggest physicians must warn prospective patients or family members about their objections before solidifying a physician–patient relationship or explain the objections to those with an established relationship and provide appropriate referrals. In the case of FGC, assuming various forms of the practice remain legal, anesthesiologists may have to decide if they can ethically agree to participate despite their strong moral opposition. If the anesthesiologist or surgeon cannot find another anesthesiologist willing to provide the requested care, the anesthesiologist will face a dilemma. She or he must compromise personal values and provide the requested service or continue to refuse to participate. The latter decision implies a philosophically problematic belief that his or her values are "better" than those of the family and should prevail.

Nonmaleficence and beneficence

Although most professional and advocacy organizations in the West strongly condemn FGC, anesthesiologists may feel conflicted because patients may end up having it done in unsanitary nonmedical settings with inadequate analgesia. FGC performed in the hands of medical professionals can reduce harms by decreasing adverse outcomes through sterile technique, increasing the skill level of the cutter, and providing appropriate pre- and post-operative care. Medical FGC may allow professionals some control over the type and severity of procedure performed. However, FGC violates the principle of nonmaleficence, the duty to do no harm. Nevertheless, physician participation may promote beneficence by reducing the harm patients would otherwise suffer in untrained hands. The case exemplifies the complexity of medical decisions we cannot reduce simply to "do no harm." The goal of harm reduction may override the physician's duty to do *no* harm.

Case analysis

The anesthesiologist must consider the medical and social risks and benefits of FGC to the patient. If he or she chooses to participate, the child may experience long-term adverse outcomes associated with FGC. However, the anesthesiologist will help the child's acceptance in her culture. The anesthesiologist must balance her or his feelings about the procedure with the parents' authority to raise their children according to their beliefs.

If the physician chooses not to participate, the child may have much greater risk for long-term adverse outcomes when performed in Somalia. Furthermore, the child will likely suffer greater procedure-associated pain. However, the anesthesiologist will be refusing to participate in a procedure contributing to the oppression of women and the rights of women to control their own bodies. The anesthesiologist may have a right to refuse to participate if he or she feels that the procedure contravenes his or her moral standards.

Key points

- FGC has wide acceptance in many cultures across the globe despite gender-related and more general human rights concerns raised by the practice.
- FGC produces adverse health outcomes, especially those arising from performance of the procedures by non-medical professionals.
- Physician participation in FGC may prevent some health consequences but also perpetuates objectionable social practices.
- FGC is particularly problematic when it involves a request from a parent for the procedure on a child, who will have to live with the long-term consequences of FGC.
- While some medical organizations, e.g., the AMA, have created guidelines for FGC, most professional societies provide only guidance, without a binding effect on members.
- Physicians' decisions to participate in FGC currently rely on personal judgments, weighing adverse medical and psychological consequences against potential cultural benefits and harms.

References

1   World Health Organization. (2009). Female Genital Mutilation. http://www.who.int/mediacentre/factsheets/fs241/en/.

2* United Nations Interagency Group. (2008). Eliminating Female Genital Mutilation. An Interagency Statement. www.unfpa.org/webdav/site/global/shared/documents/publications/2008/eliminating_fgm.pdf.

3* Nour NM. (2008). Female genital cutting: a persistent practice. *Rev Obstet Gynecol*, **1**, 135–9.

4   Brewer, D.D., Potterat, J.J., Roberst, J.M. Jr., and Brody, S. (2007). Male and female circumcisn associated with prevalent HIV infection in virgins and adolescents in Kenya, Lesotho, and Tanzania. *Ann Epidemiol*, **17**, 217–26.

5   United Nations General Assembly. Declaration on the Elimination of Violence against Women. 1993. http://www.un.org/documents/ga/res/48/a48r104.htm.

6   American Academy of Pediatrics Committee on Bioethics (1995). Informed consent, parental permission, and assent in pediatric practice. *Pediatrics*, **95**, 314–17.

7   Frader, J. and Bosk, C.L. (2009). The personal is political, the professional is not: conscientious objection to obtaining/providing/acting on genetic information. *Am J Med Genet C Semin Med Genet*, **151C**(1), 62–7.

Further reading

Cantor, J.D. (2006). When an adult female seeks ritual genital alteration: ethics, law, and the parameters of participation. *Plast Reconstr Surg*, **117**, 1158–64; discussion 1165–6.

Nour, N.M. (2004). Female genital cutting: clinical and cultural guidelines. *Obstet Gynecol Surv*, **59**, 272–9.

Obermeyer, C.M. (2005). The consequences of female circumcision for health and sexuality: an update on the evidence. *Cult Health Sex*, **7**, 443–61.

Schreiber, M., Schott, G.E., Rasher, W. and Bender, A.W. (2009). Legal aspects of ritual circumcision. *Klin Padiatr*, **221**(7), 409–14

Serour, G. I. (2010). The issue of reinfibulation. *Int J Gynaecol Obstet*, **Feb 5** [epub ahead of print]

13

Communitarian values in medical decision-making: Native Americans

Susan K. Palmer

The Case

An anesthesiologist approaches the bedside of a young Native American woman to complete a pre-anesthetic evaluation. The woman is scheduled for a lumpectomy and appears anxious. The anesthesiologist introduces herself and begins asking questions. "How long have you had diabetes? Do you measure your blood sugar at home? Why does it say here that you haven't eaten for 48 hours?" The patient does not look at the anesthesiologist nor does she immediately reply to the series of questions. She seems to be looking around the room for someone else. Three people approach the bedside. The patient looks directly at them and seems relieved, but still does not answer the anesthesiologist's questions. The three visitors stand quietly. The anesthesiologist begins again: "Have you had any surgery before today?" She is frustrated, not knowing to whom to address her questions, or when to expect answers.

There are more than 500 "tribal entities" in the US, with over 200 in Alaska alone. There are thought to be about three million Native Americans and Native Canadians. No more than 30%–40% of these individuals live on reservations or associated land trust areas.

The Indian Health Service (IHS) is a US governmental agency charged with providing preventive, curative, and community healthcare for US Native American populations throughout the US. Many Native Americans will be cared for outside of Indian Health Service (IHS) hospitals, and therefore may need care from anesthesiologists not employed by the IHS. Although most states have less than 2% of their population identified as Native Americans, some states have significant Native American populations, such as Alaska 19.0%, Arizona 5.7%, Montana 7.4%, New Mexico 10.5%, Oklahoma 11.4%, and South Dakota 9%.[1] Anesthesiologists who practice in one of

these states would be well served to acquaint themselves with the customs and cultural understandings that nearby Native Americans share. The cultural effects of Native American beliefs in the medical workplace serve to illustrate problems common to the care of patients whose cultural beliefs are significantly different from that of the traditional "health-care" culture with regard to autonomy, beneficence and informed consent.

Native Americans have populated the North American continent for at least 10 000–20 000 years – indeed, some archeologists believe it has been much longer. There is ample evidence that the tribal cultures of North America were from early times advanced in their languages, kinship systems, sacred histories, and sophisticated methods of living in sustainable ways on the land. Native Americans should not be confused with depictions of pre-historic "early man" found in many museum dioramas, which are intended to illustrate very early use of animal skins for clothing, early possible social structures, group hunting, survival behaviors, and early forms of tool-making. Confusing Native Americans with African and European evidence of early humans does a distinct disservice to Native Americans, whose history is much more recent and whose cultures are far more sophisticated than that of early man before the development of cultural identities.

Principles of respect for autonomy, respect for community, and the principle of beneficence

Communitarian values

Native American cultures are far more communitarian than mainstream American cultures. Communitarian

---

Clinical Ethics in Anesthesiology: A Case-Based Textbook, ed. Gail A. Van Norman, Stephen Jackson, Stanley H. Rosenbaum and Susan K. Palmer. Published by Cambridge University Press. © Cambridge University Press 2011.

cultures are based on the fundamental premise that the "community" is the most valued entity, with part of each individual's worth being measured by the degree to which they are able to contribute to the community's well-being. Individual members of a community have an obligation to put the community's interests before their own personal interests. In such "utilitarian" value systems, the principle of "beneficence" may therefore be practiced less in the context of individual beneficence, than in one of beneficence to the community.

Competitive white American culture often assigns social status to individuals based on their accumulation of money and possessions. Native Americans, instead, often value their ability to distribute what abundance they have to make sure that no one in their community is without necessary food, shelter, and means to care for their families. These fundamentally different value systems may lead people to make quite decisions with regard to their healthcare.

Native American views on illness

There are over 550 federally recognized Native American tribes in the US. Defining what constitutes a "tribe" would be academically difficult, but we know in general that the requirements for a distinct tribal community include: (1) having a common homeland; (2) speaking a common language; (3) having an agreed kinship system; and (4) sharing a sacred history. It would be impossible to describe the tribal customs or beliefs regarding illness and healing for each of the hundreds of federally recognized "tribal entities." There are, however, common themes among many tribes that are useful for anesthesiologists to appreciate when caring for Native American patients. What follows is a description of some features of a belief system surrounding illness and healing of one of the largest tribes in the US – the Navaho, or Dine.

Southwestern pueblo cultures, particularly the Navaho, value being in correct relationship with others in the community, with the Great Mystery, with other living creatures, with even with the features of the homeland landscapes which are thought to be part of the birthright of the tribal community. When a Navaho person becomes ill, the root cause of the illness is thought to be the loss of a "correct" relationship. Relationships must be in balance to avoid or terminate illness. Each tribal member must strive to maintain a correct relationship to other tribal members, the right relationship with spiritual forces in other life forms, and maintain respect and gratitude

to the homeland earth and climate. To restore health or "beautiful" living, the sick person may want to consult a tribal elder or a tribal member with medicinal powers. Western medical treatments may also be needed. Western medicine can be respectfully combined with tribal beliefs about restoring "right relationships" to achieve successful health outcomes for Native Americans.

Respect for the tribal homeland and designating landforms and its local flora and fauna features as sacred is part of the interrelatedness which native cultures value. The earth is often spoken of as a "mother" who nourishes and cares for the people. Traditional creation stories in many native tribes reveal that a spiritual being, the Great Mystery, preceded and then created mankind. The earth, the sun, the forces of weather, the cardinal directions, and the "brotherness" of other living creatures make everyday interactions "sacred" activities. Natives developed sustainable relationships with the flora and fauna of their homelands because they knew that the existence of their community depended on this.

The recent worldwide attention to "sustainable" living has renewed interest in the tribal ways of Native Americans. They recognized and valued sustainable living thousands of years before the emergence of the current interest in conservation of resources, preservation of species, and the development of renewable resources.

Navajo culture and informed consent

An important way in which the differences between Western and Native American values in healthcare ethics can be illustrated is through the process of informed consent. Western medical ethics place great value in "authentic" or autonomous choices of patients. In order for choices to be truly autonomous, this value system holds that a patient must be sufficiently informed and able to choose without coercion. Such information includes the nature of the treatment, risks, chances of success or failure, and alternatives to the recommended treatment.

Traditional Navajo culture, on the other hand, holds that words can change reality. A discussion of bad events, or even the possibility of them, is unwelcome, since it may actually bring the unwanted outcomes to pass. The anesthesiologist may be faced with an ethical dilemma – respect the patient's culture and withhold information out of cultural sensitivity, or fully inform the patient and reject their cultural values.

In such a dilemma, it is important to recognize that autonomy is not inextricably linked to information. In fact, patients can make completely authentic and autonomous choices by asking *not* to be informed, or by assigning the power over health care decisions to another, such as their relatives, or even the physician themselves. Furthermore, it is not the *amount* of information that is significant to autonomy, but rather what information the patient considers most important to their well-being. Therefore, we can respect autonomy, even if we do not have all of the objective information on the table, so long as we have respected the patient's values with regard to how much and what kind of information they desire and need to feel comfortable with their health care decision. The easiest way to determine this is to ask the patient what is important to her in the context of her values, choices and culture.

Ethical responsibilities of anesthesiologists caring for Native American patients (or any patient with a cultural background different from their own)

Anesthesiologists share with all other physicians the duty to be respectful to patients and their families and to put the patient's interests before their own. Learning about their culture and views on medical care is one way to demonstrate respect for our patients as individuals. Physicians are expected to act with sincere respect for our patients' beliefs, especially when we do not share similar beliefs. It would be impossible to know the cultural etiquette of all other cultures. However, it would be possible for anesthesiologists to learn some of the predominant cultural beliefs and traditional ways of Native American patients or other ethnic groups who live in their area and are likely to fall under their care. All patients are benefited by the acknowledgment of their spiritual needs. Patients who are confident that their anesthesia care is personalized are likely to be more satisfied with their care.

Further, it can be argued that physicians have a duty to examine their own background cultural influences and work to avoid de-valuing the beliefs or lifeways of patients who have a completely different value system. Negative stereotypes of those who are different need examination and revision so as not to interfere with respectful and thorough medical care. Better medical care and outcomes occur for patients, and more job satisfaction results when anesthesiologists can sincerely respect their patients.

Why should an anesthesiologist be concerned about a patient's cultural or spiritual preferences?

Apart from the humane aspect of concern for the comfort of others, scientific evidence supports the premise that a patient's psychological state affects healing, immunity, and the course of disease. Psychoneuroimmunolgy is the name used for the 20-year-old field of scientific study that acknowledges the effects that a patient's state of mind has on their neurological and immunological systems. Complex interactions between the immune system and the central nervous system, including the effects of positive and negative emotions on immunology and infection, have long been recognized and studied. Anesthesiologists have also long known that it is better to anesthetize a patient who is already calm, than to rapidly induce general anesthesia in a patient who is distraught or nearly out of control. Pre-medication can produce the picture of calmness, but may or may not produce actual psychological calm. The old saying that "patients wake up exactly as they go to sleep," is indicative of the fact that general anesthesia interrupts, but does not resolve, strong emotions. Every anesthesiologist has probably had the experience of putting a weeping patient to sleep and have them wake to continue their crying.

Cardiac rhythm, blood pressure, resistance to infection, secretion of stress hormones, and activation of endothelial reactivity are just some of the things we now know are related to patients' emotional state during emergence from general anesthesia. The phenomenon of wakefulness during apparent general anesthesia, for example, is thought to be correlated with the patient's pre-induction state of arousal.

Learning more about Native American beliefs and healthcare

A list of valuable readings regarding Native American culture and healthcare follows this chapter. Probably the single most helpful book for physicians is *The Scalpel and the Silver Bear*, by Lori Alviso Alvord. It is the story of a Navaho woman raised with traditional tribal values, who decides to pursue higher education and eventually becomes a general surgeon. Her journey away from tribal and reservation life and into the general American culture and later adoption of the prejudices which are a normal part of medical surgical training makes it clear what stresses may be affecting any of our Native American patients. Dr. Alvord's journey also illustrates a way of understanding how the strengths of Native American spiritual understandings and mainstream American views of illness and healing can be combined in a synergistic way.

> Navaho people have a concept called "Hozhone haazdlii", Walking in Beauty, but it isn't the beauty that most people think of. Beauty to Navahos means living in balance and harmony with yourself – mind, body, spirit – and having the right relationships with your family, community, the animal world, the environment – earth, air, and water – our planet and universe.
>
> Lori Arviso Alvord, M.D.

Case discussion

The patient and her family were enrolled members of the Navaho nation. This family valued tribal support, restraint in conversation, and honored the "old ways." Their understanding of disease and its treatment included respect for their tribal beliefs about the origin of disease.

Like many physicians, anesthesiologists are often unaware of the social effects and implications of their approach to patients. For example, in the interest of efficiency, anesthesiologists often begin their conversations with patients by asking questions. This has become commonplace in the hurried atmosphere of a healthcare setting, but would be considered rude in normal social situations among even non-Native Americans. It may be especially offensive and anxiety provoking for patients who come from cultures that value restraint in conversation.

Most patients, including Native Americans, appreciate it when their physicians begin a conversation by introducing themselves first, and then stating what their role will be in the patient's care. Many cultures, including those of Native Americans, prefer that the next part of the conversation includes the recognition of the patient as a unique person with important relationships. Recognizing and speaking to the patient's bedside relatives and friends is a first step in showing that the physician understands that the patient is part of an important social network, and that they and their family will be cared for in a respectful way.

The anesthesiologist should try to identify very early in the pre-anesthetic conversation what effect her conversation is having on the patient and her family. Asking the patient for guidance as to what information is important to them can be helpful when physician and patient values/beliefs diverge. Instead of the routine

pre-operative questions, one could add a question such as "What else should I know about you in order to provide comfortable care for you? Is there anything which you are concerned about in the treatment I have recommended for you?"

It is important to recognize that, for some cultures, the nature and quantity of information discussed during consent for medical care may vary. Patients have autonomous rights to limit the amount of specific information they wish to receive, and/or to designate someone other than themselves to receive information and make decisions for them. When a patient desires limited risk disclosure, the anesthesiologist should document this as part of their informed consent discussion.

Some Native Americans may wish to carry symbolic items with them during anesthesia and surgery. Provisions for safe accompaniment of symbolic items can usually be made to accommodate the patient's wishes, just as most American hospitals and most physicians allow patients and their family/pastor to complete traditional Christian prayers before whisking them off to the OR. Making time and space for tribal members and ceremonies is in the same category of respect for the healing power of Native American tribal customs.

Key points

- Native Americans have views on health or strong spiritual beliefs that should be acknowledged, respected, and safely integrated into the plan for anesthesia care.
- Native Americans have sophisticated historical spiritual belief systems that should not be confused with our understandings about pre-historic early human social organization.
- Scientific research supports the connections between spiritual and mental states and the outcomes of stressful healthcare procedures.
- Verbalizing respect for the concerns and spiritual needs of our Native American patients and their families should be a normal part of ethical anesthesia care for these patients.
- Patients of all cultures have a right to determine how much and what type of information is essential to them in making healthcare decisions. Accordingly, they may

choose to limit discussion of risks, or to designate someone else to make healthcare decisions for them.

- Anesthesiologists could benefit all their patients by beginning their conversation with an introduction of themselves and their role for the patient. Adjusting the tempo and intimacy of pre-operative questions may be necessary to accommodate social expectations and prevent anxiety for some of our patients.

References

1 Census Brief 2000. The American Indian and Alaska native popultion 2000. US Census Bureau, Washington DC. February 2002. http://www.census.gov/prod/2002pubs/c2kbr01–15.pdf.

Further reading

Alvord, L.A. and Van Pelt, E.C. (1999). *The Scalpel And The Silver Bear. The First Navaho Woman Surgeon Combines Western Medicine And Traditional Healing.* New York: Bantam Books.

D'Souza, R. (2007). The importance of spirituality in medicine and its application to clinical practice. *Med J Aust*, **21**, 186(10 Suppl): S57–9.

Fixico, D. (2003). *The American Indian Mind in a Linear World.* New York, NY: Routledge.

Hall, A. (2002). What the Navajo culture teaches us about informed consent. *HEC Forum*, **14**(3), 241–6.

Kelly, L. and Brown, J. Listening to Native Patients. (2002). *Can Fam Phys* **48**, 1645–52.

Mann, B.A. (2008). *Make a Beautiful Way. The Wisdom of Native American Women.* Lincoln, NE: University of Nebraska Press.

Martinez, D. (2009). *Dakota Philosopher: Charles Eastman And American Indian Thought.* St Paul, MN: Minnesota Historical Society Press.

McLaughlin, L.A. and Braun, K.L. (1998). Asian and pacific islander cultural values: considerations for health care decision making. *Health and Soc Work*, **23**(2), 116–26.

Nerburn, K. (1999). *The Wisdom of the Native Americans.* Novato, CA: New World Library.

Turner, N.J. (2005). *The Earth's Blanket. Traditional Teachings For Sustainable Living.* Seattle: University of Washington Press.

Utter, J. (2002). *American Indians: Answers To Today's Questions.* 2nd edn. Norman, OK: University of Oklahoma Press.

DISCOVERY LIBRARY
LEVEL 5 SWCC
DERRIFORD HOSPITAL
DERRIFORD ROAD
PLYMOUTH
PL6 8DH

14

Informed consent for preoperative testing: pregnancy testing and other tests involving sensitive patient issues

Gail A. Van Norman

The Case

A healthy 15-year-old girl presents for elective diagnostic ankle arthroscopy for ankle pain and swelling. She is accompanied by her mother. During the preoperative interview, she appears acutely uncomfortable with questions about whether she is sexually active (she denies it) and the timing of her last menstrual period. The anesthesiologist informs her that she will need to get a urine sample for a pregnancy test. The test is required by the anesthesia group's policy of pregnancy testing female patients, and members of the group will not perform elective anesthesia on pregnant patients. The patient's mother questions the necessity of the test, stating with confidence that "my daughter has never had sex." The urine pregnancy test, however, is positive. State law prevents the anesthesiologist from informing anyone but the patient of her positive test, although the mother will surely guess the test results if the case is cancelled. Furthermore, the patient is below her state's age of consent for sexual intercourse, and her pregnancy is therefore by legal definition the result of statutory rape according to state law – which also requires any doctor who suspects child abuse to notify state authorities.

While physicians often consider ethical issues concerning medical therapies, it is easy to overlook ethical issues regarding something as routine as a preoperative laboratory testing. Yet principles of beneficence (doing good) and nonmaleficence (avoiding harm) suggest that *anytime* we prescribe a medical test, ethical considerations may be relevant, since we doing such testing precisely because we hope to benefit patients and/or avoiding harm. Preoperative testing presumably benefits patients by identifying unrecognized or disguised conditions that might adversely affect anesthetic risk. But harms can also result from preoperative testing. Some harms include the risk of a false-positive test erroneously labeling a patient as

having a condition they do not have; the risk of a false-negative test falsely reassuring a patient that they do not have a condition which they in fact do; the risk that erroneous results might lead to inappropriate therapy with its attendant complications; the risk that erroneous test results might deprive a patient of important therapy they would otherwise get; and the complications of performing the test itself, and monetary cost, to name a few.

Are all preoperative tests ethically equivalent? Some of the ethical problems that face the anesthesiologist in the case introducing this chapter may be obvious, and some may not. But is there really an ethical problem with obtaining an ECG, for example? This discussion will focus on issues related to common, routine preoperative tests, and also examine two preoperative tests with special social implications: HIV and pregnancy testing.

General ethical principles regarding medical testing

Physicians have ethical obligations based in principles of beneficence and nonmaleficence to make responsible and knowledgeable decisions about whether a preoperative test is even warranted. Principles of good medical practice require that physicians balance the cost of testing against the likelihood that testing will produce more benefits than harms. Physicians are also bound by an ethical principle of fidelity to their patients. Fidelity is the concept that physicians should be faithful and committed in providing good medical care, and not compromise that care in the interests of anyone else, not even for physicians' personal interests.. This principle respects the vulnerability of patients in the doctor–patient relationship. Not only

Clinical Ethics in Anesthesiology: A Case-Based Textbook, ed. Gail A. Van Norman, Stephen Jackson, Stanley H. Rosenbaum and Susan K. Palmer. Published by Cambridge University Press. © Cambridge University Press 2011.

does the doctor have special medical knowledge and skills in which the patient must place their trust, but also the physician determines to a great degree how expensive medical testing and therapy will be.

The principle of nonmaleficence requires physicians to consider, in addition to the monetary costs of a test, both the medical and social harms that may result from unnecessary or poorly conceived testing. Medical harms include the discomfort and inconvenience of the test and the potential for false-positive or false-negative results that misdirect medical therapy in ways that create greater harms than benefits. Such misdirection can occur even with a simple ECG. Take, for example, a 40-year-old healthy man with no medical complaints who presents for knee arthromenisectomy. His surgeon orders a routine preoperative ECG as he has for the last few decades on all of his patients scheduled for surgery. The ECG demonstrates concerning but nonspecific ST segment changes, so the surgeon consults a cardiologist who orders stress cardiac imaging for further clarification. Imaging reveals a significant area of decreased apical uptake compatible with myocardial ischemia or possible attenuation artifact, so a cardiac catheterization is undertaken – which reveals normal coronary arteries. Ultimately, the patient suffers a femoral artery tear during catheterization and has to undergo emergency vascular surgery. The physical and financial cost to the patient is very high, although no medical decisions concerning the original surgery were ultimately altered and no surgical risks reduced as a result. In fact, this healthy patient's risk of a major adverse event *increased* with each test his doctor ordered. The most recent guidelines for perioperative cardiac workup now indicate questionable utility of a preoperative ECG in this case. The subsequent stress test was also not indicated because it was unlikely to reveal anything that would favorably alter outcomes for a low risk surgery.

Good medical practice, *both from ethical and medical standpoints*, includes applying evidence-based guidelines in determining if a test should be done, rather than on individual experience and beliefs. Individual experiences suffer from bias, unique confounding factors, and situational conflicts of interest. Anecdotes may be useful when no systematic investigation has been undertaken that can advise physicians about the course of action most likely to lead to the best overall outcomes. But anecdotal experience, albeit a strong tradition in medical education,

serves us best when it spurs systematic investigation that results in sound, evidence-based decision support for physicians., Once evidence-based algorithms are available, they should guide most decisions and replace "routine" or traditional patterns of ordering tests.

Preoperative HIV and pregnancy screening

Social risks associated with preoperative testing may not be as obvious as medical risks, but can be the source significant harm. Two examples of tests that can produce social harm but are of limited preoperative utility are HIV and pregnancy testing.

Adverse social consequences known to be associated with HIV seropositivity include employment discrimination, loss of insurance, and social isolation. Studies demonstrate that seropositive women experience high rates of marital break-up, abandonment, and verbal and physical violence when their HIV status is disclosed.[1] Compulsory preoperative HIV testing is known to prevent some patients from seeking medical care. Recognition of these harms has led in the US to the inclusion of AIDS patients in the protections afforded under the Americans with Disabilities Act, and has resulted in legislation specifically protecting the privacy of a patient's HIV status.

Revealing a positive pregnancy test may likewise have negative, even life-threatening consequences for vulnerable patients in social environments where their pregnancy is not accepted. Studies show that female patients and their fetuses are in some situations at risk of physical violence. Further, adolescent pregnancies are sometimes the result of child abuse, incest, and rape. Communication of a positive pregnancy test result to the parents of a pregnant minor can place the child in jeopardy of further physical harm, since it may be evidence of criminal behavior on the part of a family member, or family friend or acquaintance. Many states have statutory requirements for physicians to report evidence of child abuse, and some authorities recommend reporting pregnant minors to Child Protective Services for investigation of possible abuse.

In much of the US, a female patient of any age has the legal right to absolute privacy regarding reproductive matters. To reveal or even imply the results of a pregnancy test to a third party, even a parent or spouse, without the woman's consent, would represent an overt violation of law. The anesthesiologist who discovers a pregnancy is therefore left with few comfortable legal options if they have not first obtained the patient's voluntary informed consent for pregnancy testing and discussed both how the test results will be used and to whom they can be revealed.

Given that there are risks of both social and medical harms associated with HIV or pregnancy testing, is there evidence that routine preoperative testing for HIV or pregnancy alters outcomes in a sufficiently favorable way to justify risking such harms?

HIV testing

HIV testing is usually ordered by the surgeon or anesthesiologist to determine which patients may pose a risk to members of the operating room team, and therefore with which patients they should be particularly careful to avoid possible exposure. Studies show that most surgeons and anesthesiologists erroneously believe that: (1) compulsory routine HIV screening will reduce their personal risk of exposure; (2) ordering such tests is the prerogative of the physician; and (3) that such tests can be done without the patient's consent.

The effort to protect fellow members of the operating room team may be laudable. The doctrine of self-interest, however, is not an ethical principle, and carries little or no weight ethically when balanced against issues that affect the patient and his or her rights. This is especially true when the risk to the physician is low, and the primary method of reducing risk is applied to all patients anyway (e.g., universal precautions).

HIV testing has not been demonstrated to improve operating room safety. When applied to a low-prevalence population, positive screening tests are more likely to represent false-positive results than if testing is selectively applied to a high-risk population. False-positive results are harmful to the patient, who is unnecessarily labeled with a serious illness and may undergo further testing or treatment related to the false result. Physicians, can be harmed by false-negative test results if they are falsely reassured by the result. Furthermore, *true* negative tests can occur early in the course of HIV infection when viral titers (and infectious risks) are actually at their highest. Even a true negative test may therefore falsely reassure the operating room team that a patient represents lower risk when the opposite is actually true. If the outcome is relaxed

vigilance regarding universal precautions, such tests may paradoxically *increase* actual risk or exposure. In any case, preoperative HIV testing does not benefit the *patient*, although they will bear the monetary and social costs of the test. It is therefore difficult to justify routine unconsented preoperative HIV screening on either ethical or medical grounds.

Routine Preoperative pregnancy screening

Anesthesiologists often cite three reasons for screening pregnancy tests: (1) a desire to avoid unnecessary anesthesia exposure that may affect fetal development and/or increase the risk of spontaneous miscarriage; (2) a desire to avoid litigation for fetal anomalies or miscarriages that might occur following elective anesthesia exposure, and (3) a belief that female patients may lie to them about their pregnancy status. Are any of these fears well founded?

Despite widespread belief to the contrary, large population-based studies have failed to show definitive differences in the rates of fetal anomalies or spontaneous miscarriage following anesthetic exposure during the first trimester of pregnancy. Exposure of the fetus to anesthetic agents in early pregnancy does appear to be associated with lower birth weight.[2,3] More recently, concerns have been raised about the effects in primates of later fetal exposure to anesthetic agents and its possible effects on subsequent neurocognitive development. However, no studies have been done to test whether neurocognitive development in humans is adversely affected after fetal exposure to anesthetic agents.[4]

Preoperative pregnancy testing also does not constitute a "standard of care." In one study, only about one-third of anesthesia practices required preoperative pregnancy testing.[5] In 2003 the American Society of Anesthesiologists Task Force on Perioperative Testing and the American Society of Anesthesiologist Committee on Ethics issued a joint statement that anesthesiologists should *offer* preoperative pregnancy testing to any female patient who might desire one, but that medical evidence for *requiring* pregnancy screening prior to anesthesia and surgery was lacking.[6]

Is preoperative pregnancy testing even necessary? No study has directly tested how accurate female patients are in reporting their pregnancy status in elective conditions when patient privacy is strictly protected. A study of preoperative pregnancy testing in adolescent female patients revealed the patients were accurate in reporting if they could possibly be pregnant, and no unexpected pregnancies were detected in over 500 instances.[7] In one recent study of female patients presenting for elective surgery at a facility that performed routine pregnancy testing, the rate of "unexpected" positive pregnancy test results was < 0.2%, although one of those positive tests was actually a *false* positive.[8] Other studies have put the rate of positive preoperative pregnancy tests at between 0.9%.[9] Studies that report the results of preoperative pregnancy testing fail to distinguish between positive test results that occurred in women who claimed they were not pregnant versus those who simply didn't know and requested testing. The accuracy of urine pregnancy testing is estimated at 97%–99%. To put it another way, conducting a urine pregnancy test will result in a false negative in up to 1%–3% of cases. Asking a female patient presenting for elective surgery if she is pregnant results in a false-negative response < 1% of the time. It seems somewhat questionable whether a urine pregnancy test is actually superior to simply asking the patient whether she is pregnant. There is no evidence whatsoever that exploring a female patient's sexual and menstrual history has any influence on pregnancy test outcomes, much less anesthesia and surgical outcomes, despite the bizarre invasion of privacy these questions represent.

Is undetected pregnancy a major litigation issue in the practice of anesthesiology? As of 2003, two cases had been described in the ASA Closed Claims database related to spontaneous miscarriage of a previously undetected pregnancy following elective anesthesia.[10] In one case, the patient prevailed against her surgeon when it was determined that the patient should have had a pregnancy test prior to deciding to proceed to surgery, since a positive test would have explained her medical condition and eliminated the need to operate. In the second, the anesthesiologist prevailed against the patient, because the patient failed to demonstrate that anesthesia was the cause of a later miscarriage, or even that preoperative pregnancy testing by anesthesiologists was a standard of care.

The ethical principle of respect for patient autonomy requires physicians to respect the decisions of competent patients once they have been properly informed of the risks. In most studies of preoperative pregnancy testing, the finding of a positive test was highly correlated with a woman's decision to postpone surgery, indicating that the test results represented important information most of the women considered relevant in deciding whether to have surgery. Anesthesiologists therefore have an ethical duty to explain what is known and what is *not* known about the risks of anesthesia and surgery in early pregnancy, and to offer pregnancy testing to women, in case their decision to have surgery would be affected by the information. An autonomous woman who is properly informed of these largely theoretical risks has the right to refuse testing, both by law and ethical principles. Coercing such a patient into having a test against her wishes violates patient autonomy, and in general, refusal to have a test should not result in a cancellation of anesthesia or surgical care.

Case discussion

The anesthesiologist in our case presentation faces several serious ethical and legal problems: (1) The laws of her state afford an absolute right to privacy for females of any age with regard to reproductive status. To reveal, or even imply to anyone other than the patient that she is pregnant is an explicit violation of state law and the patient's rights. (2) It is impossible for the anesthesiologist to know if revealing the information will expose the patient or her fetus to risk of serious physical harm from others. (3) The anesthesiologist has no practical way to discuss the results without the mother's knowledge, and simply canceling the surgery will certainly clue the patient's mother in to the test results. (4) To make matters worse, state law also requires the anesthesiologist to report her findings to Child Protective Services as evidence of sex with a minor, which is illegal under child abuse statutes. (5) Failure to obtain informed consent for the test is also a *separately actionable legal claim* in that state, even if no medical harm occurs. Instead of reducing the possibility of litigation, the anesthesiologist's management of this case has actually opened an entirely separate avenue of litigation against her.

As is often the case when a situation gets off to such a bad start, there is no simple way to easily extricate our anesthesiologist from the ethical and legal mess in which she finds herself. But this situation might easily have been avoided if ethical principles had been followed from the outset. In the first place, a policy of requiring routine preoperative pregnancy testing is questionable at best and based on little or no supportive medical evidence. It creates ethical and legal dilemmas and potential social harm, while failing to provide proven improved outcomes to patients. Because not everything is known, or likely will ever be known, about the effects of anesthesia on a developing fetus, patients should be privately informed of the theoretical concern that pregnancy outcomes could be affected by surgical stresses and anesthetic exposure. They should also be informed that true risks are unknown, and they should be offered pregnancy testing if they desire it. The practitioner should also determine how the patient wishes test results to be handled, whether positive or negative. The informed consent process requires respect for informed refusal, and with rare exceptions patients should not be coerced into undergoing screening pregnancy testing by threatening to cancel the case if they refuse.

Whether or not routine pregnancy testing is mandated by group policy, preoperative pregnancy testing requires informed consent. The anesthesia practice should have policies and procedures that at minimum assure the following; (1) reproductive information will be elicited in private; (2) if the patient refuses testing, the anesthesiologist will have a response to third parties (such as parents) that respects the patient's right to privacy; and (3) the consent process includes a private discussion with the patient about to whom she wants test results to be revealed. Anesthesiologists need to be aware of the social and legal consequences of discovering a pregnancy in a minor female patient, and group practices should have a process in place to refer appropriate patients for counseling and prenatal care. In some cases, if the patient is a minor, Child Protective Services may need to be involved if a test returns positive. Finally, if a group practice does decide despite these difficulties to mandate pregnancy testing, it would be wise to provide that information prior to the day of surgery to all female patients contemplating anesthesia with that practice, so that patients can incorporate this information in their decision of whether to have the surgery done at their institution, or go elsewhere.

Key points

- Good medical practice, *both from ethical and medical standpoints*, includes applying evidence-based guidelines in determining if a preoperative test should be done.
- Social risks associated with preoperative testing may not be as obvious as medical risks, but can be the source significant harm – and may well outweigh any potential medical benefit.
- Pregnancy testing and HIV testing are examples of two tests with significant social implications, but little proven medical benefit as screening tests. Policies requiring such tests should be reconsidered in light of the ethical principles respecting patient autonomy and striving for beneficence and nonmaleficence.
- Patients should be informed of the risks and benefits of preoperative testing; informed refusals should in general be honored.
- If socially sensitive preoperative tests are mandated by policy, patients should be informed at the time of scheduling of surgery and anesthesia that these tests are required, so that they can make a determination whether, in the interest of their own privacy, they wish to have care elsewhere.

References

1* Lester, P., Partridge, J.C., Cheesny, M.A., and Cooke, M. (1995). The consequences of a positive prenatal HIV antibody test for women. *J Acquir Immune Defic Syndr Hum Retrovirol*, **10**, 341–9.

2* Mazze, R.I. and Kallen, B. (1989). Reproductive outcomes after anesthesia and operation during pregnancy: A registry study of 5405 cases. *Am J Obstet Gynecol*, **161**, 1178–85.

3 Reedy, M.B., Kallen, B. and Kuehl, T.J. (1997) Laparoscopy during pregnancy: A study of five fetal outcome parameters with use of the Swedish Health Registry. *Am J Obstet Gynecol*, **177**, 673–9.

4* Loepke, A.W. and Soriano, S.G. (2008). An assessment of the effects of general anesthetics on developing brain structure and neurocognitive function. *Anesth Analg*, **106**(6), 1681–707.

5* Kempen, P.M. (1997). Preoperative pregnancy testing: a survey of current practice. *J Clin Anesth*, **9**, 546–5.

6* Practice Advisory for PreAnesthesia Evaluation. (2003) ASA Task Force on Preanesthesia Evaluation, Revised. American Society of Anesthesiologists, Park Ridge, IL.

7* Malviya, S., D'Errico, C., Renolds, P., *et al.* (1996). Should pregnancy testing be routine in adolescent patients? *Anesth Analg*, **83**(4), 854–8.

8 Kahn, R.L., Stanton, M.A., Tong-Ngork, S., *et al.* (2008). One-year experience with day-of-surgery pregnancy testing before elective orthopedic procedures. *Anesth Analg*, **106**(4), 1127–31.

9 Hennrikus, W.L., Shaw, B.A., and Gerardi, J.A. (2001). Prevalence of positive pregnancy testing in teenagers for orthopedic surgery. *J Pediatr Orthop*, **21**(5), 677–9.

10 Personal communication to the author from ASA Closed Claims Database analyst.

Further reading

Lawerence, V.A., Gafni,, A., and Kroenke, K. (1992). Preoperative HIV-testing: is it less expensive than universal precautions? *J Clin Epidemiol*, **46**, 1219–27.

Nyrhinen, T. and Leino-Kilpi, H. (2000). Ethics in the laboratory examination of patients. *J Med Ethics*, **26**(1), 54–60.

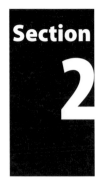

Section 2

End-of-life issues

15

The principle of double effect in palliative care: euthanasia by another name?

Denise M. Dudzinski

The Case

Mrs. Ryan was a 58-year-old woman with widely meta-static breast cancer. She entered a hospice a month prior to this hospital admission. A Do Not Attempt Resuscitation (DNAR) order had been written 2 months ago at her request. Per her living will, she was willing to forgo artificial nutri-tion and hydration when she was no longer able to take food and water by mouth. Her pain and symptoms were well con-trolled on an outpatient regimen of celecoxib, amitriptyline, lorazepam, oxycodone hydrochloride, and morphine sulfate. After 2 weeks on this regimen, she was admitted to the hospi-tal due to unbearable pain in her back, pelvis, and shoulders (presumed due to bone metastases). In order to relieve pain and symptoms, intravenous fentanyl and lorazepam were administered and titrated up when Mrs. Ryan exhibited ver-bal or physical signs of distress or pain. She was receiving 700 mcg/h of fentanyl with 100 mcg boluses every hour for break-through pain. In keeping with Mrs. Ryan's wishes, her physi-cians achieved their therapeutic goal of relieving her pain and symptoms, but they knew there may be a "double effect." The medications could suppress respiration and hasten her death.

What is the ethical rationale for allowing physicians to take this risk?

The principle of double effect (DE)

St. Thomas Aquinas first used the term "double effect" to refer to "the duality of results of a single human action" in discussing killing in self-defense.[1] If one attempts to defend oneself, and the assailant is killed, it does not mean that death was the defender's intention. Catholic moral theology distinguishes what someone intends and the side effect ("foreseen but unintended conse-quences"), suggesting that people remain responsible for, but are less culpable for, such double effects.

A modern formulation of DE is:

(T)he traditional rule of double effect specifies that an action with two possible effects, one good and one bad, is morally permitted if the action: (1) is not in itself immoral; (2) is

undertaken only with the intention of achieving the possible good effect, without intending the possible bad effect even though it may be foreseen; (3) does not bring about the pos-sible good effect by means of the possible bad effect; and (4) is undertaken for a proportionately grave reason.[2]

In the context of caring for a terminally ill patient, DE allows healthcare providers to: (1) provide adequate pharmacological pain and symptom management (a good action) knowing that (2) the foreseen but unin-tended consequence is that the medications may sup-press respirations and hasten death. The provider must intend only good pain management. She may not hope to save the patient from suffering by causing the patient's death, as this would constitute euthana-sia which is illicit in this moral framework. (3) Death (the bad effect) is not a means to alleviate suffering (the good effect). (4) Pain and suffering at the end of life is a "proportionately grave reason" to justify the use of opioids, but the risk of hastening death is only ethically justified if the patient is terminally ill.

Preconditions and components of DE

Certain virtues and prohibitions are taken for granted in the employment of DE. For example, alleviating pain at the end of life is morally virtuous, and inten-tionally killing or assisting in the death of another person is always prohibited. Physicians need not hold these beliefs. There are a myriad of other ethical frameworks that may inform moral behavior, such as maximizing benefit and minimizing harm (utility) or acting according to duty (deontology). For example, if a competent, terminally ill patient requested euthan-asia by means of high doses of opioids, one could argue this is morally permissible because it is consistent with the patient's wishes, the patient is dying, and euthan-asia will mercifully end her suffering in the manner she chooses. This is a legitimate ethical argument, but it is

---

Clinical Ethics in Anesthesiology: A Case-Based Textbook, ed. Gail A. Van Norman, Stephen Jackson, Stanley H. Rosenbaum and Susan K. Palmer. Published by Cambridge University Press. © Cambridge University Press 2011.

not an argument based in DE. Ultimately, each physician must decide if he finds DE reasoning persuasive, and to do so he should understand both the preconditions necessary for an appeal to DE and its specific components.

Proportionality

Prior to invoking DE, the patient must be dying and there must be evidence that the patient's pain and suffering cannot be managed using less risky means, which always include non-pharmacological management such as spiritual and social support. The expert management of pharmacological and non-pharmacological treatments is essential to the concept of proportionality. Jansen and Sulmasy describe proportionality: "A physician's therapeutic response to terminal suffering is justified, even if it imposes a high risk of hastening the patient's death, if and only if (1) the measures implemented are directly proportionate to the intensity of the patient's suffering; [and] (2) the measures implemented are appropriate for the type of suffering the patient is experiencing …"[3] In addition, we must exhaust all "equally efficacious alternatives with fewer side-effects."[4] For example, if Mrs. Ryan was receiving moderate doses of narcotics and anxiolytics but was still in pain and her doctor chose to suddenly administer an extremely high dose of fentanyl, DE could not legitimately be invoked. There is no medical or ethical justification to leap to such a high dose of fentanyl without first testing accelerated but intermediate doses, and therefore no "proportionately grave reason" (e.g., unremitting pain despite carefully titrated analgesia). *An appeal to DE can only be made after the patient is receiving expert pain and symptom management.* One cannot rely on DE to justify poor clinical care.

The principle of DE does not address the issue of consent

In cultures where respect for autonomy is a legal and ethical priority, the patient or legal surrogate should understand and accept the risks of pain management. Patients and surrogates consent to all medical interventions, so palliative care should be no exception. However, we respect patient autonomy due to obligations that are independent of DE. DE is silent on consent. Instead, DE revolves around intention.

Intention

Doctors who want to appeal to or better understand DE should be able to distinguish between the intention of the *act* and the intention of the *actor*. The intention of the act is the goal of an action and should be discernible by looking at the drugs and dosage increments as well as the way pain and symptoms are assessed. For example, lorazepam, oxycodone hydrochloride, morphine sulfate, and fentanyl effectively alleviate pain and anxiety. However, the administration of potassium chloride, under the auspices of analgesia, would be impermissible because, under the principle of DE, therapy must still be governed by the standard of care, and potassium chloride cannot alleviate pain.

In the interest of good palliative care, pain and symptoms should be assessed frequently so that the patient can receive additional medication if she needs it and so that the dosage can be maintained if pain relief has been achieved. When physicians use appropriate analgesics and write orders to titrate medication based on evidence of pain and suffering, such as groaning, agitation, verbal complaints, diaphoresis, hypertension, or unexplained tachycardia, they demonstrate that the intention of the act is geared toward alleviating pain. Unmonitored continuous infusions or orders to titrate up irrespective of signs of pain, anxiety, or dyspnea may suggest poor clinical management or a covert intention to hasten death. Neither is acceptable under DE. Expert clinical management and exhaustive efforts to avoid risks of respiratory depression are *preconditions* of DE. Pre-emptive dosing in anticipation of signs and symptoms of suffering is not forbidden under DE, provided it meets all DE criteria, is proportional, incremental, and in keeping with expert clinical management and monitoring.

The motives and intentions of the actor (the physician ordering medication, nurse administering the medication, etc.) are more difficult to ascertain. The physician should aim only to alleviate the patient's suffering, not to hasten death. DE asks physicians to carefully examine their motives and assumes that one's private moral intentions are morally relevant, even though we can never be certain of another's intentions. Put simply, we trust the stated goals and motivations of providers, unless there is good reason or evidence to question them.

DE permits extremely high opioid doses

DE places no upper limit on opioid or other medication dosages. The patient's narcotic tolerance, age, underlying diseases and organ dysfunction, current level of sedation, and previous alcohol or drug use account for pronounced variations in narcotic and benzodiazepine requirements. An experienced anesthesiologist might be astounded by the dosages a patient requires and may continue to titrate up, provided she doses based on *ongoing clinical assessments* to alleviate *targeted* distressing symptoms such as dyspnea, agitation, and pain, and provided narcotics are not increased after symptoms are relieved. DE unquestionably supports this clinical approach, because it meets the proportionality condition.

Double effect reasoning, physician aid-in-dying and euthanasia

DE is invoked when physician aid-in-dying (a.k.a. physician-assisted suicide) and euthanasia are illegal and/or deemed immoral. Washington and Oregon Death with Dignity Acts allow competent adults residing in those states who "have been determined by the attending physician and consulting physician to be suffering from a terminal disease, and who … voluntarily expressed their wish to die, may make a written request for medication that the patient may self-administer to end his or her life in a humane and dignified manner."[5] These Acts describe physician aid-in-dying (PAD) as practiced in the US. Even outside the specific provisions of state Death with Dignity Acts, physician aid-in-dying occurs when the physician complies with a competent patient's request for a prescription for lethal medication and the physician understands that the patient intends to *self-administer* the medication for the purpose of ending his or her life. It is not PAD when a patient hoards medications prescribed for therapeutic purposes and overdoses, provided the physician was not aware of the patient's intention.

In contrast, "euthanasia occurs when a third party administers medication or acts directly to end a person's life."[6] It is the action of another person that causes the patient's death, and he acts out of mercy to end the patient's suffering. Physicians may feel they are on the cusp of euthanasia when treating pain and symptoms in dying patients. Granted, in some cases, the line between the two may not be clear, but certainty is not required, even were it possible. DE addresses this concern and helps to distinguish "slow euthanasia" from the DE of effectively treating terminal pain and suffering.

Billings and Block describe one example of slow euthanasia as the practice of "hanging the morphine drip" without adjusting medications for targeted symptoms.[7] Because the dying process tends to be slower, those involved might feel that death is simply the DE of aggressive comfort care measures, however the interval between treatment and death is irrelevant in DE. One can intend to hasten death slowly or quickly. For reasons already outlined, DE does not support hanging the morphine drip, failing to monitor the patient's symptoms, and succumbing to pressures from family or providers to end the anguishing experience of witnessing a longer-than-anticipated dying process. These pressures should be addressed in other ways such as educating the family and providing emotional and spiritual support to the family and providers.

Legal and professional appeals to double effect reasoning

In the interest of good anesthesia practice, physicians widely hold dual commitments to relieve pain at the end of life and to minimize respiratory depression and other undesired side-effects of analgesia. This professional obligation does not rely on the principle of DE. However, when this balancing act is no longer sustainable, both medical societies and courts seem to support DE reasoning. The American Medical Association states that "physicians have an obligation to relieve pain and suffering and to promote the dignity and autonomy of dying patients in their care. This includes providing effective palliative treatment even though it may foreseeably hasten death."[8] Similarly, laws distinguish intended versus unintended action. For example *mens rea* crimes, crimes of direct intent, result in stricter punishments than crimes of neglect. Intention is relevant to culpability, because "we can refuse to cause harm intentionally, but can't avoid all harm that occurs as a side effect."[9]

In Vacco v. Quill, the United States Supreme Court responded to the argument that ending or refusing life-saving medical treatment is "nothing more nor less than assisted suicide."[10] Chief Justice William Rehnquist wrote that that the distinction between withdrawing or withholding medical interventions and assisted suicide "comports with fundamental legal principles of causation and intent." "When a patient refuses life-sustaining medical treatment, he dies from an underlying fatal disease or pathology; but if a patient ingests lethal medication prescribed by a physician, he is killed by that medication."[10] Indeed, it is precisely uncertainty concerning cause of death that raises the ethical dilemma: Am I hastening death by adequately treating pain? DE permits death as a side effect not because we assert, without proof, that the underlying disease was the cause of death, but because the physician is not culpable even if the medications he administered were the cause of death.

The Supreme Court seems to concur. "(I)n some cases, painkilling drugs may hasten a patient's death, but the physician's purpose and intent is, or may be, only to ease his patient's pain. A doctor who assists a suicide, however, "must necessarily and indubitably, intend primarily that the patient be made dead."[11] In Vacco v. Quill, Justice Rehnquist wrote "Just as the State may prohibit assisting suicide while permitting patients to refuse unwanted lifesaving treatment, it may permit palliative care related to that refusal, which may have the foreseen but unintended 'double effect' of hastening the patient's death."[10]

Criticisms of DE

DE's emphasis on intention invites criticism. Timothy Quill, Rebecca Dresser, and Daniel Brock write, "(A)ccording to modern psychology, human intention is multilayered, ambiguous, subjective, and often contradictory. The rule of double effect does not acknowledge this complexity; instead, intention is judged according to the presence or absence of a clear purpose. Clinicians familiar with the requirements of the rule may learn to express their intentions in performing ambiguous acts … in terms of foreseen but unintended consequences …"[12] On the contrary, DE does acknowledge the complexity of human intention, but still requires moral honesty and integrity, not perfection, in examining private intentions. Under virtue-based traditions, the fact that human psychology and motivation is complex and sometimes ambiguous – that we often have mixed intentions – does not exempt one from setting morally appropriate goals, examining mixed intentions, and acting in good faith. Certainly, a physician can appeal to DE to justify his intention to hasten death and none may be the wiser. DE does not "let him off the hook" simply because it has no mechanism to objectively test for dishonesty. Rather, his intentions never met criteria for DE despite his claim.

Key points

- Until relatively recently, dying patients were routinely undertreated for pain because physicians feared that the treatment would hasten death.
- The principle of double effect permits aggressive treatment of pain when death may be an *unintended* effect of that treatment.
- DE requires that the therapy in question be within the standard of care for treating the targeted symptoms.
- DE does not provide moral justification for poor clinical care.

References

1 Summa Theologica of St. Thomas Aquinas, I–II.

2* Sulmasy, D.P. and Pellegrino, E.D. (1999). The rule of double effect: clearing up the double talk. *Arch Intern Med*, **159**(6), 545–50.

3* Jansen, L.A. and Sulmasy, D.P. (2002). Proportionality, terminal suffering and the restorative goals of medicine. *Theoret Med Bioeth*, **23**(4), 321–37.

4* Young, R. (2007). *Medically Assisted Death*. Cambridge, UK: Cambridge University Press. p. 251.

5 Revised Code of Washington, 70.245.020.

6* Braddock, C. and Tonelli, M.R. (2009). Physician Aid in Dying. Ethics in Medicine Website, University of Washington, Seattle WA. http://depts.washington.edu/bioethx/topics/pas.html

7* Billings, J.A. and Block, S.D. (1996). Slow euthanasia. *J Palliative Care*, **12**(4), 21–30.

8* Council of Ethical and Judicial Affairs. (1992). *Decisions Near the End of Life*. Chicago, IL: American Medical Association.

9* Hawryluck, L.A. and Harvey, W.R. (2000). Analgesia, virtue, and the principle of double effect. *J Palliative Care*, **16 Supplement**, S24–30.

10 *Vacco v. Quill*, 521 US793 (1997).

11 *Washington v. Glucksverg*. 521 U.W. 702 (1997).

12* Quill, T.E., Dresser, R. and Brock, D.W. (1997). The rule of double effect – a critique of its role in end-of-life decision making. *N Engl J Med*, **337**(24), 1768–71.

Further reading

Battin, M. (2008). Terminal sedation: pulling the sheet over our eyes. *Hastings Ctr Rep*, **38**(5), 27–30.

Boyle, J. (2004). Medical ethics and double effect: the case of terminal sedation. *Theoret Med Bioeth.* **25**(1), 51–60.

Hawryluck, L.A., Harvey, W.R., Lemieux-Charles, L, and Singer, P.A. (2002). Consensus guidelines on analgesia and sedation in dying intensive care unit patients. *BMC Med Ethics,* **3**(3): E3.

Jansen, L.A. (2010). Disambiguating clinical intentions: the ethics of palliative sedation. *J Med Philos,* **35**(1), 19–31.

Surgical interventions near the end of life: "therapeutic trials"

Carl C. Hug, Jr.

The Case

An 86-year-old retired accountant was experiencing worsening symptoms and signs of congestive heart failure. He was particularly frustrated by generalized fatigue and dyspnea on excretion, which severely limited his functionality. Cardiac catherization and echocardiography revealed calcific aortic stenosis (0.8 cm²), significant occlusions of his coronary arteries (>95% LAD, >75% circumflex and RCA), global hypokinesis (EF 0.25), 2+ mitral regurgitation, dilated left ventricle, and pulmonary artery hypertension (70/35 mmH)g. Co-morbidities included non-insulin diabetes mellitus and right ocular blindness. The cardiac surgeon estimated a 20%–30% operative mortality and a 30%–40% chance of reducing his debilitating symptoms. The patient declined surgery initially, but returned 3 months later stating he would "rather die than go on in his present condition."

He underwent aortic valve replacement and coronary artery bypass grafting during 3 hours of cardiopulmonary bypass after which an intraaortic balloon pump and multiple inotropic drugs were required to sustain marginal cardiac function. Platelets were required to treat his coagulopathy.

His 26-day stay in the intensive care unit required treatment for bacteremia and pneumonia, tracheotomy, and peritoneal dialysis. Fluctuating mentation, persistent low-grade fever, and two failed attempts of tracheal extubation indicated insertion of a percutaneous endoscopic gastric (PEG) feeding tube and a percutaneous intravenous central catheter. On the 27th postoperative day he was transferred to a long-term acute care facility.

On the 33rd postoperative day he suffered a massive GI bleed and systolic blood pressures in the 50's. He was transferred to the hospital ER, then to the ICU with continuing requirements for transfusions, inotropic vasopressors, and mechanical ventilation to stabilize his vital functions. Two days later, profuse bleeding recurred and after 45 minutes of cardiopulmonary resuscitation (CPR) death was declared.

Ethical considerations: should the operation have been offered?

The patient clearly understood and accepted the balance of benefits versus risks, and gave informed consent to the procedure. Offering the operation is respectful of the ethical principle of autonomy. On the other hand, a surgeon might consider the balance of the principles of beneficence and nonmaleficence to be unacceptable, and as an independent moral agent, could justifiably refuse to perform the operation.[1]

Patients should carefully consider three specific questions before undergoing an intervention with substantial risks of bad outcomes:

(1) What are my goals for the intervention?
(2) What disabilities are unacceptable to me?
(3) What are my alternative options?

The patient's primary goals were to improve his functionality and to reduce his symptoms even in the face of a substantial risk of dying. It is not clear that he fully understood that he might incur disabilities beyond those he was experiencing preoperatively. It is almost certain that the alternative option to surgery was palliative care and hospice either at home or in a hospice facility.

Interventional trials

Medicine has been described as the science of uncertainty and the art of probability. There is never 0% or 100% benefit or risk. Sir William Osler said, "Every treatment is an experiment."[2] An interventional trial with both potential benefits and recognizable risks of death is neither euthanasia nor physician-assisted suicide. Statements by ethicists include: "only after starting treatments will it be possible in many cases … to

Clinical Ethics in Anesthesiology: A Case-Based Textbook, ed. Gail A. Van Norman, Stephen Jackson, Stanley H. Rosenbaum and Susan K. Palmer. Published by Cambridge University Press. © Cambridge University Press 2011.

balance prospective benefits and burdens";[3] "…trial interventions, coupled with hard-nosed clinical realism, may appropriately balance the possibilities for good or ill…";[4] "…The moral burden of proof often should be heavier when the decision is to withhold than it is to withdraw treatments."[3]

However, an interventional trial has important requirements in the case of surgical operations with substantial risks of serious disabilities and death. Some time will be required to allow recovery from the operation. With evidence of progressive improvement over days (with transient ups and downs) support of vital functions should be continued. But there should also be an understanding and willingness to discontinue vital function support if:

(a) It is unlikely that the patient's goals will be achieved,

(b) There is worsening of the patient's condition despite continuing or even increased supportive therapy, and most assuredly,

(c) If multiple organ systems fail.

Ideally, all these possibilities should be discussed with the patient and his/her family well in advance of undertaking the operation.

Does this case represent surgical "euthanasia?"

On the basis of the principle of double effect, the answer to that question depends on the intentions of the patient and the surgeon.[3] Although the patient and the surgeon recognized death as a possible outcome of surgery, it is clear that they accepted this possibility and had the intention of improving the patient's status. The patient never stated a wish for euthanasia or assisted suicide.

What roles should the patient's living will and durable power of attorney for healthcare (DPAHC) decisions have played?

The restrictions on interventions expressed in his living will (dated several years earlier) would have to be suspended for any patient undergoing cardiac surgery, because resuscitation measures such as mechanical ventilation, defibrillation, etc. are routinely used in the conduct of cardiac operations. His specific instructions to his primary (wife) and secondary (son who is an obstetrian/gynecologist) surrogates, if any, are unknown. Both were supportive of his decision to have the operation. It is doubtful that the issues of

suspending his living will and the timing of reinstating it were ever discussed.

Several questions need to be addressed when the outcome of the intervention is poor and the possibilities of achieving the patient's stated goals are virtually nil:

(1) When should the primary emphasis of care be changed from restorative to palliative? Both are intimately part of patient care throughout the intervention,[5] but the restorative measures may become ineffective and burdensome to the patient and even to his family and friends. The burdens may include pain and discomfort as analgesic and sedative drug doses are reduced in attempts to wean the patient from mechanical ventilation. Examples of burdens to his family and friends include perceiving the patient as suffering, the uncertainty about the degree and duration of his dependency on continuing interventions and life supporting measures, the escalation of continuing costs of care, and the possibility that the patient would never be able to return to his home.

(2) What are the options for decelerating vital function support? First of all, the family should receive regular and *realistic* updates on the patient's progress, or lack thereof, toward achieving the patient's stated goals for the operation. The focus should be on the overall trend and not the minor ups and downs of vital signs, drug infusion rates, ventilatory settings, etc. It is important to recognize that it will take time, perhaps days, for the family to grasp the lack of improvement or deterioration in the patient's condition.

Decelerating and discontinuing vital function support [6]

When it becomes clear to the physicians that the patient is failing to respond to maximum therapy, and deterioration of one or more vital organ functions is occurring, it is appropriate to approach the patient (if able to comprehend) and family members on the issues of decelerating vital function support while continuing to keep the patient comfortable. *Never say: "There is nothing more we can do."* Rather, assure the family that "we can keep the patient comfortable."

Recognizing the family's need for time to accept and adjust to the circumstances, deceleration may take a stepwise course. Often, the first step is to establish a do-not-resuscitate (DNR) order, while reassuring the family that all other therapies will be continued for the present time. Assure the family that the patient's needs will not be ignored. The patient will not be abandoned. To the author, DNR has two meanings: **Do Not Resuscitate. Do Not Relax!**

Subsequent discussions may include discontinuation of one or more vital function supporting measures (e.g., dialysis). Sometimes a family will agree to discontinue all vital function supports with the exception of one particular measure which may be symbolic to them. When the ultimate decision is to discontinue all vital function supports, the family should be reassured that the patient will not be allowed to suffer. For that reason, an intravenous infusion of fluids should be continued, and drugs administered to prevent agonal respiration, which is most distressful to the family (e.g., morphine infusion at 2–5 mg per hour), and a drying agent (e.g. scopolamine 0.2 mg iv) along with oral pharyngeal and tracheal suction to prevent the "death rattle." Intensivists differ on the maintenance or removal of the endotracheal tube to prevent these distressing signs.

Transferring the patient from the ICU

If the patient is stable but in need of continuing life-supporting measures, discussions with the family about transferring the patient from the ICU to another facility (e.g., long-term acute care) should be outlined in some detail and assurances given that there will continuity of care by virture of direct communication with the physicians and nurses at that facility.

Social Services can be very helpful in locating the appropriate facility that is satisfactory to the family. Most importantly, there should be assurances that communications with the physicians in that facility will include specific information about any limitations on further interventions (e.g., DNR order) to which the patient and family have agreed.

If the patient requires only moderate assistance with the activities of daily living, adhering to the prescribed schedule of medications, and a proper diet, the transfer sequence may be from the ICU to a private room in the hospital and then to a rehabilitation facility and then to a nursing home-type facility.

Given the stress of caring for such a patient in a private home the family should think long and hard about the burdens of providing 24/7 continuous care,

especially if that burden will fall primarily on one person. [7]

Dealing with demands that "everything" be done

This case is typical of the cases most commonly brought to an ethics committee of an acute care hospital today. Acute care hospitals are primarily involved with surgical and other types of invasive interventions sometimes followed by intensive care. Fortunately, most patients are successfully discharged from the hospital in stable condition, but some have varying degrees of disability and continuing requirements for assistance with their convalescence.

Aging draws on physiologic reserves (see Fig 16.1) to maintain independent function, and for some, the functional level is amazingly good as they compensate for accumulating chronic diseases. But when a significant hurdle is imposed, even apparently very fit patients may have too little additional reserves to clear the hurdle.[8] This fact of life is not recognized or accepted by the general public in the US, especially by those "baby boomers" who strive to live "forever." And discussions of death are taboo in most families and among friends.

In addition, the ideas of "medical miracles" in the news media coupled with television situations in which resuscitation virtually never fails, the common expectations are that "doing everything" will successfully restore any patient. Obviously, the truth is otherwise for many cases.

Suggestions of what physicians and nurses can do when faced with a family who demands that everything be done to save their loved one who is deteriorating include:

(1) Consistently state the truth about the patient's condition in a compassionate manner and do not suggest there is hope based on minor, usually transient, changes in vital functions.

(2) Ideally, agree to have a single physician communicate with the family to avoid their impressions that the care team is divided because different physicians use different words and have different body language that are interpreted as different conclusions.

(3) Constantly refer to what the goals of the patient were in consenting to the intervention. Of course it is important to have the goals explicitly stated and recorded in advance.

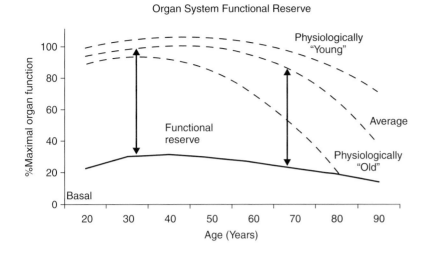

Organ System Functional Reserve

Figure 16.1 Functional reserve is needed when a person faces a stressful situation. As persons age, they draw on their functional reserve to maintain relatively normal function, and as a consequence, they have less reserve to meet a new, stressful challenge such as a major surgical operation and the demands of recovery.

(4) Remind all involved that it is one thing to keep a heart beating, but quite another to restore a meaningful life as defined by the patient's previous statements.

(5) Distinguish prolonging death from extending life.

(6) Involve pastoral services to help the family deal with their dread and grief. For many people, there is belief that death is a transition to another (better) existence.

Case resolution

As a therapeutic trial, the lengthy and complex operation initially had limited success in so far as the patient made slow progress. When it became evident that his situation remained tentative with virtually no chance that the patient could tolerate any major set back, consideration of initiating DNR would have been appropriate for two purposes: (a) it was in line with the patient's advance directives; and (b) it would have been a clear signal to his surrogate-family members that expectations for reaching his stated goals were diminishing day by day.

Most importantly, the failure to have a DNR order in place at the outside facility resulted in an inappropriate transfer back to the hospital and futile attempts to salvage what clearly was a fatal event given his already extremely limited reserves.

Key points

- In end-of-life care, focus on the patient's goals, not merely the individual procedures involved.

- Be willing to discontinue aggressive care if the goals cannot be achieved.
- Recognize that "comfort care" is an important and continuous form of caring.
- Deal with the demand that "everything be done" sympathetically but realistically.

References

1* Code of Medical Ethics. Termination of the physician–patient relationship. American Medical Association, Chicago, IL 2008–2009 edition, Section 8.115, p. 261–263; Section 8.20, p. 289, and Section 10.05, p. 354.

2* Jonsen, A.R. (2000). *A Short History of Medical Ethics.* New York: Oxford University Press, p. 89.

3* Beauchamp, T.L. and Childress, J.F. (2001). Non-maleficence. In *Principles of Biomedical Ethics*, 5th edn, New York: Oxford University Press, pp. 113–64.

4* McCullough, L.B., Jones, J.W., and Brody, B.A. (1998). *Surgical Ethics.* New York: Oxford University Press, pp. 152–70.

5* Statement on clinical practice guidelines for quality palliative care. (2006). American Academy of Hospice and Palliative Care. Glenview, IL. www.nationalconsensusproject.org.

6* Truog, R.D., Cist, A.F.M., Brackett, S.E. *et al.* (2001). Recommendations for end-of-life care in the intensive care unit: the Ethics Committee of the Society of Critical Care Medicine. *Crit Care Med*, **29**(12), 2232–48.

7* Mittelman, M. (2005). Taking care of the caregivers. *Curr Opin Psychiatry*, **18** (6), 633–9.

8* Muravchick S: (2000). Anesthesia for the elderly. In *Anesthesia* 5th edn. Miller, R.D., ed. Philadelphia, PA: Churchill Livingstone, p. 2141.

Further reading

Ethical guidelines for the anesthesia care of patients with do-not-resuscitate orders or other directives that limit treatment (2008). ASA Standards, Guidelines and Statements, American Society of Anesthesiologists. Park Ridge, IL.

http://www.asahq.org/publications and services/ sgstoc.htm

McCullough, L.B., Jones, J.W., and Brody, B.A. (1998). *Surgical Ethics*. New York: Oxford University Press, p. 182.

Troug, R.D., Campbell M.L, Curtis J.R. *et al.* (2008) Recommendations for end-of-life care in the intensive care unit: a consensus statement by the American College of Critical Care Medicine. *Crit Care Med*, **36**(3), 953–63.

Withholding and withdrawing life support in the intensive care unit

Mark D. Siegel and Stanley H. Rosenbaum

The Case

Mrs. Jones is an 88-year-old woman with a history of diabetes, stable coronary artery disease, and hypertension. She lives independently in her own home, with weekly visits from a housekeeper. Three grown children live nearby, and one of her children (a son, age 54) lives out of state.

The housekeeper discovers Mrs. Jones unconscious in the hallway of her home after an obvious fall that is believed to have occurred sometime in the preceding several days. Mrs. Jones is intubated, and admitted to the ICU. She has a broken hip, severe dehydration, and aspiration pneumonitis. Shortly after admission, she is diagnosed with a subdural hematoma and proceeds to surgery for emergency evacuation of the subdural. She never regains consciousness.

Postoperatively, she remains ventilator dependent with significant hypoxemia requiring 100% oxygen and PEEP. She develops sepsis, with hypotension, tachycardia, and myocardial ischemia. After resuscitation from a cardiac arrest due to ventricular tachycardia, she develops acute renal failure that requires hemodialysis. Liver function tests demonstrate elevated transaminases.

Discussions with the family about withdrawing life supporting therapy begin. While the three local children are in favor of limiting treatment to comfort care, the son from out-of-state wants to continue invasive treatments.

More than one-fifth of deaths in the US follow intensive care unit (ICU) admission, usually after decisions to forgo life support.[1] Each day, intensivists must decide whether to start or continue life sustaining therapies such as cardiopulmonary resuscitation, mechanical ventilation, or hemodialysis. Often, the decision to forgo treatment may protect a dying patient from ineffective care and suffering, but sometimes the decision may determine if a patient lives or dies.

End-of-life care in the ICU has many shortcomings. For example, patients with similar illnesses receive highly variable care and end-of-life decisions may be more closely related to the country, hospital,

and physician in charge rather than to the patient's wishes or disease. In many cases, treatment is exceedingly unlikely to confer benefit and resources expended could be better directed elsewhere. Dying patients often endure needless pain and suffering, while family members experience severe psychiatric symptoms. Families participating in end-of-life decisions often describe conflict with the medical team, a potential source of dissatisfaction.[2]

Several comprehensive reviews offer guidance to physicians and other caregivers seeking to optimize end-of-life care and are included in the "Further reading" at the end of this chapter. This chapter will consider an ethical framework to guide decision making, to explore frequently encountered obstacles, and to offer practical suggestions to enhance care for patients dying in the ICU.

Ethical framework for end-of-life decision-making

Four basic ethical principles should guide end-of-life decision-making in the ICU: (1) respect for the patient's autonomy; (2) the duty of beneficence; (3) the duty of nonmaleficence; and (4) the obligation to ensure just distribution of care. Day-to-day dilemmas in the ICU frequently bring these principles into tension. Patients may exercise their autonomy by refusing recommended care or requesting treatments that physicians believe they should forgo. Alternatively, resource limitations may force caregivers to deny care, even if desired or potentially beneficial. Negotiating these tensions is a challenge for physicians seeking to providing ethically appropriate care.

End-of-life decisions fall broadly into two categories depending on the degree to which available choices are constrained. Constrained choices include those affected by triage or futility considerations. For

---

Clinical Ethics in Anesthesiology: A Case-Based Textbook, ed. Gail A. Van Norman, Stephen Jackson, Stanley H. Rosenbaum and Susan K. Palmer. Published by Cambridge University Press. © Cambridge University Press 2011.

Table 17.1. An example of a triage scoring system*

Level 1 – Patient requiring life support and with potential to benefit

Level 2 – Patient requiring close monitoring with potential to benefit

Level 3 – Patient requiring life support with minimal potential to benefit

Level 4 – Patient requiring close monitoring with minimal potential to benefit

Level 5 – Patient does not meet standard ICU criteria

example, when the demand for ICU beds exceeds capacity, physicians may have to deny admission to patients who might benefit.[3] Similarly, physicians may not be able to provide requested care because desired outcomes cannot be achieved, which, by definition, limits options.[4] Most end-of-life decisions in the ICU, however, are less constrained, leaving patients or surrogates with treatment options to consider.

Triage

With increasing frequency, physicians are forced to choose among multiple patients vying for a limited number of ICU beds. Contributing factors include growth in the critically ill population, increasing recognition of better outcomes associated with ICU admission, and concerns about bioterrorism and pandemics. As a result, ICU administrators and physicians are obligated to implement effective, fair triage plans to optimize bed use.

By definition, triage implies that patients who might benefit from the ICU may be denied admission. The decision to deny admission could bring harm, including death, to the patient. Hospitals should seek to avoid the need to triage by investing sufficiently in resources to meet demand by ensuring a sufficient supply of qualified staff, beds, and equipment. In addition, steps should be taken to safely decrease ICU length of stay by promoting good practices, such as timely weaning from mechanical ventilation, making timely end-of-life decisions, and encouraging efficient throughput by transferring patients out of the ICU as soon as they are eligible. Institutions should maximize their ability to care for patients outside the unit, for example by increasing skills and staffing of non-ICU personnel. Denying ICU admission should not be equated with the decision to forgo life support, although sometimes that may be the implication.

The goal of triage is to maximize utilization of the ICU by patients most likely to benefit (Table 17.1). In choosing among patients, two key factors to consider are severity of illness and potential to benefit. Patients requiring life support technology such as intubation and mechanical ventilation, continuous renal replacement therapy, or left ventricular support devices generally have a more compelling need for ICU care than those requiring monitoring alone. At the same time, factors such as severity of the acute illness and chronic comorbidities strongly influence the likelihood of benefit. Patients who are moribund and unlikely to survive despite aggressive care are often less likely to benefit than those that are less ill. The same holds for patients with severe underlying illnesses, like advanced cancer, in whom the prognosis is likely to be poor regardless of the intervention provided.

Basic principles of fairness should govern triage. It is inappropriate to discriminate on the basis of race, gender, sexual orientation, ability to pay, or political connections. Whether to discriminate on the basis of age or functional status is controversial. Objective scoring systems should be used to maximize fairness. To minimize conflicts of interest, triage responsibility should be delegated to physicians not directly involved in patient care. Physicians responsible for triage require institutional support to support their authority while the hospital administration, attorneys, and ethics committee should be enlisted to provide oversight and guidance. Finally, when admission is denied, decisions must be made to determine if life saving efforts will be attempted outside the ICU or whether the focus should shift to palliation alone.

Futility

In the context of decision-making, futility refers to care that cannot achieve a desired end point.[4] How often futile care is requested or provided is unknown; however, the frequency undoubtedly depends on the definition used. Both quantitative and qualitative criteria for futility have been proposed, although consensus is lacking. In general, agreement is more easily achieved when situations are extreme, for example, when the patient is moribund.

At least in theory, identifying futility should transform decision-making and relieve families from considering treatments that cannot alter outcome, shifting the focus to those that can. Offering futile care makes little ethical sense: it cannot help, it may cause harm, and it may waste resources and deny other patients access to care.

Surrogate decision makers will occasionally request care that physicians consider futile. Professional societies have opined that physicians are not obligated to provide care that cannot achieve treatment goals, even if requested.[5] Careful, informative, empathic discussions will generally resolve most disputes. In the minority that persist, a deliberate approach that incorporates second opinions and opportunities to transfer care may ultimately lead to unilateral decisions to forgo treatment. However, not all physicians agree that unilateral decisions are appropriate and some suggest deferring to families in the small minority where impasse cannot be resolved.[4]

For practical reasons, the futility rationale should probably be curtailed for all but the most obvious cases. Physicians and nurses are often unable to accurately identify futility, raising the possibility of error. Concerns about self-fulfilling prophecies suggest that poor outcomes may occur simply because physicians consider the prognosis poor. Finally, survival appears to be improving for some patients with traditionally devastating illnesses, such as stem cell transplant recipients with respiratory failure, suggesting that prior beliefs about futility may be obsolete. For these reasons, we believe futility designations should be limited to obvious cases, while favoring traditional approaches that balance risk, benefit, and patient preferences when there is doubt.

Unconstrained decision-making

Surrogate decision-making

Most decisions in the ICU are unconstrained by triage and futility concerns, leaving physicians and surrogates with options to consider. Respect for the patient's autonomy should dictate most decisions. Unfortunately, most critically ill patients cannot represent themselves due to cognitive impairment resulting from their acute illness, delirium, sedation, or dementia. Surrogate decisions-makers, usually family members, must speak for them.[6]

Ideally, surrogates may be able to articulate patients' previously documented wishes, for example if relevant advance directive are available. If no explicit direction is available, surrogates may be able to provide substituted judgment, indicating what they believe the patient would choose, for example, on the basis of prior discussions or what is known about the patient. If no

information is available to guide these judgments, surrogates may be left to choose treatment they believe to be in the patient's best interest.

Several factors are likely to increase the burden faced by surrogates. Decision-making subjects family members to enormous stress. Many family members experience severe anxiety and depression during the ICU stay, which could interfere with their ability to be effective surrogates.[7] Some may not know the patient well enough to feel comfortable making decisions. Although they are probably more accurate than physicians, family members may not reliably make the same choices the patient would.[2] Even if past discussions occurred, patients' wishes may not be static – prior conversations and advance directives may not accurately portray what patients would choose under the circumstances encountered.

Certain observations may be helpful. The willingness of individual patients to endure aggressive therapy should not be underestimated. Many patients with severe underlying diseases are willing to choose aggressive ICU care, particularly if there is a chance for functional survival. In contrast, patients tend to be less willing to undergo ICU care if the likely outcome is functional or, especially, cognitive impairment.[8]

Family meetings

The primary purpose of family meetings is to choose treatments best suited to meet the patient's goals. Effective family meetings can increase family satisfaction and may mitigate long term psychiatric complications during bereavement. At its core, appropriate family meetings include all the components of any other discussion devoted to informed decision making. Physicians must ensure that surrogates are in a position to make decisions most likely to meet the patient's goals. Surrogates must have the capacity to make informed decisions and physicians must give them the information required, including descriptions of the patient's illness, available treatments options, and the risks, benefits, and likely outcomes of each option. Most surrogates want physicians to contribute to decision-making[9] and physicians should provide input to the degree that families desire.

Unfortunately, family meetings are often poorly run.[1] Many are led by physicians with little experience and tend to emphasize procedural details (e.g., intubation and CPR) without adequately discussing likely outcomes, risks, and alternatives. There is often undue focus on "code status," rather than appropriate treatment goals, which should, in turn, guide decisions. Families are often asked to decide upon major interventions with insufficient information to guide them.[10]

Many families have limited understanding of their loved ones' illnesses and prognoses. Many know relatively little about life-sustaining technologies and often overestimate the likelihood of success.[10] Many express a fear, not entirely misplaced, that a do not resuscitate (DNR) decision will lead to less aggressive care overall.[1] Language barriers when families do not speak English and also when imprecise terminology and jargon are used may compromise communication. An undue burden is often placed on families to make decisions independently, even though most would prefer to share responsibility with physicians.[9] Physicians often miss opportunities to let families speak or to share emotional support and empathy, which, in turn, could undermine negotiation.[11]

Several reviews have highlighted the features of successful family meetings.[1,5,11] Key among these are meeting early in the ICU stay, planning in advance, following a structured but flexible format, allowing time for family members to speak and ask questions, avoiding undue pressure to make decisions, and showing empathy. Families show greater satisfaction when they are assured that their loved one will not suffer or be abandoned, and when they receive support for their decision.[11]

Under the best of circumstances, physicians and family members may not be able to agree on decisions. Families may choose treatments that differ from those physicians recommend. Physicians are obliged to ensure that families understand treatment options and that coherent decisions are made in accord with the patient's wishes, if known, or best interest, if not. Physicians may choose to gently disagree and negotiate with families. However, in most cases, they should defer to families, as long as the choices are well considered and are limited to options consistent with standard medical care.

Families will occasionally request treatment that arouses misgivings among team members. In some cases, physicians may feel that the requested care is likely to cause excessive suffering and little good; alternatively, physicians may be concerned that families are refusing potentially effective care and putting patients at risk. Ultimately, physicians are obligated by basic ethical principles to avoid causing pain and

suffering if there is no reasonable associated treatment benefit.

Most perceived impasses and conflicts between family members and caregivers are actually due to identifiable problems that can be readily addressed (Table 17.2). Different perceptions regarding prognosis may respond to open, patient discussion. Many perceived sources of conflict such as anger, distrust, and unrealistic expectations may simply be the manifestations of grief associated with the trauma of hearing bad news and may dissipate if caregivers show empathy. Various cultural barriers may impose obstacles, particularly when physicians and families are from different racial, religious, ethnic, or cultural backgrounds or speak different languages.[12] Families from non-Western backgrounds may not share standard beliefs regarding patient autonomy, delivering bad news, or the family's appropriate role in decision-making. Families from traditionally oppressed groups may be less inclined to trust that physicians have the patient's best interest at heart. Families from some religious backgrounds may believe in miracles and may not be inclined to consider the physician's prognostic estimates relevant. Sensitivity to these potential sources of conflict and input from allied personnel such as professional interpreters, chaplains, and social workers may help identify and overcome barriers. Finally, it is important to recognize that most families experience anxiety and depression when faced with losing a loved one. Patience, empathy, and willingness to share in the burden of decision making may prove valuable. In the setting of a trusting relationship, physicians should rarely feel the need to override families' choices. Negotiation, education, and good communication about prognosis and treatment options should eliminate or minimize barriers to consensus.

Withholding and withdrawing life support

If the decision is made to withhold or withdraw life support, it is generally appropriate to proceed expeditiously, while allowing time for family and other visitors to gather. When appropriate, local organ banks should be notified so that donation options are pursued – often local policy may require notification, particularly in the setting of brain death.

The patient's physical comfort must be assured prior to withdrawing life support, particularly when intubation and mechanical ventilation are discontinued. Families may differ regarding their preference

Table 17.2. Sources of conflict in end-of-life decision-making and potential solutions

Nature of conflict	Potential solutions*
Religious	Input from clergy
Unrealistic expectations	Teaching, time-limited treatment trials
Lack of trust	Build rapport, emphasize mutual desire to help patient
Cultural barriers	Input from interpreters or caregivers from similar background
Irrational thinking	Consider cognitive impairment and/or psychiatric symptoms, consider input from social work, take a gentle approach, be patient
Anger	Build rapport, redirect emotions

* Suggested solutions are not meant to imply that conflicts raised have easy or predictable solutions, nor that the cause is always easily identified. The nature of the dispute cited by the family or identified by caregivers may mask deeper conflicts requiring further exploration.

for removing the endotracheal tube and their wishes should generally be respected as long as the patient's comfort is paramount. Withdrawal of life support is best approached as a procedure with specific, necessary components. Medications should be targeted to ensure comfort. To achieve symptom control, the dosing of some medication, particularly opiates, may lead to respiratory depression or even quicken death in some cases. From an ethical perspective, such dosing is acceptable (i.e., the principle of "double effect" – see Chapter 15) as long as the primary purpose is to alleviate discomfort and not primarily to suppress respiration or hasten death. In most cases, however, opiates do not shorten time to death and sometimes symptom management may lead to a period of temporary stabilization.

Families require substantial support during and after withdrawal of life support. Physicians may offer reassurance by visiting the patient's room intermittently, answering questions about the dying process, reinforcing their support for the decision, and expressing empathy and support. It may be helpful to explain the role of medications to treat distressing symptoms. Similarly, it may be helpful to explain the dying process, particularly agonal breathing, and reassure families that symptoms will continue to be effectively managed. Recognizing that family members, particularly spouses, are at significant risk for developing psychiatric disorders during bereavement, plans for follow-up care and appropriate referrals might be considered.

If the bed is available and death is imminent, patients should be kept in the ICU and families should be allowed to spend time with the body afterwards if they wish. However, if process is likely to be prolonged,

transfer to a hospice unit or a floor able to provide continue expert care may be necessary, particularly if ICU beds are in short supply.

Case resolution

Mrs. Jones failed to improve. Her physicians saw death as inevitable and tried to persuade the family to withdraw life support. Three children embraced these recommendations, but the son from out of town did not. Over the next 2 days, the medical team met frequently with the family, accompanied by ICU nurses, a social worker, and a chaplain. During these meetings, the son acknowledged a strained relationship with his siblings and expressed regret that he had not visited his mother more often. He ultimately acknowledged that his mother was not improving and came to support his siblings' view that she would not want to remain on the ventilator given the poor prognosis. Consensus was soon reached to switch the focus to palliation. A morphine infusion was started for pain and dyspnea and the ventilator was disconnected. Mrs. Jones died peacefully several minutes later, surrounded by her family and the ICU team.

Key points

- End-of-life care, particularly making decisions to withhold or withdraw life support, is a fundamental component of critical care practice.

- Appropriate end-of-life decision-making hinges on the intensivist's understanding of key ethical principles. In some cases, decisions are constrained by limits in available

ICU resources, particularly beds; in other cases, decisions are constrained by limitations imposed by the patient's disease.

- Careful, deliberate, and empathic explanations and negotiation usually lead to choices acceptable to both family members and the medical team. Impasses may occasionally arise, although most are likely to resolve with patience and identification of the barriers preventing agreement.
- When life support is discontinued, it is crucial to providing ongoing care both to patients and their newly bereaved families.

References

1* Siegel, M.D. (2009). End-of-life decision making in the ICU. *Clin Chest Med*, **1**, 181–94.

2* Way, J., Back, A.L., and Curtis, J.R. (2002). Withdrawing life support and resolution of conflict with families. *BMJ*, **325**, 1342–5.

3* Guidelines for intensive care unit admission, discharge, and triage. (1999). Task Force of the American College of Critical Care Medicine, Society of Critical Care Medicine. *Crit Care Med*, **27**(3), 633–8.

4* Burns, J.P. and Truog, R.D. (2007). Futility: a concept in evolution. *Chest*, **132**(6), 1987–93.

5* Truog, R.D., Campbell, M.L., Curtis, J.R., Haas, C.E. *et al.* (2008). Recommendations for end-of-life care in the intensive care unit: a consensus statement by the American College [corrected] of *Critical Care Medicine*. [erratum appears in *Crit Care Med*. 2008 **36**(5), 1699]. *Crit Care Med*, **36**(3), 953–63.

6* Berger, J.T., DeRenzo, E.G., and Schwartz, J. (2008). Surrogate decision making: reconciling ethical theory and clinical practice. *Ann Intern Med*, **149**(1), 48–53.

7* Pochard, F., Azoulay, E., Chevret, S., *et al.* (2001). Symptoms of anxiety and depression in family members of intensive care unit patients: ethical hypothesis regarding decision-making capacity. *Crit Care Med*, **29**(10), 1893–7.

8* Fried, T.R., Bradley, E.H., Towle, V.R., and Allore, H. (2002). Understanding the treatment preferences of seriously ill patients.[see comment]. *N Engl J Med*, **346**(14), 1061–6.

9* Heyland, D.K., Cook, D.J., Rocker, G.M., *et al.* (2003). Decision-making in the ICU: perspectives of the substitute decision-maker. *Intensive Care Med*, **29**(1), 75–82.

10* Heyland, D.K., Frank, C., Groll, D., *et al.* (2006). Understanding cardiopulmonary resuscitation decision making: perspectives of seriously Ill hospitalized patients and family members. *Chest*, **130**(2), 419–28.

11* Curtis, J.R. and White, D.B. (2008). Practical Guidance for Evidence-Based ICU Family Conferences. *Chest*, **134**(4), 835–43.

12* Kagawa-Singer, M. and Blackhall, L.J. (2001). Negotiating cross-cultural issues at the end of life: "you got to go where he lives." *JAMA*, **286**(23), 2993–3001.

Further reading

Beauchamp, T.L. and Childress, J.F. (2009). *Principles of Biomedical Ethics*. 6th edn. New York: Oxford University Press.

Medical futility in end-of-life care (1999). Report of the council on ethical and judicial affairs. *JAMA*, **281**, 937–41.

Ratnapalan, M., Cooper, A.B., Scales, D.C., and Pinto, R. (2010). Documentation of best interest by intensivists: a retrospective study in an Ontario critical care unit. *BMC Med Ethics*, **11**, 1.

18

Discontinuing pacemakers, ventricular assist devices, and implanted cardioverter-defibrillators in end-of-life care

Cynthiane J. Morgenweck

The Case

Mr. K is a 59-year-old who was diagnosed with idiopathic ventricular tachycardia at age 50. He had an implantable cardioverter defibrillator (ICD) placed at that time. Within a month of placement, Mr. K experienced his first shock and described it as a 'sledgehammer to my chest.' He became afraid of further shocks and limited his activities in the hopes of avoiding them. The ICD was reprogrammed, his medications were readjusted and he underwent cognitive behavioral therapy to lessen his fears of the shocks. With these changes in place Mr. K was able to resume several activities. He now returns requesting that his ICD be turned off because he has been diagnosed with unresectable cancer. He had undergone some palliative chemotherapy but has decided that he does not want more chemotherapy because it makes him so ill that he cannot focus on getting his affairs in order before he dies.

Are there ethical arguments for keeping the ICD activated?

Some practitioners will not disable any cardiac devices – pacemakers, ICDs or ventricular assist devices (VADs), citing several potential ethical arguments for leaving the device intact and functioning. One argument is that the device has become part of the patient's physiology. It is a "biofixture" and to disable it is to interfere with the patient's current physiologic functioning in a negative manner.[1] Physicians should not be a part of actions that diminish patients' health, because it would violate the principle of non-maleficence or "do no harm." A second argument is that disabling the device constitutes euthanasia in that without the device, the patient will have a cardiac event that is no longer readily reversible, as it would probably be were the device active. The physician who writes the order for disabling the device writes an order that is the potential cause of the patient's death. A third argument is that disabling a cardiac assist device could be construed as physician-assisted suicide because the order to disable the device must be written by a physician in response to a patient request. What could such an order be but an agreement to help the patient to commit suicide?

In a recent survey of physicians and their attitudes towards device deactivation, 46% of respondents believed it was illegal or were unsure if it is illegal to disable a device. Once they were reassured that it is legal, 91% of the respondents indicated that they would be willing to discuss disabling cardiac devices under certain circumstances.[2]

Responses to arguments against disabling cardiac devices

The biofixture analysis is adapted from legal concepts and is not a fully analogous argument. Devices are inserted and removed from patients throughout their lifetimes. For example, intraocular lenses and artificial joints are implanted in patients and explanted if not functioning properly. The device does not contain the patient's DNA or other attributes that identify it as uniquely specific to a particular patient. Further, disabling a cardiac device does not entail its removal, so the patient is not at risk for further surgery.

When it is argued that disabling a cardiac device will harm a patient, it is important to remember that harm assessments ought to come from the patient, particularly if the therapy has been ongoing. The physician must educate the patient about the potential

Clinical Ethics in Anesthesiology: A Case-Based Textbook, ed. Gail A. Van Norman, Stephen Jackson, Stanley H. Rosenbaum and Susan K. Palmer. Published by Cambridge University Press. © Cambridge University Press 2011.

benefits and burdens of disabling the device, but it is the patient who decides whether or not to accept the benefits and burdens. In this case the patient initially accepted the benefits and burdens of his ICD; however, as the patient's life circumstances changed, those benefits no longer outweighed the burdens in his view.

The writing of an order to disable a device should not be viewed as euthanasia. In general, euthanasia is considered to be an act on the part of a healthcare provider that intentionally hastens the death of a patient. A physician may believe that the lack of countershock will inevitably hasten the death of the patient; however, this may also be an overestimate of the value of the ICD. Not all delivered shocks are appropriate, there are nonfatal arrhythmias, and death may occur from other causes. Also, disabling the device is merely the removal or forgoing of a therapy that is no longer requested by a patient rather than a further intervention that is designed to hasten the death of the patient.

Disabling a device is not physician-assisted suicide. The requests for disabling cardiac devices are generally made in the context of other life-limiting diseases where the benefit of a device that causes the heart to function while the rest of the body is failing is no longer acceptable. If a practitioner is uncertain about the mental health of a patient, it is reasonable to consult with a psychiatrist or psychologist.

The doctrine of "double effect" may help in analysis of this issue. (For more about Double Effect, refer to Chapter 15). If the intention of the physician is to relieve suffering that the device is causing, and the death itself is unintended, then disabling may be ethically permissible. It is important to remember that disabling the device does not inherently cause the death of the patient – there are patients who have devices implanted who have never been shocked. Alternatively, shocking a dying patient may unnecessarily prolong death and cause further discomfort.

The rationale for disabling the device are based on a fundamental notion of patient autonomy, informed by patient awareness and acceptance of the consequences of the choices made. This set of conditions is analogous to the withdrawal of other medical therapies such as ventilatory support or dialysis. A debate about disabling cardiac devices has arisen in part because these devices are relatively new, because they literally support the symbolic organ of life (the beating heart), and because true to the technological imperative, health care providers rush to support those with debilitating diseases with less thought to the limits and burdens of the technology.

Distinguishing characteristics of current cardiac devices

Each of the three types of currently used cardiac devices has different functions and a different mix of harms and benefits. These differences may impact the decision to disable the device. Each device may be disabled by simply "deprogramming," or by battery pack disconnection.

Pacemakers

Pacemakers are the oldest of the devices, having been used since the early 1960s. There are risks with implantation. There can be infection, lead fractures, and inability to place the leads in a satisfactory manner with a resultant inability to pace. If the patient is able to have a pacer placed successfully, there appears to be minimal downside. It is a small device with little disfigurement of the patient and it performs its function without patient awareness. By maintaining an adequate cardiac rhythm, a pacemaker can help a patient to have a nearly normal life with few restrictions.

When a patient is dying, continued pacing may be seen as a burden. The pacing can be viewed as a mandatory continuation of one physiological system that is out of sync with the overall condition of the (dying) patient. But exactly what happens if a pacemaker is discontinued is of concern. A slower heart rate may cause congestive heart failure with shortness of breath, pulmonary edema, and an inability of the patient to enjoy the last days of life. These symptoms may be ameliorated with good palliative care. It might also be that the patient's intrinsic rate is sufficient to maintain the limited activities of a bedridden, dying patient.

There are few stories available for review of what happens to patients when their pacemakers are disabled and so it is hard to predict what will happen. If the device is disabled within the context of multiple lethal diseases, there is little reason to fix blame for all of the patient discomfort on that action alone. It is important to remember that good palliative care can ameliorate the symptoms that the patient might experience during the dying process when the pacer is disabled. If the patient is completely pacer dependent – i.e., there is no underlying cardiac rhythm – death will likely occur shortly after the pacer is disabled. Obviously, specific plans should be made regarding do-not-resuscitate orders prior to disabling such a device.

Implantable cardioverter defibrillator (ICD)

Today, pacemaker technology is usually enveloped in the ICD so that one device functions as a pacemaker or ICD or both. This section will focus on the ICD function of the device. The initial placement of the device has the risks of inability to place, infection, and lead fracture. Recovery time from the placement is short, if the device is functioning well. It is a relatively small device with minimal disfigurement. However, once the ICD is in place and functioning, it may not be as benign as a simple pacemaker. Patients are frequently aware of the firing of the device and describe the shock as traumatic. These experiences create anxiety, depression, and panic states in some patients. They may self-impose activity limitations in the hope of avoiding being shocked. Thus, patients may have a greater interest in ICD removal than with simple pacemakers in which awareness of function is not an issue. If there are other disease states that are not reversible or controllable, the patient may decide that the burden of ICD shocks added to the incurable illness creates a quality of life that is unbearable and ask for disabling of the device.

Disabling an ICD in a patient with a terminal diagnosis creates the potential for a more peaceful death. With no ICD function, death will occur either as the result of a fatal arrhythmia or as a result of the terminal illness. Shocks that would occur if the device were not disabled might prevent a peaceful death that is being sought by many patients. Patients who accept their imminent death may desire comfort care only and might actually prefer a sudden cardiac death to a more prolonged dying with its attendant diminution of functioning.

When discussing ICD disabling with a patient (and/or surrogates), it is necessary to describe the possibility of arrhythmias that do not cause the death of the patient, but do create increased disability. Further, it is important to point out that disabling the device does not guarantee a sudden cardiac death. This may also be the time to initiate a do-not-resuscitate (DNR) order. (See Chapter 2.)

Ventricular assist device (VAD)

VADs are the most recently developed cardiac assist devices, with clinical trials ongoing to determine the best design and most appropriate candidates for VADs. VAD placement is a more invasive surgical procedure with a longer in-hospital recovery time. VADs are more noticeable than pacers or ICDs. VADs were initially viewed as "bridging devices," that is, placed until the patient was able to either undergo definitive therapy (cardiac transplantation) or recover from the cardiac illness. Currently, VADs are being used as destination devices, i.e., they are implanted with the understanding that they will remain in place as long as the patient is alive. Patients who receive a destination VAD are very ill – they have refractory Class IV heart failure and systolic dysfunction. Even with a properly functioning VAD, a patient may decide after living with the device that the quality of life improvement is not sufficient to continue. The patient may experience neurologic complications, repeat infections, thromboembolic complications, and bleeding problems with recurrent hospitalizations. When a VAD is disabled, patient death is likely to occur within a short period of time, although this is sometimes hard to predict. Currently most VADs have external battery packs, and the VAD can be disabled by simply disconnecting the battery. Again, plans should be made regarding do-not-resuscitate orders prior to disabling the device.

"Preventive" ethics

The decision to disable a cardiac device can be wrenching for the patient, for family members and for healthcare providers. Preventive ethics may ease some of the emotions that are experienced when such a request is made.[3] Physician self-knowledge, communication with patients at the time of placement, and anticipation of points of dispute can diminish some of the anxiety about such decisions.

Physicians should reflect on their own responses to such requests before they are made.[4] These responses must be communicated to the patient. If the physician would never honor such a request, the patient ought to be informed at the beginning of the patient/physician relationship. If the physician is willing to consider patient-initiated requests for disabling the device, a great opportunity for conversation is when the device is placed. Discussion should include the circumstances under which the physician would recommend disabling or when the patient might request that the device be disabled. Patients should be encouraged to fill out advance directives if they have not already done so.

Sometimes the decision to disable a cardiac device may be advocated by all parties involved in the healthcare of the patient. At other times, there may be disputes that will have to be resolved so that the most appropriate care of the patient can be rendered with the best possible understanding of the choices made in the treatment plan.

In the ICU environment, it is perhaps more difficult, but still important to develop as complete an understanding of the patient's goals and values as possible. Knowing the patient's goals and values will enable the physician to craft a plan of care that is respectful of the patient's life views. It is nearly always helpful to involve the patient's family to the extent that the patient will permit such involvement. A family member usually provides a broader understanding of the patient's life and can become a reflective sounding board for decisions. This may minimize disputes.

What to do if a request is made to disable a device

When a request to disable a cardiac device is made, it is important to assure the patient that the request is being taken seriously, but also to inform the patient that disabling the device will not occur immediately, because the potential irreversibility of the disabling necessitates assessment of the request. Conversation with the patient, exploring the reasons for the request is the starting point for the evaluation the request. The dialogue may not be long, since there may be obvious reasons that need little explanation. In other cases, review of the patient's overall disease state with an emphasis on the prognosis may help to determine if disabling of the device will meet the patient's real goals.

It is important to determine if the patient has "decisional capacity" (the capacity to make decisions). Elements of "decisionality" include the patient's abilities to comprehend information, to consider the information in the context of the patient's preferences, and to communicate a decision that is consistent over time. It is imperative that the physician recognize and accept that decisional patients may refuse any and all therapies, even ones that have been instituted years ago. If there are unanswered questions about the patient's decisionality, formal psychiatric or psychologic evaluation will be beneficial.

The physician should also consider the request in the context of prior knowledge of the patient. If this request seems consistent with the patient's previous choices in healthcare, then the request is likely to be valid. If the patient has an advance directive, the request can be evaluated against the choices made in the document and in conversation with the appointed agent.

If the reasons do not appear sound, then discussion with colleagues as well as the patient's family and friends (assuming patient permission) is reasonable. Ethics consultation may also be of value. If the physician, as a moral agent, finds herself incapable of honoring a valid request, the physician must assist in the transfer of care of the patient to another physician who is willing to honor the request.

A palliative care consultation may also be helpful when a patient requests that their cardiac device be disabled. The focus of this consult will be to anticipate and alleviate uncomfortable symptoms that may occur when the device is disabled, to describe the timeline of the patient's death as well as the possibility of continued life, and to prepare the patient, family, and friends for the death.

It is vital to document the conversation and the plan developed for disabling the device. Sometimes, an outside technician is needed to disable the device. They may seek greater understanding of the physicians order for disabling the device before carrying out such an order. A well-written note will prevent miscommunications. This is also true for all other healthcare providers who may be cross-covering or coming on service shortly after the decision was made.

> ### Key points
>
> - Refusal of standard medical care, even if life threatening, is within a patient's right to personal autonomy.
> - Pacemakers, ICDs, and VADS represent forms of cardiac-supportive therapies that patients may legitimately forgo or discontinue as part of end-of-life decision-making.
> - In situations where the benefit vs. burden balance of medical care does not seem appropriate to medical personnel, additional psychological or ethics team consultation may be helpful.
> - Discontinuing cardiac device therapy should be accompanied by thoughtful discussion, discernment of patient goals, and plans for appropriate palliative care.

References

1* Paola, F.A. and Walker, R.M. (2000). Deactivating the implantable cardioverter-defibrillator: a biofixture analysis. *So Med J*, **93**, 20–3.

2* Sherazi, S., Daubert, J.P., Block, R.C., *et al.* (2008). Physicians' preferences and attitudes about end-of-life care in patients with an implantable cardioverter-defibrillator. *Mayo Clin Proc*, **83**, 1139–41.

3* Wiegand, D.L. and Kalowes, P.G. (2007). Withdrawal of cardiac medications and devices. *AACN Adv Crit Care*, **18**, 415–25.

4* Mueller, P.S., Jenkins, S.M., Bamstedt, K.A., and Hayes, D.L. (2008). Deactivating implanted cardiac devices in terminally ill patients: practices and attitudes. *Pacing Clin Electrophysiol*, **31**, 560–8.

Further reading

Ballentine, J.M. (2005). Pacemaker and defibrillator deactivation in competent hospice patients: An ethical consideration. *Am J Hosp and Pall Med*, **22**, 14–19.

Berger, J.T., Gorski, M., and Cohen, T. (2006). Advance health planning and treatment preferences among recipients of implantable cardioverter defibrillators: an exploratory study. *J Clin Ethics*, **17**, 72–8.

Dudsinski, D.M. . (2006). Ethics guidelines for destination therapy. *Ann Thorac Surg*, **81**, 1185–8.

England, R., England, T., and Coggon, J. (2007). The ethical and legal implications of deactivating an implantable cardioverter-defibrillator in a patient with terminal cancer. *J Med Ethics*, **33**, 538–40.

Goldstein, N., Carlson, M., Livote, E., and Kutner, J.S. (2010). Brief communication: management of implantable cardioverter-defibrillators in hospice: a nationwide survey. *Ann Intern Med*, **152**(5), 296–9.

Goldstein, N.E., Lampert, R., Bradley, E., *et al.* (2005). Management of implantable cardioverter defibrillators in end-of-life care. *Ann Int Med*, **141**, 835–8.

Goldstein, N.E., Mehta, D., Siddiqui, S., *et al.* (2008). "That's like an act of suicide." Patients' attitudes toward deactivation of implantable defibrillators. *J Gen Intern Med*, **23 Suppl 1**, 7–12.

Kirkpatrick, J.N., Fedson, S.E., and Verdino, R. (2007). Ethical dilemmas in device treatment for advanced heart failure. *Current Opin Support Palliat Care*, **1**, 267–73.

Lewis, W.R., Luebke, D.L, Johnson, N.J., *et al.* (2006). Withdrawing implantable defibrillator shock therapy in terminally ill patients. *Am J Med*, **119**, 892–6.

Manganello, T.D. (2000). Disabling the pacemaker: the heart-rending decision every competent patient has a right to make. *Health Care Law Mon*, **Jan**, 3–15.

Rizzieri, A.G., Verheijde, JL., Rady, M.Y., and McGregor, J.L. (2008). Ethical challenges with the left ventricular assist device as a destination therapy. *Phil, Ethics, Humanit Med*, **3**, 20.

Zellner, R.A., Aulisio, M.P., and Lewis W.R. (2009). Should implantable cardioverter-defibrillators and permanent pacemakers in patients with terminal illness be deactivated? Deactivating permanent pacemaker in patients with terminal illness. Patient autonomy is paramount. *Circ Arrhythm Electrophysiol*, **2**(3):340–4.

DISCOVERY LIBRARY
LEVEL 5 SWCC
DERRIFORD HOSPITAL
DERRIFORD ROAD
PLYMOUTH
PL6 8DH

End-of-life issues

Brain death

Robert B. Schonberger and Stanley H. Rosenbaum

The Case

A 35-year-old patient is comatose following a drowning. The treating neurologist has found the patient to be irreversibly unconscious with absent brainstem reflexes and no respiratory effort during an apnea test. Because of persistent limb movements thought to be most likely spinal in origin, the primary team elects to get a confirmatory EEG that indicates no brain activity. At the conclusion of EEG testing, the attending neurologist writes in the chart, "3/15/09 20:00. The patient is now deceased." The next of kin decide the following morning not to donate the organs, and respiratory support is promptly removed with an accompanying chart note saying, "3/16/09: The patient has died. Time of death 0700." Two weeks following this incident, the state medical examiner contacts the care team and inquires as to the proper time of death.

The historical development of a neurological standard of death

While the determination of death among many traditions has for thousands of years relied on the cessation of the pulse or respirations, twentieth-century medical care brought about both new possibilities and incentives for redefining death in terms of a neurological standard. The possibility of brain death in the presence of continued cardiovascular function emerged during the 1950s, largely as a consequence of new developments in the medical care of the critically ill. Shortly thereafter, the incentives for a new definition of brain death expanded and took on new practical urgency with the advent of deceased-donor organ transplantation.

Among the medical developments that led to the possibility of a new concept of brain death was the improvement in techniques of pulmonary support via mechanical ventilation during the polio epidemics of the 1940s and 1950s.[1] Other techniques of cardiovascular support soon followed, including the development of cardiopulmonary bypass in the 1950s and the formalization of cardiopulmonary resuscitation in the late 1950s and early 1960s. As society was confronted with the possibility of an apparently alive body in an irreversibly brain dead patient, medicine was ripe for a neurologically based definition of death that could guide the ethical discontinuation of cardiopulmonary support in such patients. In 1959, the concept of irreversible coma was introduced by Mollaret and Goulon in France. However, it may have been the subsequent development of organ transplantation, and the accompanying increase in the practical import for determining brain death, that led 10 years later to the creation of the first widely accepted standard of brain death.

In 1968, 1 year after the first successful heart transplant, a well-publicized effort in the United States to reexamine the definition of death in terms of a neurological standard was conducted by a committee at Harvard Medical School.[2] This committee, lead by the chairman of Anesthesiology at Harvard Medical School, Henry Beecher, MD, published what subsequently became known as the Harvard Criteria for determination of brain death which included: (1) unreceptivity and unresponsivity; (2) no movements or breathing; and (3) no reflexes (including deep tendon reflexes). The criteria also suggested checking an electroencephalogram (EEG) when available for its "great confirmatory value."[2] An isoelectric EEG should demonstrate no brain activity, and there should be no muscle movement. The Harvard Criteria mandated these tests be done twice separated by 24-hours. In addition, it was necessary to confirm that the patient was neither sedated nor hypothermic. While the Harvard criteria would be modified by various authorities over the subsequent four decades as described below, these guidelines represented the inaugural moment for a neurological standard of death into medical practice.

Clinical Ethics in Anesthesiology: A Case-Based Textbook, ed. Gail A. Van Norman, Stephen Jackson, Stanley H. Rosenbaum and Susan K. Palmer. Published by Cambridge University Press. © Cambridge University Press 2011.

Current international neurological standards for determination of death

The whole brain death standard

While the concept of brain death is now well established, the specific criteria for its determination vary among different countries. The legal brain death standard that has been adopted in the majority of the United States is based on the advice of the National Conference of Commissioners on Uniform State Laws[3] which formed a model of brain death legislation in 1980 that was subsequently adopted by both the American Medical Association and the American Bar Association as well as a large majority of state legislatures. This standard requires the determination of "irreversible cessation of all functions of the entire brain, including the brain stem." Similar so-called "whole brain death" standards have also been adopted in Canada, Australia, and South America, as well as most European countries with the notable exception of the United Kingdom (see below).

East Asian countries have seen more recent acceptance of a neurological standard, with brain death criteria analogous to the US standards having been adopted in Japan in 1997[1] and in South Korea in 2000. A major meeting of Chinese officials to discuss the establishment of neurological standards of brain death occurred in 2008, but no English language summary of their findings was located by the present authors.

The determination of whole brain death, when made on clinical grounds, requires the demonstration of three things: (1) an irreversible comatose state; (2) the loss of brainstem reflexes; and (3) brainstem inactivity leading to apnea. After reversible causes of apparent coma, such as hypothermia, intoxication, severe metabolic derangement, or residual neuromuscular blockade have been ruled out or otherwise corrected, a patient meets the standard by demonstrating the absence of responses to painful stimuli including to cranial nerve territories (coma), the lack of all cranial nerve reflexes (brainstem areflexia), and the absence of respiratory efforts in the face of a hypercarbic challenge (brainstem inactivity). Of note, the whole brain death standard differs from the Harvard criteria in making no mention of spinal cord function or the total absence of muscle movements. This standard also requires no documentation of hypothalamic failure. Although hypothalamic dysfunction including diabetes insipidus is often seen in patients diagnosed as brain dead, both hypothalamic and pituitary function as well as spinal reflexes are commonly found to continue in patients who meet the current whole brain death criteria.

Protocols for the clinical determination of brain death vary among institutions but must generally be made by more than one doctor in one of several relevant specialties (usually some combination of neurology, neurosurgery, trauma, or anesthesiology). In some institutions, most commonly in reference to pediatric patients, clinical assessment must be repeated over various intervals of time before the declaration of death can be properly made.

Sufficiency of the clinical diagnosis of brain death versus neurophysiologic testing

The majority of the US as well as most European Union countries have followed the lead of the Harvard committee in specifying that the clinical diagnosis of brain death in adults is sufficient in itself for the determination of death, without the need for confirmatory neurophysiologic testing. In these jurisdictions, neurophysiologic assessment is reserved for young pediatric patients as well as for circumstances in which there is an inability to perform any of the required clinical tests of brain death or where, for whatever reason, some doubt exists about the clinical diagnosis of brain death. For example, a patient too unstable to tolerate an apnea test, may instead undergo alternative neurophysiologic testing. Exceptions to the sufficiency of the clinical standard in adults include France, Italy, Luxembourg, and the Netherlands, each of which requires some type of confirmatory neurophysiologic testing even in the presence of clinical brain death.[4]

Neurophysiologic testing generally falls into two categories that serve either "to confirm the loss of bioelectrical activity of the brain" or to "demonstrate cerebral circulatory arrest."[4] Confirmation of brain death via examination of bioelectrical activity can itself be conclusive via the finding of an isoelectric EEG in the absence of other causes for central neurological depression. The absence of brainstem auditory evoked potentials or somatosensory-evoked potentials can also be useful in certain circumstances. These tests have the advantage of being less susceptible than EEG to distortion by sedative drugs, but evoked potential monitoring, while suggestive, cannot in isolation conclusively determine whole brain death.

Neurophysiologic determinations of cerebral circulatory arrest include four-vessel cerebral angiography as well as various scintigraphic perfusion studies. Angiography demonstrating absence of blood flow to the brain is widely accepted throughout Europe and the US as a valid standard, while scintigraphic perfusion studies, which may be less sensitive markers for the absence of brain perfusion, are accepted in some United States institutions as well as in Germany and Switzerland.[4] Finally, transcranial Doppler may be used as a valid confirmatory test of brain death only in Germany but is not in itself sufficient for the diagnosis of brain death due to the possibility of an insufficient bone window for valid blood flow determinations.[4]

The brainstem death standard

The UK and India are unique in having a neurological standard of death that specifically focuses on brain stem dysfunction. In 2008, the UK's Academy of Medical Royal Colleges published its "Code of Practice for the Diagnosis and Confirmation of Death."[5] (UK) The authors reaffirm the UK's original 1976 neurological standard of death which was based on "the irreversible cessation of brainstem function." In India, a similar declaration was part of the Transplantation of Organs Act of 1994. The Academy of Medical Royal Colleges argues that loss of brainstem function entails both apnea as well as the loss of consciousness and therefore suffices for the determination that the "death of the individual" has occurred. For the exclusively clinical diagnosis of brain death, there is little practical difference between the UK definition and a whole brain definition of death. If neurophysiologic testing is used, however, patients with continued cortical EEG activity or cortical blood flow could still be considered dead according to the UK and Indian standards but not by the other countries considered in this review.

Practitioners involved in brain death determinations or engaged in the care of deceased organ donors would be well advised to familiarize themselves with their own institutional guidelines as well as the laws of their particular jurisdiction, as the nuances and procedural requirements for determination of brain death may be critical in determining the status of suspected brain dead patients. Moreover, some jurisdictions give the next-of-kin the right to deny that a neurological standard of death be used at all.

The ethical foundations for a neurological standard of death

Philosophical underpinnings of differing neurological standards of death

The philosophical question of why brain death should be equated with the death of a patient has been answered largely either in terms of sociological traditions or bio-philosophical arguments. Several arguments have been made in support of a neurological standard, and they have great import for the resultant neurological standard, if any, that is advocated. The current review will focus briefly on three common ethical foundations used in support of a neurological standard of death.

Formulations of a neurological standard based on a reliance on cultural traditions

Defenders of various formulations of the neurological standard of death sometimes reference or explicitly rely on sociological traditions for their justification of a particular standard. For example, neurologist Christopher Pallis,[6] one of the early developers of the UK standard, justified his country's standard in reference to a tradition that equates both breathing and consciousness to the existence of the human soul. The tradition focusing on apnea and unconsciousness does indeed have quite a strong history within the Judeo-Christian framework of which Pallis was a part.

Genesis 2:7 recounts "and the Lord God formed man of the dust of the ground and breathed into his nostrils the breath of life, and man became a living soul."[7] This tying together the idea of breath – albeit a positive pressure breath! – with the essence of life has resonated deeply through Western culture. The Christian doctrine that the soul departs the body at the time of death has been interpreted by many theologians, Pope Pius XII among them, as meaning that the soul leaves the body at the time of irreversible loss of consciousness. It is of interest to note that the sole reference listed in the Harvard committee's original report was a speech by Pius XII.

It is, of course, possible to advocate an apnea and unconsciousness standard on non-religious grounds. In addition, it is possible to advocate for other neurological standards – or none at all – based on tradition. Any standard thus formulated is subject to all the strengths and weaknesses of all arguments from tradition. Some thinkers might argue that all neurological standards share at some level such a philosophical foundation.

Formulations of the neurological standard based on "loss of personhood:"

Some justifications for a neurological standard resort to a "loss of personhood" argument, asserting that the absence of a particular set of functions – often permanent lack of consciousness and reasoning ability – even when they occur independently from the death of the human organism, may nevertheless suffice for the ethical and legal determination of death of the person.

Such a theory finds resonance in the Western canon at least as far back as Aristotle who argued that the rational soul was the unique and essential characteristic of man. Some argue that an individual who lacks such capability has lost his or her essential claim to personhood. This stance may have provided the ethical foundation for a decision by the American Medical Association Council on Ethical and Judicial Affairs in 1995, that advocated for the use of anencephalic neonates as organ donors.[1] Such neonates are born without a brain cortex and could reasonably be assumed to lack the possibility of a meaningfully conscious life.

In accord with the AMA council's philosophical view of personhood, it might have been reasonable to assume (though the council disputed this suggestion) that not only anencephalic newborns, but any persistently vegetative patients who lacked function beyond primitive brainstem activities might reasonably qualify to be considered dead-as-people. The council subsequently reversed their stance regarding anencephalic babies,[1] presumably concluding that denying personhood based on an ill-defined threshold of higher order brain functions was a hopelessly messy enterprise, with possibly untoward slippery slope implications. As a matter of law, there is no jurisdiction that currently equates persistently vegetative states with death.

Loss of personhood arguments, however, can also be used to advocate for other standards, including the whole brain death standard. In separating the death of the person from the ultimate death of the patient, such a formulation resonates with the common desire to call a person with a beating heart still living. In doing so, however, such arguments shy away from advocating for a truly neurological standard of death equivalent to the cardiovascular standard. It may be this argument that has prevailed in some jurisdictions where next-of-kin may refuse a neurological standard altogether. If the neurological standard of death were truly equivalent to a cardiovascular death in the eyes of the legislators who passed such laws, it would be difficult to imagine that they could grant a family the right to consider a dead patient alive, no matter what the family's beliefs.

Foundations specific to the whole brain death neurological standard

So far in this discussion, we have seen that even among people who agree that a neurological standard of death should exist, the specifics of what such death should entail as well as the arguments used in their support can be vastly different. Of the few positions outlined above, one relies on an exclusively brainstem-based standard while another relies on an exclusively cortical standard. We will now turn to an ethical foundation that may be specific to the whole brain death standard.

The bio-philosophical position that was expounded by some members of the United States President's Council on Bioethics in their 2009 report advocates for the whole brain death standard. In contrast to the "loss of personhood" standard, they dispute that there can be the death of the person independent from some more fundamental phenomenon of organismal death.

Specifically, they assert that there is only one death, and that permanent and total brain failure, including both cortex and brainstem, is its necessary harbinger. Underlying their stance is the argument that a living human organism must of essence exhibit "self-preserving commerce with the world" including some inchoate expression of neediness and actions to satisfy those needs. The necessary qualities for human organismal life have been expressed by one author as "openness to the surrounding environment, ability to act upon that environment, and inner experience of need."[6]

In accord with this philosophical position, the neurological standard that would warrant a declaration of death is more stringent than both a "loss of breath and consciousness" standard as well as most incarnations of a "loss of personhood" standard. This philosophical stance requires that function of the entire brain – including cortical and brainstem activity – cease prior to the determination of death. The majority of the Presidential council that delineated this standard supported the current United States standard of whole brain death even as they provided a new philosophical grounding for it.

They rejected an exclusive reliance on brainstem death – the apnea and unconsciousness standard of England and India – largely based on epistemological grounds. The principal objection was that the inner state of a person with cortical electrical activity after brain stem death is fundamentally unknowable, and it would therefore be problematic to conclude that there was a definitive lack of consciousness in cases of continued cortical activity. There may be good reason for such doubt, given recent strong evidence for the preservation of higher-order consciousness in some patients previously considered to be in persistently vegetative states.[8]

By their standard, they also would reject a purely cortical definition of brain death, since in their view a spontaneously breathing but unconscious person would still possess a primitive neediness, openness to the world, and ability to act and would thus fulfill the criteria for continued life. It is notable that hypothalamic activity was not addressed in detail by the President's council in their report, which leads to the question of why temperature autoregulation (a feature of hypothalamic activity) would not also qualify as an inchoate self-preserving commerce with the world that was worthy of being called life.

The whole brain death standard – with slight variations – has come to be the most widely held international neurological standard of death. While the philosophical foundations underlying the whole brain death standard may include arguments from tradition, loss-of-personhood arguments, or other arguments not described here, it seems that the "self-preserving commerce with the world" stance may be most specific to a whole brain death standard.

Case resolution

Determining the time of death – the essence of the neurological standard

From a legal standpoint, most jurisdictions hold that when the neurological standard of death has been satisfied, it is legally equivalent to a declaration of death based on cessation of cardiovascular function. Such jurisdictions would hold that the neurologist's first declaration of death was the correct one.

From an ethical standpoint, according to the "self-preserving commerce with the world" stance, as well as many arguments based on sociological tradition, a brain dead patient is fundamentally equivalent to a corpse. As such, a person fulfilling the whole brain

death criteria should be considered not just dead as a person, but dead as an organism. Such an ethical standpoint therefore would agree that the neurologist's original declaration of death was correct and that the subsequent declaration the following day misunderstood the essence and practical import of a neurological standard of death.

In this regard, the "loss of personhood" stance fundamentally differs from the other philosophical stances since it maintains a distinction between death of the person and death of the organism. Although few jurisdictions follow this distinction, an argument could be made under the loss of personhood standard that both declarations of death in the case above were correct – the neurologist's declaration of death was in reference to the death of the person and second declaration was in reference to the death of the organism. Such a distinction is still widely held in the public and the press as evidenced by frequent reports of brain dead patients "being kept alive" on life support pending final care decisions. For most advocates of a neurological standard, such a statement is accurate only in reference to persistently vegetative patients.

Whether or not a ventilator remains on or off and whether or not there is a blood pressure, most jurisdictions hold that a brain dead patient is a corpse. This is the essence of the neurological standard of death, and both doctors and society at large continue to struggle with its justification.

Key points

- Advances in medical technology and transplantation lead to the re-defining of death to include not only cardiopulmonary death, but death by virtue of "brain death."
- The medical and legal definitions of brain death vary slightly among countries – with some using a "whole brain" definition of death in which no cortical activity may be present, and some relying on a "brainstem" standard, in which some cortical activity may be detectable.
- In all countries where brain death is recognized legally, the diagnosis rests with physical examination, at times supported by further medical testing.
- Philosophical arguments for the integrity of brain death as a definition of death rest

in historic religious and social concepts of what constitutes life, or with ideas that loss of "personhood" may be equivalent to, or another form of, death.

- Because of differences in social, religious and cultural beliefs, "brain death" is by no means universally accepted, and continued debate can be expected regarding what, if any, neurological standard of death should be recognized.

References

1* Van Norman, G.A. (1999). A matter of life and death: what every anesthesiologist should know about the medical, legal, and ethical aspects of declaring brain death. *Anesthesiology*, **91**(1), 275–87.

2* A definition of irreversible coma: a report of the ad hoc committee of the Harvard Medical School to examine the definition of brain death. (1968). *JAMA*, **205**, 337–40.

3* Uniform Determination of Death Act. (1980). National Conference of Commissioners on Uniform State Laws. Chicago, IL. http://www.law.upenn.edu/bll/archives/ulc/fnact99/1980s/udda80.htm

4* Haupt, W.F. and Rudolf J. (1999). European brain death codes: a comparison of national guidelines. *J Neurol*, **246**(6), 432–7.

5* A Code of Practice for the Diagnosis and Confirmation of Death by the Academy of Medical Royal Colleges. (2008). http://www.aomrc.org.uk/aomrc/admin/reports/docs/DofD-finalpdf 2008.

6* Controversies in the Determination of Death: A White Paper by the President's Council on Bioethics. (2009) http://www.bioethics.gov/reports/death/ 2009.

7   Holy Bible, King James version.

8* Owen, A.M., Coleman, M.R., Boly, M., *et al.* (2006). Detecting awareness in the vegetative state. *Science*, **313**, 1402–3.

Further reading

Aita, K. (2009). Japan approves brain death to increase donors: will it work? *Lancet*, **374**(9699), 1403–4.

Ethical issues in organ donation after cardiac death

Richard L. Wolman

The Case

Mr. Gift is a 59-year-old man who is permanently quadraplegic and ventilator dependent due to a C2–3 fracture dislocation following a fall during an equestrian competition 8 weeks ago. Since the accident he has undergone several surgeries, including C-spine stabilization, tracheostomy, jejunostomy tube placement, and intramedullary fixation of a femur fracture. He is scheduled for a tracheostomy revision tomorrow, due to intermittent partial obstruction of the trachea and tracheal stenosis.

Mr. Gift is awake, alert, and finds life intolerable in his dependent state. He does not want the scheduled surgery. He views his situation as both emotionally and financially draining for his family. In the event of a cardiac arrest, he has stated he does not want to be resuscitated, and he has a Do-Not-Resuscitate (DNR) order in his chart. Mr. Gift has further requested that his ventilator support be terminated, that he be given comfort measures only to relieve dyspnea and anxiety, and that his organs be donated for transplantation after his death. He has read that sometimes life-supporting therapy can be withdrawn in an operating room, and organ procurement carried out immediately after death. In order to provide the greatest possible number of organs, he has talked to an organ procurement organization (OPO) representative, and requests that this be arranged. His family is supportive of the DNR order, but unsure about withdrawal of life-supporting therapy and organ donation.

While discussions are ongoing, Mr. Gift is accidentally extubated while being turned in bed. Attempts to replace the tracheostomy tube fail. By the time the resuscitation team arrives, Mr. Gift is unconscious, hypoxemic, and hypotensive. Physicians are unsure of whether to attempt intubation, given the DNR order. The OPO representative, who happens to be on the unit when these events unfold, demands that they continue to attempt to intubate Mr. Gift and initiate cardiopulmonary resuscitation despite his DNR order, so that arrangements can be made for a controlled cardiac arrest in the OR followed by organ donation per his wishes.

The transplantation program in the US is an altruistic program based on the premise that organ donation is a gift, and relying on ethical principles of autonomy, respect for persons (beneficence, nonmaleficence), and justice. Public confidence in this system assumes obligations of grateful use, grateful conduct, and reciprocation, and the core shared societal values of voluntarism, respect for family preferences, promotion of a sense of community through generosity, and improving the quality of life for others.[1] The legislative basis of this system of transplantation is the 1968 Uniform Anatomical Gift Act (UAGA) that defined the ability of individuals to donate their organs via an opt-in approach to organ donation that honored the free "autonomous" choice of individuals to donate their organs via a "first person consent" or "donor designation" process.

Since the early days of organ transplantation, there has been general acceptance of the dead donor rule, an ethical axiom that states it is unethical for organ procurement to cause death or injury and, except in the case of living donation, it is unethical for organ procurement to precede death. This rule illustrates society's respect for the donor as a person (autonomy), the donor's interests, and life (nonmaleficence). It was also necessary to safeguard and protect the interests of vulnerable populations, avoid "slippery slope" situations, and to insure public support for a voluntary system of organ donation.[2] Adherence to the "dead donor rule" presupposes an acceptable, stringent definition of death.

Defining death

Initially, the only accepted definition of death was cardiopulmonary death, and organs were only procured from nonheartbeating donors. This placed practical limitations on transplantation of many organs, such as

---

Clinical Ethics in Anesthesiology: A Case-Based Textbook, ed. Gail A. Van Norman, Stephen Jackson, Stanley H. Rosenbaum and Susan K. Palmer. Published by Cambridge University Press. © Cambridge University Press 2011.

hearts, lungs and livers, whose viability declines rapidly with circulatory arrest. In the meantime, redefining death became important for the ever-increasing population of unconscious patients being subjected to aggressive and potentially non-beneficial life-supporting medical therapies. Such patients not only presented ethical and medical dilemmas (resource utilization, futility, end-of-life care and right to die decisions), but were also a potential source of organs for transplantation. In 1968, Henry K. Beecher and the ad hoc committee of the Harvard Medical School defined clinical criteria for "brain death" or death of the whole brain and brainstem.[3] (See Chapter 19.)

A legislative "stringent" definition of death in the US was provided by the 1980 Uniform Determination of Death Act (UDDA), which defined death as either cardiopulmonary death (irreversible cessation of circulatory and respiratory function) *or* brain death (irreversible cessation of all functions of the entire brain and brain stem). Despite this broadening of the definition of death, the shortage of viable organs has remained a problem, and transplant waiting lists continue to grow.[a] The shortage of organs for transplantation resulted in renewed interest in vital organ procurement from non-heartbeating donors (donation after cardiac death or DCD) in 1992.[4]

Donation after cardiac death (DCD)

A non-heart-beating organ donor is "[a] cadaver, whose death was determined by demonstrating irreversible cessation of cardiopulmonary function (simultaneous and irreversible unresponsiveness, apnea, and absent circulation) from whom organs are procured."[5] DCD may be "uncontrolled" or "controlled." *Uncontrolled* DCD may follow, for example, a failed cardiopulmonary resuscitation. *Controlled* DCD occurs when organ donation follows death after a planned withdrawal of life support that is expected to result in rapid death (either in the operating room or intensive care unit).

In order for controlled DCD to be ethically acceptable, three independent discussions and questions need to be answered by the prospective donor and/or surrogates without coercion from conflicted parties. Each discussion must be separated from the others by a functional "firewall". The first is a discussion and decision to forgo resuscitation in the event of cardiopulmonary arrest. Then, a discussion and decision to withdraw life-sustaining therapies with continuation of comfort care can be reached. Finally, and only after the first two decisions have been made, a discussion and decision regarding organ donation can occur. Important procedural questions regarding controlled DCD may only be discussed after a decision regarding organ donation is made. These include where and by whom withdrawal of life-sustaining therapies will occur and informed consent for premortem procedures to promote organ viability – such as placement of vascular cannulae to allow premortem administration of medications to enhance organ preservation, and the infusion of preservative solutions at the time of death.

Life-sustaining therapy may be withdrawn in the intensive care unit or in an operating room with family present. After diagnosis of pulmonary and circulatory arrest, the family, if present, leaves the operating room. A waiting period of 2 to 10 minutes, depending on institutional protocol and national standards, is observed prior to declaring death. Organ procurement can begin once death is declared. In the event that cardiopulmonary death does not occur within a reasonable period of time, often defined as 1–2 hours, the patient is returned to the ICU or to a palliative care unit, and is no longer considered a potential donor.

It was hoped that DCD would significantly reduce the shortage of viable organs for transplantation, as well as provide closure and meaning to patients and their families who wished to donate organs after death. The concept of DCD was supported by the Society of Critical Care Medicine,[5] Opinion 2.157 of the AMA's Code of Medical Ethics,[6] the Institute of Medicine (IOM),[7] and a national conference on organ donation after cardiac death.[8] However, despite increasing annual numbers of DCD donors, they still represented less than 11% of all deceased donors in 2008.[9] Attempts to increase the number of DCD donors have included relaxation of the strict criteria for donation after cardiac death, and administrative, legislative, and social changes to the organ donation process. These measures have resulted in ethical and moral controversies and have only increased the public's preexisting misperceptions and fears regarding organ procurement and DCD. These fears include those of physicians' potential conflicts of interest favoring donation over saving the life of a "potential donor" or over end-of-life care for the "potential donor". Other fears include worries that physicians will hasten the death of potential donors to facilitate organ transplantation and fears of not being dead at the time of organ donation. Such fears could potentially result in a decrease in agreements to sign donor cards and increased unwillingness to donate under DCD protocols.[10]

Legal precedents

Legislative precedents in the United States are unambiguous, allowing any competent or previously competent individual to exercise their autonomous decision to withdraw what they believe are non-beneficial life-sustaining therapies and donate their organs. These autonomous rights to have non-beneficial life sustaining therapies withdrawn in favor of comfort care are supported by the AMA Code of Medical Ethics,[11] the American Thoracic Society,[12] and a Task Force on Ethics of the Society of Critical Care Medicine.[13] Some jurisdictions in the United States do limit the ability to withdraw care in incompetents without clear (advance) directive who are not in a persistent vegetative state.[14]

Ethical controversies

Ethical dilemmas in DCD are confounded by the fact that DCD combines two morally complex events – decisions and care of the donor at the end of life, and the gift of organ donation. Dilemmas include conflicts of interest in the separation between end-of-life care and donation, use of the presumptive approach to consent (in which the donor is *presumed* to consent unless concrete proof exists to the contrary), possible violations of the donor's autonomous wishes when consent is presumed or obtained from surrogates, supremacy of donation over the donor's advance directives and end-of-life care wishes, the determination of who withdraws life-sustaining therapies, the appropriateness of premortem use of organ protection agents, and the irreversibility of circulatory arrest in the age of cardiopulmonary resuscitation (CPR).

The *practice* of DCD has been even more ethically problematic than the *concept* of DCD. In 1998, the Department of Health and Human Services, Health Care Financing Administration (HCFA) changed the Medicare (Hospital) Conditions of Participation (COP) rules to require that a member of the Organ Procurement Organization (OPO) or an OPO trained "designated requestor" initiate the request for organ donation.[15] This breached the firewall between end-of-life care and organ donation and presented an extreme conflict of interest, since employees of organizations whose livelihood is to obtain organs for transplantation can clearly not be assumed to represent the donor's interests first and foremost. The breaking down

of barriers between the three critical decisions necessary in DCD – to forgo resuscitation, to end life-sustaining treatments, and to donate vital organs – raises the potential for intended or unintended coercion of the potential donor or their family.

With the change in COP rules, OPOs began to adopt a "presumptive approach" to organ donation, in which it is presumed that patients want to donate organs unless proven otherwise. OPOs justified an aggressive approach by promulgating the belief that everyone *should* donate organs, since it is the right thing to do, and therefore any approach that leads to increased organ donation may be justified by the beneficent end of more organ availability.[16] Since the "rightness" of organ transplantation is far from a universally accepted concept, and even in some cases may violate cultural and religious beliefs of individuals, such beliefs by organ transplant agencies are at the least insensitive, and may at times frankly violate ethical principles of respect for individuals. Many have concluded that this approach is misleading, manipulative and/or coercive, undermines some of the core elements of informed consent, and is ethically questionable under the principle of nonmaleficence.[17, 18] Others point out that the involvement early in the process of professionals knowledgeable and involved in organ donation (OPO personnel) may result in a "dual advocacy" that considers the interests of both the donor and their family and the transplant recipient.[19]

Truog compares organ donation with participation in research, involving altruistic gifts, benefits to others, potential risk or harm to the patient or family, and obligations of clinicians to support the desires of patients.[17, 18] He notes that the meticulous safeguards present in research consent are absent in the presumptive approach to consent for organ donation. Clearly, under the principle of nonmaleficence, a potentially coercive, conflicted, and presumptive approach would not be tolerated in research-informed consent. Ultimately, the presumptive approach has the potential to undermine the public's confidence in the organ procurement process and further decrease the donor pool.

Families that revoke a donor's autonomous intention to donate present additional practical, ethical, and possibly legal challenges to those involved in organ procurement. In 1998, the Center for Organ Recovery and Education (CORE), an OPO in regions of New York, Pennsylvania, and West Virginia, began a controversial policy of respecting and acting on the documented wishes of the patient to donate independent of the family's consent. This shifted the approach to families from one of seeking consent, to one of informing that the individual's documented decision to donate would be respected. It rarely resulted in opposition to the donation by the families. As discussed by May and colleagues,[20] there was a firm ethical basis for this policy shift that was morally permissible and morally required. The CORE policy respects: (1) the autonomous rights of patients to donate their organs (respect for persons) by adhering to a donor directive that is definitive and applicable; (2) patients by having their interests survive their death by the fulfillment of their wishes; (3) the grieving families by relieving them of a burdenous decision at a time of loss; and (4) the caregivers, by moving them out of a possible conflict between opposing viewpoints.

Other attempts to increase the donor pool have not been so enthusiastically supported in the United States. Pressure from advocacy groups, such as the *Presumed Consent Foundation*,[21] to shift the national organ transplant system to an opt-out program in which an individual would be required to register opposition to avoid automatically becoming an organ donor upon death, is extremely controversial. Although considered by national organizations such as the American Medical Association, the Health and Human Services Advisory Committee on Organ Transplantation, and UNOS as a means of increasing organ donation, well accepted as national policy in some European countries, and supported by British Prime Minister Gordon Brown, a shift in US national organ donation policy to that of presumed consent was neither supported by a 1994 US survey (71% of those opposed the practice)[22] nor a 2006 IOM report.[23] Differences in primary ethical priorities from autonomy and beneficence in the United States to beneficence and social justice in the European Union may account for this. Concerns in such an opt-out system include the protection of vulnerable populations such as non- or poorly English speaking persons, the young, elderly, and those who are educationally, economically, or socially disadvantaged. Such populations may neither be aware of the need to actively "opt-out" nor have access to resources to make sure that they can exercise such options.

A more recent legislative attempt to increase the number of organ donors included the 2006 revision of the UAGA,[24] which had both unintended and unacceptable consequences for end-of-life care. The ethical and legislative problems for end-of-life medical decision-making that were raised by UAGA 2006 are discussed in detail in Chapter 21.

Beneficence and nonmaleficence require that to avoid even the *perception* of conflict of interest, the person withdrawing life-sustaining therapies should not be involved in the transplantation process. In addition, the person withdrawing life-sustaining care should have expertise in palliative care, should participate voluntarily, and have an established patient–physician relationship with the patient. Withdrawal of life-sustaining medical therapies is complex, requires special knowledge or training, and lack of knowledge may result in suffering by patients and their families and therefore, harm.[25] Participation by other physicians, e.g., noncritical care anesthesiologists, is improper and may raise misconceptions regarding the priority of care. The involvement of operating room anesthesiologists may further foster the misperception that anesthesia is needed because organs are actually being removed prior to death, or that anesthetics are needed for the purpose of killing the donor.

Hastening death and declaring death

Two of the most controversial questions in the practice of DCD are: (1) whether premortem administration of organ preservation agents is acceptable, since they do not benefit the donor, and may hasten death; and (2) how long the interval must be between the onset of circulatory arrest and the declaration of death. A 2005 National Conference on DCD[8] supported both the administration of organ preservation agents and a very short time interval for declaration of death, noting that the intent of the patient and/or their family is to donate viable organs and therefore, practices to improve this goal are in the best interests of the patient's/family's goals. However, the ethical concerns regarding both practices bear some review.

Organ preservation and the potential to hasten death

Heparin and phentolamine are examples of two drugs which might hasten death in violation of the dead donor rule, and are therefore not generally used in non-donors who suffer from conditions similar to those of DCD donors, e.g., intracranial pathology or trauma, or other conditions in which enhanced bleeding might be fatal. The argument that the unintended "evil" that might occur is balanced by the potential "good" of increasing organ viability superficially sounds like the principle of double effect, which is even invoked by some of its proponents. However, the principle of double effect refers to a treatment that is intended to benefit a patient (and does), but also causes harm as an unintended side effect to that patient. Administration of organ preservation drugs has no potential benefit for the donor, and *therefore can only have no effect, or will actually harm the donor.* The principle of double effect therefore does not apply. Although a utilitarian philosophy might support administration of such drugs under a principle of beneficence, because it helps the recipient, the practice would not be supported from a deontological perspective, because it clearly treats the donor as a means rather than an end unto themselves. (For more on the principle of double effect, see Chapter 15.)

Declaring death … a matter of timing?

The timing of the declaration of death in DCD is extremely controversial, both legally and ethically. For death to be declared, circulatory arrest must be irreversible, in compliance with the UDDA's definition of cardiopulmonary death. A primary goal in DCD is to minimize warm ischemic time – the time between cessation of circulation and organ reperfusion in the recipient. However, the time between circulatory arrest and declaration of death cannot be so short that irreversibility is not established, lest the patient be killed in the organ donation process. The University of Pittsburgh decided to set the appropriate duration of asystole at two minutes prior to declaration of death, based upon controversial evidence from 180 patients that autoresuscitation (spontaneous return of pulse and circulation) did not occur after that time. However, Adhiyaman and colleagues dispute the claim that there is no autoresuscitation after 2 minutes, noting reported survival of patients following much longer periods of cardiac arrest.[26]

In order to counter concerns that 2 minutes of asystole is not long enough to assure that circulatory arrest is "irreversible," some have argued that, for a patient who will not be resuscitated, "irreversible" and "will not be reversed (or resuscitated)" are ethically identical. However, these situations are clearly *not* equivalent ethically, at least under deontological principles. In deontological reasoning, actions are determined to be "right" or "wrong" independent of their outcomes. This is because the actor does not have control over all of the consequences of an action, and accountability

is therefore difficult to assign when based on the outcomes alone. Under deontological reasoning, the morality of an action is dependent on the *intent* of the actor, as much if not more than the outcome, because *intention* is more likely than outcome to be under the actor's control.

Inability to reverse a cardiac arrest although one intends to do so is not morally the same as never intending and not even attempting to reverse a cardiac arrest even though one *might be able to do so if they tried.* A potential rescuer who fails in their efforts to save a drowning person is not morally equivalent to someone who might be able to save the victim if they try, but intentionally stands by and watches them drown.

Moreover, a drowning person who is struggling in the water but who will not be rescued is not "dead," but rather is "going to die". *Prediction* of death must not be confused with a *diagnosis* of death. By such flawed reasoning, anyone who is ever *going to die* would have to be defined as *already dead.* The controversial definition of "irreversibility" creates an irresolvable paradox, because death describes a state that, biologically, socially, or morally, is exclusive of life in whatever way we might choose to define life. Under the proposed definition in which irreversibility is equivalent to "will not be reversed," an individual is at once both living (as an integrated organism) and dead (because they will not be rescued) immediately preceding and immediately following a cardiac arrest, even though they can only be either dead or alive, but not both, at any given time. Clearly, when the definition of death depends on the intentions and motives of a third party and not the physical state of the person whose heart has stopped, then pronouncement of death represents a social construct and not a biological fact.

The dead donor rule presents major conceptual and procedural ethical problems in DCD, and limits this method of organ donation. Importantly, however, society seems willing to accept violations of this rule without compromising the trust necessary for our voluntary system of organ donation. In a survey of 1351 Ohio residents, 45% of those with consistent answers were willing to violate the dead donor rule and donate organs of patients they considered to be alive.[27] Furthermore, a survey of terminally ill adult cystic fibrosis patients found that one-third desired to donate their kidneys under anesthesia and be allowed to die when admitted for terminal care.[28]

Solutions to the lack of donor organs are neither clear nor without political and ethical controversy. We must decide whether as a society we should accept the concept that the dead donor rule is a violation of autonomy, or whether we should ignore the dead donor rule and allow donation from patients who have lost personhood (irreversibly neurologically impaired but do not reach the definition of brain death) or those who have decided that they wish to donate organs prior to their death or submit to other nontherapeutic procedures – whether or not these invasions result in death. Alternatively, society can abandon our strong emphasis on autonomy and develop more communitarian principles, a difficult political shift in a country founded under concepts espoused by the Enlightenment of individual life, liberty and the pursuit of happiness. The conflict arises when one pits the individual's rights (autonomy, personal beneficence, nonmaleficence, and justice) against the welfare of society, and utilitarianism cannot solve this conflict.

Ethical frameworks

Individualism: utilitarian and deontological perspectives

Liberal individualism may be supported by both utilitarian and Kantian (deontologic) ethical concepts. Steinbock, Arras, and London note that "[w]hether ethical norms are conceived in terms of enlightened self-interest, maximized utility, or the recognition of autonomy and human rights, they are applicable to all times and places."[29] Thus, looking at the most controversial suggestion, the right of a person to donate vital organs prior to death (and thus be killed by organ donation) or submit to nontherapeutic invasion (whether or not these actions result in their death), utilitarianism would support such rights under appropriate safeguards. Utilitarian theory, as espoused by Mill, would support the ethical right of persons with decisional capacity as well as those with precedent autonomy (advance directives) to make this autonomous decision, based on their values, desires, and wants, irrespective of harm to self.[30] Mill values the ability of persons to choose and follow their own life plans with little interference. If the decision to donate vital organs and die as a result is based upon reason and rationality (e.g., the patient is terminal and certain to die and their current suffering is worse than

death) then, the patient has made a moral decision. If the decision results in the most happiness (greatest happiness principle) then it is morally correct based on utilitarian concepts.[31] Here, the only harm is to self and that is morally permissible because "the individual is not accountable to society for actions, in so far as these concern the interests of no person but himself."[30]

On first glance, deontologic (Kantian) ethics would forbid patients to donate organs for the good of society if such donation resulted in their death, as the patients would be treated as means rather than as ends.[32] However, if *a priori*, patients decide that their duty is not to burden themselves, their families or society with continued life, then the decisions are morally correct based on Kantian concepts as long as patients treat themselves as ends and not means. They are judged by their intentions and not the consequences of their decisions. Based upon these concepts, the state or any other power structure (medical profession, judiciary, etc.) has no right to interfere. Coercive or paternalistic disruption of the patient's autonomous decision is unacceptable to both Kant and Mill. For Kant, *refusing* to allow the donation might be to treat the patient (potential donor) as a means and not an end. For Mill, the interference would also be morally unacceptable. According to Englehardt, "it is not medicine's responsibility to prevent tragedies by denying freedom, for that would be the greater tragedy."[33]

In contrast, if patients are incompetent and without reason, they cannot be autonomous and Kantian theory is not applicable. Utilitarianism also falls by the wayside if patients are unable to define what grants them the greatest happiness. In this model of principlism, decisions based on beneficence, nonmaleficence, and justice (best interests) would trump nonexistent autonomy. Decisions based upon the best outcomes (consequences) would pass moral muster, and controlled paternalism, with interest only for the patients, would be acceptable.

Communitarianism

In the situation where there is no autonomy and no precedent autonomous choices, communitarianism may provide the moral answer. Individual account of a good life will not resolve the problem of what care to give patients who are not and never were competent. Moving beyond individualism and autonomy, toward an ethic of interdependence, may provide the moral and ethical answers to these dilemmas.[34] According to Emanuel,[35] the principles of autonomy do not apply in the care of incompetent patients because they have no choice, decisions are made by another person (surrogate), the question of treatment is procedural, and we have avoided the question of what treatment incompetent patients should receive. Emanuel recognizes the substantive standard of best interests and realizes the multifactorial ways of determining what is best for the patient. He bases his solution on the development of democratically determined community consensus that defines the substantive content of best interests based on particular conceptions of the good life. In contrast, Callahan[36] recognizes that there is inherent conflict between the individual's best interests and what is best for society as a whole. His criteria for deciding on healthcare priorities give priority to the good to society over the good to individuals. Therefore, Callahan's version of communitarianism, with prohibitions protecting vulnerable groups, would support the ability of persons to donate their organs, even if the donation resulted in their death. He would also support the changes in Centers for Medicare and Medicaid Services (CMS) regulations and presumed approach for obtaining consent for organ donation, concepts of presumed consent, and therefore, the unconsented perfusion of organs following uncontrolled cardiac death. Kantian (deontologic) and utilitarian theory, while supporting some of the 2006 revisions of the UAGA that enforced the patient's right to donate over the objections of the family, would find most of the other revisions (e.g., Section 21), as well as the changes in CMS regulations, the presumed approach for obtaining consent, presumed consent, and the unconsented perfusion of organs following uncontrolled cardiac death morally unacceptable.

We live in a pluralistic liberal society, with no privileged perspective of the good, where respect for individual autonomy trumps the other principles of beneficence, nonmaleficence, and justice. These individual positive and negative liberty rights, imprinted in our Constitution and enforced by statutory and common law, allow self-harm but prohibit harm to others, and form the basis of our moral thought. Respect for autonomy involves respect for the legal and moral right to be free of nonconsensual interference. Therefore, it is just as unethical to force a person to become an organ donor as it is not to allow them the opportunity to become one,

so long as the individual's actions are free of harm to others. Respecting the ethical and judicial rights of both donors and recipients in DCD may require moving beyond the dead donor rule to accommodate the informed wishes of dying patients.

Key points

- Organ donation after cardiac death (DCD) is controversial because it combines two ethically complex events: withdrawal of life-supportive therapies as part of end-of-life care of the dying patient, and the altruistic gift of organ donation.
- The dead donor rule presents ethical problems for expansions of DCD, and some legislative and practice changes to counteract these limitations may have presented even greater ethical problems than the dead donor rule itself.
- DCD by its very nature incorporates conflicts of interest between the care of the donor and the needs of the recipient.
- Firewalls should separate the three key decisions involved in DCD: the decision to forgo resuscitation, the decision to withdraw life-sustaining therapies, and the decision to donate organs after death.
- Physicians involved in DCD should have expertise and special training in end-of-life care – involvement of general anesthesiologists can be harmful, and may lead to the mistaken belief that donors may be alive and/or suffer during vital organ procurement.
- Administration to the donor of drugs for the sole purpose of organ preservation is ethically problematic when those drugs may hasten death.
- The timing of declaration of death is also controversial, since the point of "irreversibility" of cardiac arrest has not been defined.
- Resolving conflicts in the DCD process may require revisiting the dead donor rule.

Notes

a According to data from www.unos.org and www.optn.transplant.hrsa.gov in 2009 there were 14 632 donors (8 021 deceased and 6611 living) resulting in 28 465 transplants (21 854 from deceased donors and 6 611 from living donors). As of June 2010, there were 107 970 patients on waiting lists and up to 30% will incur significant morbidity or mortality while waiting for transplantation.

References

1 Murray, T.H. (1987). Gifts of the body and the needs of strangers. *Hastings Cent Rep*, **17**(2), 30–8.

2 Robertson, J.A. (1999). The dead donor rule. *Hastings Cent Rep*, **29**(6), 6–14.

3* A definition of irreversible coma. (1968). Report of the Ad Hoc Committee of the Harvard Medical School to examine the definition of brain death. *JAMA*, **205**(6), 337–40.

4* University of Pittsburgh Medical Center policy and procedure manual. (1992). Management of terminally ill patients who may become organ donors after death. *Kennedy Inst Ethics J*, **3**, A1–15.

5 Ethics Committee, American College of Critical Care Medicine, Society of Critical Care Medicine. (2001). Recommendations for nonheartbeating organ donation. *Crit Care Med*, **29**(9), 1826–31.

6 Council on Ethical and Judicial Affairs, American Medical Association. (2008). Opinion 2.157: Organ donation after cardiac death. *Code of Medical Ethics of the American Medical Association: Current Opinions with Annotations, 2008–2009 Edition*. Chicago, IL, American Medical Association, p. 71.

7* Institute of Medicine National Academy of Sciences. *Non-Heart-Beating Organ Transplantation: Medical and Ethical Issues in Procurement*, 1997 and *Non-Heart Beating Organ Transplantation: Practice and Protocols*, 2000, both Washington, DC, National Academy Press.

8 Bernat, J.L., D'Alessandro, A.M., Port, F.K., *et al.* (2006). Report of a national conference on donation after cardiac death. *Am J Transplant*, **6**(2), 281–91.

9 www.unos.org.

10 Sanner, M. (1994). A comparison of public attitudes towards autopsy, organ donation, and anatomic dissection. A Swedish study. *JAMA*, **271**(4), 284–8.

11 Council on Ethical and Judicial Affairs, American Medical Association (2008). Opinion 2.20: Withholding or withdrawing life-sustaining medical treatment. *Code of Medical Ethics, Current Opinions with Annotations*, 2008–2009 Edition. Chicago, American Medical Association, pp. 82–3.

12 American Thoracic Society. (1991). Withholding and withdrawing life-sustaining therapy. *Am Rev Respir Dis*, **144**(3 Pt 1), 726–31.

13 Task Force on Ethics of the Society of Critical Care Medicine. (1990). Consensus report on the ethics of forgoing life-sustaining treatments in the critically ill. *Crit Care Med*, **18**(12), 1435–9.

14 *In re Guardianship of L.W.* Wis. Supreme Court, Case No. 89–1197 (1992) and *In re Edna M.F.* 210 Wis.2d 557, 563 N.W.2d 485 (1997).

15 Medicare and Medicaid programs; hospital conditions of participation; identification of potential organ, tissue, and eye donors and transplant hospitals' provision of transplant-related data – HCFA. Final rule. (1998). *Fed Regist*, **63**(119), 33856–75 and CFR Section 482.45 Medicare and Medicaid Programs: Conditions of Participation: Identification of Potential Organ, Tissue and Eye Donors and Transplant Hospitals' Provision of Transplant-Related Data.

16 Zink, S. and Wertlieb, S. (2006). A study of the presumptive approach to consent for organ donation: a new solution to an old problem. *Crit Care Nurs*, **26**(2), 129–36.

17 Truog, R.D. (2008). Consent for organ donation-balancing conflicting ethical obligations. *N Engl J Med*, **358**(12), 1209–11.

18 Waisel, D.B. and Truog, R.D. (1997). Informed consent. *Anesthesiology* **87**(4), 968–78.

19 Luskin, R.S., Glazier, A.K., and Delmonico, F.L. (2008). Organ donation and dual advocacy (Correspondence). *N Engl J Medicine*, **358**(12), 1297–8.

20* May, T., Aulisio, M.P., and DeVita, M.A. (2000). Patients, families, and organ donation: who should decide? *Milbank Q*, **78**(2), 323–36.

21 http://www.presumedconsent.org.

22 Seltzer, D.L., Arnold, R.M., and Siminoff, L.A. (2000). Are non-heart-beating cadaver donors acceptable to the public? *J Clin Ethics*, **11**(4), 347–57.

23 Childress, J.F. and Liverman, C.T., eds. (2006). Committee on Increasing Rates of Organ Donation of the Institute of Medicine of the National Academies. *Organ Donation: Opportunities for Action*. Washington, DC: National Academy Press, pp. 1–358, available at http://www.nap.edu.

24 http://www.anatomicalgiftact.org.

25* Van Norman, G. (2003). Another matter of life and death: what every anesthesiologist should know about the ethical, legal, and policy implications of the non-heart-beating cadaver organ donor. *Anesthesiology*, **98**(3), 763–73.

26 Adhiyaman, V., Adhiyaman, S. and Sundaram, R. (2007). The Lazarous phenomenon. *J R Soc Med*, **100**(12), 552–7.

27 Siminoff, L.A., Burant, C., and Youngner, S.J. (2004). Death and organ procurement: public beliefs and attitudes. *Kennedy Inst Ethics J*, **14**(3), 217–34.

28* Fost, N. (2004). Reconsidering the dead donor rule: is it important that organ donors be dead? *Kennedy Inst Ethics J*, **14**(3), 249–60.

29 Steinbock, B., Arras, J.D., and London, A.J. (eds.) (2003). *Ethical Issues in Modern Medicine.* Boston, MA, McGraw Hill, p. 26.

30 Mill, J.S. (1986). *On Liberty.* Amherst, NY, Prometheus Books, pp. 106–129.

31 Mill, J.S. (1987). *Utilitarianism.* Amhurst, NY, Prometheus Books, pp. 16–7.

32 Kant, I. (1988). *Fundamental Principles of the Metaphysic of Morals.* Amherst, NY, Prometheus Books.

33 Englehardt, H.T. Jr. (2003). Commentary. In *Ethical Issues in Modern Medicine.* Steinbock, B., Arras, J.D., and London, A.J. (eds.). Boston, MA, McGraw Hill, pp. 307–8.

34* Gaylin, W. and Jennings, B. (2003). *The Perversion of Autonomy: Coercion and Constraints in a Liberal Society.* Washington DC, Georgetown University Press, pp. 251–68.

35* Emanuel, E.J. (1991). *The Ends of Human Life: Medical Ethics in a Liberal Polity.* Cambridge, MA, Harvard University Press.

36* Callahan, D. (1990). *What Kind of Life: The Limits of Medical Progress.* Washington DC, Georgetown University Press, pp. 103–34.

Further reading

Arnold, R.M. and Youngner, S.J. (1993). The dead donor rule: should we stretch it, bend it, or abandon it? *Kennedy Inst Ethics J*, **3**(2), 263–78.

Fost, N. (1999). The unimportance of death. In *The Definition of Death: Contemporary Controversies.* Youngner, S.J., Arnold, R.M., and Schapiro, R. (eds.). Baltimore, MD, Johns Hopkins University Press, pp. 161–78.

Joffe, A.R. (2007). The ethics of donation and transplantation: are definitions of death being distorted for organ transplantation? *Philos Ethics Humanit Med,* **2**, 28.

Robertson, J.A. (1988). Relaxing the death standard for organ donation in pediatric situations. In *Organ Substitution Technology: Ethical, Legal, and Public Policy Issues.* Methieu, D. (ed.). Boulder, CO, Westview Press, pp. 69–76.

Volk, M.L., Warren, G.J., Anspach, R.R., *et al.* (2010). Attitudes of the American public toward organ donation after uncontrolled (sudden) cardiac death. *Am J Transplant,* **10**(3), 675–80, Epub 2010 Feb 1.

Revising the Uniform Anatomical Gift Act – the role of physicians in shaping legislation

Gail A. Van Norman and Michael DeVita

The Case

In Pennsylvania, a man lies in critical condition. He has indicated in his living will that he would not want his life maintained "on machines." He has a do-not-resuscitate (DNR) order. He has also designated on his driver's license that he wishes to be an organ donor. His physicians are prevented from discussing of palliative care options by a new state law based on the new Uniform Anatomical Gift Act (2006). The new law prioritizes management of potential organ donors to promote organ viability, even if it compromises palliative care. According to the new law, the family may not intervene when, despite his DNR order, the patient is resuscitated from a hypotensive arrest and mechanical ventilation is continued. After evaluation for organ donation, he is taken to an operating room for withdrawal of life-sustaining treatment. Shortly thereafter he dies and his organs are procured for transplantation.

In Washington State, an anesthesiologist who is unaware of these events discovers that adoption of a state law based on the new UAGA (2006) is about to pass out of committee in the state senate and will likely be signed by the governor. She is troubled by several problems with the legislation, one of which is that it would permit organ procurement agencies to override a patient's living will and continue or even initiate life-sustaining treatments to promote organ viability, without the agreement of the patient or the patient's surrogate decision-makers.

The original Uniform Anatomical Gift Act (UAGA) is model legislation for states to emulate, and to promote uniform laws among states. It was enacted in 1968 and revised in 1987, assuring patients of their rights to donate their organs for transplantation after death. More than 40 years later, organ transplantation is a fixture in modern health care in developed countries. But controversies in organ transplantation persist: particularly those involving rights of donors versus the needs of recipients, the balance between end-of-life (EOL) care and preservation of transplantable organs, and concerns for vulnerable populations who may experience either barriers to organ donation or, alternatively, become the victims of rules that do not fairly recognize their rights and desires to refuse organ donation.

The original version of the 2006 revision of the UAGA and its consequences is an object lesson in how well-meaning experts unintentionally crossed critical ethical boundaries in their desire to improve organ donation. It is also a story of how legislative actions can profoundly affect clinical practice in anesthesiology, and an illustration that clinical practitioners have important roles to play in promoting ethical legislation. A revised version of the UAGA 2006 has now been adopted in most of the US, but the story still serves to remind us that our ethical responsibilities do not end at the hospital doors, but include a duty to help shape healthcare legislation.

The 1987 revision of the original UAGA never achieved national ratification and was only adopted by 26 states.[1] Organ donation and transplantation often transcends state boundaries, and the US needed uniform rules for organ donation and transplantation that could be adopted in all 50 states. In addition, despite a seemingly clear mandate in the first UAGA to protect the rights of persons to donate organs, the decisions of donors to make their organs available were often being treated by physicians and families as though they were merely suggestions rather than formal mandates. It is still common for donors' wishes to be countermanded once they have died or can no longer speak for themselves, because of family objections to organ donation.[2] Some physicians are reluctant to proceed with organ donation over family objections, even when the donor's wishes are clear – in part out of fear of litigation, in part due to uncertainty about legal obligations. This is occurring while demand for transplantable organs far outstrips supply, and loss of organs from

Clinical Ethics in Anesthesiology: A Case-Based Textbook, ed. Gail A. Van Norman, Stephen Jackson, Stanley H. Rosenbaum and Susan K. Palmer. Published by Cambridge University Press. © Cambridge University Press 2011.

willing donors because of objections of third parties is perceived as a barrier to increasing organ availability.

The UAGA (2006) sought to accomplish several explicit goals set forth in the preamble, among them: (1) to address the critical organ shortage by providing additional ways to make donations; (2) to strengthen language barring others from overriding a donor's decision to donate organs; (3) to broaden opportunities for organ donation by expanding the definition of persons who could agree to donate a patient's organs when the patient could not do so for him or herself to non-family members, such as "an adult who exhibited special care and concern for the decedent;" (4) to provide an explicit way for persons who did not wish to donate organs to refuse to do so; and (5) to expand the number of transplantable organs by promoting processes biased toward preserving organ viability.[1]

Respect for patient autonomy

A major flaw in the UAGA revision was the manner in which it dealt with conflicts between provisions of living wills and procedures to promote organ donation. UAGA 2006 permitted, even required, institution of measures to "ensure the medical suitability of the organ for transplantation," stating that "therapy may not be withheld or withdrawn from the prospective donor, unless the declaration [of a desire to be an organ donor] expressly provides to the contrary."[1] The National Conference of Commissioners on Uniform State Laws (NCCUSL) assumed that organ donors always want to prioritize organ donation over other EOL decisions, although they had no empiric evidence for this presumption. There is evidence that the major concerns of patients at the EOL are control over the timing and location of death, relief of symptoms including pain, dyspnea, anxiety and depression, avoidance of a prolonged death, and preservation of therapeutic options including withdrawal of life-sustaining measures and terminal sedation.[3] The lack of basis for prioritizing organ donation ahead of other EOL concerns led to criticism of the original UAGA 2006.[4] Critics of the original UAGA 2006 point out that, even if a majority of dying patients would agree to suspend their living wills in order to become donors, the ethical principle of respect for autonomy demands that we respect the rights of patients who do not agree, and are seeking EOL care that conforms with different goals. Thus a more flexible approach would be warranted.

The UAGA (2006) provided that once a person had designated that they are an organ donor, there were only limited ways in which their wishes could be countermanded. The donor could rescind their agreement by executing a new legal document of recission, they could destroy the original document agreeing to organ donation, or they could provide verbal rescission of the agreement to donate. Each of these measures required two witnesses, one of whom "could not be an interested party," such as a family member or transplantation representative.[1] These provisions were intended to promote respect for the wishes of donors, but they failed to adequately respect the autonomy of persons whose wishes regarding organ donation change with time and circumstance. They also failed to take into account practical aspects of EOL decision-making. Donors may lack the opportunity or be unable to execute new legal documents as EOL approaches and they become incapacitated. Many depend on family members to represent them in medical decision making when they are unable to make or express decisions for themselves. Legal and ethical principles in surrogate decision-making have traditionally recognized the legitimate role of family, since they presumably share common elements of culture, upbringing, values, and religious beliefs. And there may be no non-family members present when a last-minute rescission is expressed by a dying patient. Without the presence of such a "disinterested party," late changes of heart would not necessarily be followed under the new law.

Respect for patient autonomy requires that patients be fully informed about implications that organ donation may have for other aspects of EOL care. UAGA 2006 required no such discussion, even though in its original form, its mandates clearly could be interpreted to say that EOL decisions to forgo life-saving interventions must be rescinded, and measures to promote organ viability must be initiated if a patient states that they want to be an organ donor. It is reasonable to assume that most patients do not understand that their EOL preferences and organ donation decisions impact each other, although the model law assumed that the potential conflict *is* understood and this prioritization has been made when an organ donor designation is created. A common way in which many people express their interest in becoming organ donors is to sign a statement on the back of their driver's license, where there is no opportunity for "informed consent" about how that signature could potentially alter their other options for EOL care.

The principle of beneficence

The NCCUSL intended to assure patients who wished to donate organs that their desires would be carried out at EOL. By resolving ambiguities in favor or organ donation, they also hoped to increase the supply of organs for transplantation. However their approach fostered an either-or process instead of a collaborative decision making process. Organ donation is an important part of EOL planning that should be honored by physicians and family.

Organ donation may provide meaning for patients and families at EOL. On the other hand, unwanted resuscitation can cause physical suffering for the patient, and has emotional implications for families. The balance of benefits and harms for dying patients is complex, with highly individual considerations. An absolute solution that fits the needs of all patients and is of sufficient moral accountability in all cases is probably impossible to legislate. Instead, it is better for it to rest in the dialogue between patients, their families, and their physicians.

The principle of nonmaleficence

The UAGA (2006) sought to end a potential harm to organ donors – the risk that their wishes, even if clear, might be rescinded at EOL and their gift not accepted or honored. But the model statute failed to recognize two important things about dying patients. The first is that donors can and do sometimes change their minds at EOL, when they may be both vulnerable and have limited capacity to express their change of heart.[5] Meaningful EOL care involves managing and facilitating – not hindering – a wide array of decisions to meet the changing needs and wishes of dying patients. The second is that patients may truly have conflicting desires as EOL approaches: the desire to donate viable organs, and the desire to forgo life-sustaining interventions that would make such a donation possible. These seemingly conflicting goals may not be entirely resolvable. We propose that consideration of organ donation is an important component of good EOL care, but that organ donation does not trump EOL care. Society and physicians have generally chosen in circumstances where a clear resolution of conflicting goals is not obvious, to "err" on the side of asking the patient or their surrogate decision-makers to clarify their priorities, since the goal of care is to promote beneficence and nonmaleficence first and foremost for the patient, and not for third parties such as organ procurement agencies, transplant teams and organ recipients.

The principle of justice; fair distribution of burdens and benefits

Principles of justice require that equal persons be treated equally. The NCCUSL based their resolution of conflicting EOL decisions in favor of organ donation on the fact that often donor wishes are ignored even if there is no conflict about EOL management. The most common situation is after death determination using neurological criteria where the wishes of up to 20% of potential donors are ignored.[6] Nevertheless, when there emerges a situation where EOL care and organ donation have to be prioritized, there is not evidence to support that most dying patients would prefer one or the other priority.

By not creating clearer processes to firmly establish that in the setting of needed EOL care a patient did or did *not* want to be an organ donor, the model law had the potential to disproportionately harm vulnerable populations. Economically disadvantaged patients, minority populations, and those who do not speak English as a first language are least likely to be informed about such procedures, or to have means to carry them out. Organ distribution in the US is already known to suffer from imbalance: minority patients are less likely to receive vital organs than Caucasian men, for example.[7] The concern, accurate or otherwise, is that the organ donation "system" takes organs from the poor, and unfairly benefits the wealthy. It is one of the reasons cited for why organ donation from minority populations remains low.[8] Legislation that even has the appearance of unfairly treating vulnerable populations may foster mistrust in the transplant system, and therefore could adversely affect future organ donations.

Several factors likely contributed to the fact that original UAGA 2006 got so far, even being enacted in eighteen states, before the flaws became obvious. First, of all the numerous "stakeholders" identified by the NCCUSL in its preamble to UAGA 2006 did not include any physician group traditionally associated with end of life care in the intensive care unit, such as the American Academy of Hospice and Palliative Medicine, or the Society of Critical Care Medicine.[1] Physician specialists in end-of-life have a critical understanding of complex end-of-life issues, and are arguably *the most important physicians* to involve in any discussions surrounding medical issues at end-of-life. Second, the implementation of the legislation was poorly publicized, both nationally and locally. Many physicians involved in organ transplantation were unaware that UAGA was being revised. In Washington State there had been no widespread public announcement of the adoption of the legislation. Indeed, the witnesses at Senate hearings were for the most part organ transplant recipients and representatives of the local organ procurement network. As a result, the committee members were under informed and perhaps not well positioned to assess unintended consequences of the wording of the UAGA.

Ethical obligations in promoting healthcare legislation

Physician advocacy for patient rights is not only the responsibility of a few politically interested parties; patient advocacy is a founding principle in medical practice, and is a specific duty of every physician in practice. Such advocacy can take many forms; from supporting individual patients in their endeavors to seek health benefits owed to them, to developing and advocating for positive changes in health care legislation.

Physician professional organizations acknowledge that ethical obligations of physicians extend beyond those between individual doctors and patients. The AMA's "principles of medical ethics" states that, "A physician shall respect the law and also recognize a responsibility to seek changes in those requirements which are contrary to the best interests of the patient."[9] The AMA Code of Medical Ethics goes on to say that: "Whenever engaging in advocacy efforts, physicians must ensure that the health of patients is not jeopardized and that patient care is not compromised."[10] When doctors engage in legislative efforts, they are therefore obliged to look at all of the benefits and harms that might result from such rules.

The AMA Principles of Medical Ethics form a foundation upon which the American Society of Anesthesiologist basis its own Guidelines for Ethical Practice of Anesthesiology, first adopted in 1992, and reconfirmed in 2008.[11] Anesthesiologists who recognize special concerns in health care legislation and who have special knowledge to inform lawmakers should step forward when needed to help assure that laws and regulations do not result in unintended negative outcomes for patients.

The end of the story and Its "morals"

The case summarized at the beginning of this chapter was reported by Drs DeVita and Caplan in 2007 in the Annals of Internal Medicine.[4] It was their intention to point out the flaws in UAGA 2006 with regard to end-of-life care for dying patients, flaws in the NCCUSL process and its consequences, and to promote passage of significantly amended UAGA model legislation in its place. The "revised" UAGA 2006 (the "New Section 21") was proposed by the NCCUSL and contained patient-centered rather than organ-centered resolution when conflicts between living wills and donation declarations occurred.[1] DeVita and Caplan further suggested that states that had passed the original UAGA 2006 should amend their legislation to include this critical change.[4]

In Washington State, the anesthesiologist partnered with a community opinion leader to contact and inform state legislators about flaws in the legislation which was based on the original UAGA 2006. They placed an editorial in a local leading newspaper, urging voters to contact their legislators.[12] The anesthesiologist solicited letters to the legislators from national opinion leaders in anesthesiology and critical care who supported amending the legislation. She then met with the governor's legislative aide on healthcare issues and urged that the governor not sign the legislation until it was amended to contain the revised wording of Section 21. Despite strong opposition from the local organ procurement agency, the bill was placed on hold for one year until more informed discussion could occur. A revised UAGA 2006 was ultimately passed, containing the critical amendment protecting patient rights and options regarding EOL care.

Key points

- Laws can significantly impact individual patient care. Without input from physicians of all involved specialties, including anesthesiology, legislators may inadvertently create rules and regulations that lead to unintended negative consequences for patients.
- Anesthesiologists have ethical duties to understand legislation that may affect their patients, to publicize concerns, and to press for legislation that adequately and protects the rights of all patients.

- Decisions regarding organ donation are critical in EOL planning, and when patient wishes produce contradictory instructions, physicians have a duty whenever possible to discuss and resolve those contradictions with the patient or their legal surrogates. Such resolutions should represent the patient's priorities with regard to his or her own healthcare, and should not be guided exclusively by the interests of third parties, such as organ procurement agencies.

- Legislative change requires the actions of just a few knowledgeable persons. Individual physicians should not be discouraged from trying to effect positive change when misinformation or lack of debate may lead to the adoption of flawed regulations or laws that are detrimental to patient care.

References

1* National Conference of Commissioners on Uniform State Laws. (2006). Revised Uniform Anatomical Gift Act with Prefatory Note and Comments. South Carolina; National Conference of Commissioners on Uniform State Laws.

2* Christmas, A.B., Burris, G.W., Bogart, T.A., and Sing, R.F. (2008). Organ donation: family members not honoring patient wishes. *J Trauma*, **65**(5), 1095–7.

3* Truog, R., Cist, A.F.M., Brackett, S.E., *et al.* (2001). Recommendations for end-of-life care in the intensive care unit: The Ethics Committee of the Society of Critical Care Medicine. *Crit Care Med*, **29**, 2332–48.

4* DeVita, M. and Caplan, A. (2007). Caring for organs or for patients? Ethical concerns about the Uniform Anatomical Gift Act (2006). *Ann Int Med*, **147**, 876–9.

5* Ditto, P.H., Jacobson, J.A., Smucker, W.D., *et al.* (2006). Context changes choices: a prospective study of the effects of hospitalization on life-sustaining treatment preferences. *Med Decis Making*, **26**, 313–22.

6* Barber, K., Falvey, S., Hamilton, C., *et al.* (2006). Potential for organ donation in the United Kingdom: audit of intensive care records. *BMJ*, **332**, 1124–7.

7* Siminoff, L.A., Burant, C.J. and Ibrahim, S.A. (2006). Racial disparities in preferences and perceptions regarding organ donation. *J Gen Intern Med*, **21**, 995–1000.

8* Siminoff, L.A. and Sturm, C.M.S. (2000). African-American reluctance to donate: beliefs and attitudes aobut organ donation and implications for policy. *Kennedy Inst Ethics J*, **10**, 59–74.

9* American Medical Association. (2001). Principles of Medical Ethics. American Medical Association, Chicago, IL.

10* American Medical Association. (2004) AMA Code of Medical Ethics, Opinion 9.025. American Medical Association, Chicago, IL.

11* American Society of Anesthesiologists. (2008). Guidelines for the Ethical Practice of Anesthesiology. Adopted 2003; amended 2008). American Society of Anesthesiologists, Highland Park, IL.

12* Van Norman, G, and Brown, S. (2007). Organ donation a personal decision. Opinion, *The Seattle Post Intelligencer*, March 20.

Further reading

Beacuhamp, T. and Childress, J.F. (2009) Justice. In *Principles of Biomedical Ethics*, 6th edn. New York, NY: Oxford University Press.

Physician aid-in-dying and euthanasia

Alex Mauron and Samia Hurst

The Case

Mr. B., a successful 79-year-old scientist, has a very aggressive malignancy, is no longer able to work or function independently and is weakening rapidly. Oral medication helps somewhat with his bone pain but does not alleviate his severe dyspnea. He asks his physician for medication to "put him out of his misery", but is told that such treatment is "illegal." The day before his planned admission to a nursing facility for hospice care, Mr. B., with a final surge of energy, goes to the shed behind his house and shoots himself fatally. His written farewell note to his family ends with "it is a shame that a man has to do this for himself."

This case occurred 50 years ago; what would have happened today?

Should physicians end a patient's life at his or her request (as in euthanasia), or otherwise collaborate with the ending of life at a patient's initiative (as in assisted suicide)? This question unavoidably raises two separate ethical issues. One regards the general prohibition of killing, its justifications, and possible exceptions; the other concerns the specific obligations of physicians and healthcare personnel in this respect. This question also demands a consideration of historical context, since the phenomenology of dying has changed a great deal over time. For centuries "natural death" was conceived of by physicians and lay people alike as an experience that was at once tamed by familiarity, and yet utterly unavoidable. Dealing with death had much to do with social mores and religious rituals, little with medical interventions, which were in any event quite incapable of forestalling an inevitable demise. Modern medicine, especially emergency medicine and critical care, has changed all that and often made impending death the locus of complex decisions and choices. Research, including the classical ETHICUS study,[1] has shown conclusively that for a majority of patients dying in a Western intensive care unit, treatment limitations were in force, albeit with significant variations according to culture and religion.[2] Foregoing life-sustaining treatment on account of futility and/or patient wishes has become standard procedure and there is a vast literature discussing how to do it in an ethically defensible way.

The fatality of impending death has been replaced by what is aptly called "end-of-life *decisions*." Do-not-resuscitate (DNR) orders, advance directives, practice guidelines and the like are tools for choosing and deciding where formerly no choice existed and no decision was required. This shift has implications for the way physicians should classify their death-related actions. The smug distinction between "letting nature take its course" (innocent) and "active killing" (guilty) is no longer tenable once it is clear that acceptable forms of treatment limitation are causally connected to the patient's death. That does not necessarily mean that the traditional distinction between killing and letting die is moot, but it does imply that the relevant distinctions are more subtle and go beyond a mechanical analysis of causes and effects, actions and omissions.

The intentional ending of a human life at this person's request thus raises two distinctive ethical issues. It is obvious that the moral and legal permissibility of voluntary death, be it at another's hand, or with another's help, or wholly self-administered, has been a topic of philosophical and religious controversy for millennia. The debate still goes on and is reflected in the heterogeneity of legislation concerning euthanasia, assisted suicide (with or without physician involvement), and even suicide itself. At the same time, there has been a parallel debate in medical ethics, which is about the professional duty of physicians: does it necessitate the preservation of life no matter what? If not (as nearly everybody agrees), what are the sorts of end-of-life

Clinical Ethics in Anesthesiology: A Case-Based Textbook, ed. Gail A. Van Norman, Stephen Jackson, Stanley H. Rosenbaum and Susan K. Palmer. Published by Cambridge University Press. © Cambridge University Press 2011.

management strategies that are ethically acceptable? Do they include physician-assisted suicide and voluntary active euthanasia? What about terminal sedation? Both the broader societal discussion and the debate within medical ethics are important. They are related, to be sure, but must not be confused.

Definitions

"Physician aid-in-dying" is a somewhat ambiguous term, requiring clarification. Although general questions regarding end-of-life care and decision-making are related to our topic, not all of them are part of it. This chapter is not about interrupting life support, DNR orders, or palliative care, but about the wilful termination of a patient's life by a physician and the willing collaboration of a physician to the patient's suicide. The term "physician-assisted death" used by some authors is clear and covers our subject matter. Some practices may be seen as borderline, such as terminal sedation, and we will therefore discuss it also since it is a specific concern of anesthesiologists. The issue of the withdrawal of food and hydration from comatose patients, or from dying patients who request it, is often drawn into the legal controversy on physician-assisted death. Examples are the case of Terry Schiavo[3] or the very recent case of Eluana Englaro in Italy (a bill currently before the Italian senate would make hydration and alimentation compulsory).[4] In fact, these broader end-of-life issues have a way of spilling over into the debate on physician-assisted death, in part because similar arguments have been used in both areas. As noted by Dworkin in 2007:

> When these practices (i.e., withdrawal of life-support, accepting a refusal of artificial hydration and alimentation, etc.) were proposed by physicians, and when they were sanctioned by the courts, there were the same kinds of prediction made by opponents as are now made about physician-assisted suicide. Patients would be manipulated or coerced into making, or agreeing, to such practices. Patients who might be cured by new discoveries would mistakenly request to be removed from life-support. The slippery slope from voluntarily requesting DNR to having such orders entered on their chart without consent would be traversed.[5]

Nevertheless, we will largely limit ourselves to a consideration of voluntary active euthanasia and physician-assisted suicide. As regards euthanasia, this means that both nonvoluntary and involuntary euthanasia are outside our remit (and universally seen

as beyond the pale). We will also focus on *physician-assisted suicide*, even though we have to broaden our perspective occasionally, as in discussing the Swiss legal situation.

Ethical arguments and legislation

Physician-assisted death harks back to a general debate on voluntary death that has been going on for millennia, and some of the arguments given today have been present throughout this history. They closely parallel arguments made in favor of or against euthanasia and assisted suicide.[6]

Arguments against euthanasia and assisted suicide

(1) That although respect for autonomy is important, it should not extend to euthanasia or assisted suicide. For long periods of history, lives were considered to belong to God, or the State, or both. In monarchies, suicide was a common law felony against the king. More recently, philosophers have argued that suicide cannot be autonomous because it ends the possibility of autonomy. Nor can a request for assisted death be considered autonomous if it is a symptom of a disease, such as depression: if this is always the case, these requests are never autonomous.

(2) That beneficence does not necessarily extend to authorizing assisted death, and should concentrate exclusively on the use of alternatives and the promotion of well-conducted and universally available palliative care. Furthermore, requests for assisted suicides are often cries for help, which should be answered with appropriate understanding and care, rather than assisted death. This is part of suicide prevention, a major public health goal.

(3) That although we allow withdrawal or withholding of life-sustaining interventions, this is significantly different from allowing euthanasia or assisted suicide. The actual acts are different: injecting a lethal medication, or removing an invasive apparatus, are not the same. Moreover, physicians who withdraw treatment do not intend to end the patient's life, but to put aside a medical intervention which could itself be the cause of further suffering.

(4) That allowing euthanasia or assisted suicide would have severe adverse consequences, such as a trivialization of suicide, or a "slippery slope"

leading to cases of euthanasia without patients' consent. Opponents point to data suggesting that such involuntary euthanasia takes place in the Netherlands. They fear that patients may sometimes choose euthanasia under pressure, or to avoid becoming a burden on loved ones.

Arguments in favor of euthanasia and assisted suicide:

(1) That respect for autonomy does support allowing voluntary death, because autonomy means self-ownership of persons and the right to pursue our own goals in life, as long as we harm no one else. If autonomy means control over how we live, it also entails control over the way we die, which has been considered since Antiquity to be the one undeniable human freedom, and must be authorized as a liberty-right in a liberal polity. Decriminalization of suicide also recognizes that choosing to die can be a reasonable option, and makes assisted suicide a victimless crime.

(2) That even alleviation of physical pain has a failure rate, and even well developed palliative care cannot address all types of suffering with equal success. Sometimes, living with a painful disease may reasonably be seen as worse than death, we should therefore allow euthanasia or assisted suicide in cases where palliation is ineffective. The epidemiology of legal assisted suicide is very different from that of suicide generally, so it is possible to allow the first without jeopardizing public health efforts to prevent the latter. Although some requests for assisted death are cries for help, this is not always the case: attempting to understand all such requests in this way would represent "hermeneutic obstinacy" similar to the "therapeutic obstinacy" involved in persisting with life sustaining treatment over a patient's refusal.[7] The possibility of assisted death also reassures many people who are healthy, but know that they could become terminally ill someday, and that this could involve intractable suffering. The possibility of euthanasia or assisted suicide can alleviate some of their fears.

(3) That euthanasia and assisted suicide are not significantly different from practices such as withdrawal of life sustaining treatments at the end of life, which are broadly accepted as ethically justified. In both types of cases the patient requests to die, the physician intends to end the patient's life, and the patient indeed dies. The only difference is the "proximate cause": when life-sustaining treatment is removed, the patient is killed by his disease. In the case of euthanasia, the direct cause of death is the physician's act, in the case of assisted suicide, it is the patient's act. Proponents of voluntary euthanasia question the moral significance of this distinction.

(4) That "slippery slope" arguments are not valid: controversial practices can be regulated and controlled. It would be surprising if we were able to abide by a rule forbidding euthanasia, but not by a rule limiting the circumstances where it can take place. Countries where assisted suicide and/or euthanasia are legal have not experienced a slippery slope; since legislation authorizing euthanasia and assisted suicide often comes with stricter requirements for notification, it is difficult to know whether cases of involuntary euthanasia increase or decrease following the legislative change.

The ethical status of physician participation in euthanasia and suicide assistance is a distinct point in this debate. Opponents highlight the tension between assisting death and duties to preserve life, and risks to the physician–patient relationship. Proponents view assisting death as an intrinsic part of a humane response to suffering, and a form of the respect owed to patients' self-determination. Moreover, the idea that the physician–patient relationship would suffer from allowing euthanasia or *physician* assisted suicide is speculative, and data suggests that legalizing aid-in-dying would not affect patients' trust in their physician negatively.[8]

Currently, assisted suicide is legal in the US states of Oregon, Washington and Montana, and in Switzerland, Luxemburg, Belgium, and the Netherlands. Euthanasia is legal in the last three countries. All but one of these legislations provides a detailed description of the circumstances where assisted death is permissible, require physician involvement, and mandate notification. The exception is Switzerland, where nonphysicians can assist suicide and where the only legal requirements are that the patient be capable of decision-making and perform the lethal act himself, and that the helper be motivated only by altruistic motives. Typically, requirements for legal euthanasia or assisted suicide include that patients need to be capable of decision-making and persistently requesting death, and that there be otherwise intractable suffering.

Attitudes and practices

Public attitudes

Public attitudes toward assisted death vary between countries and with the sort of situation considered. In the US two-thirds of surveyed members of the general public favor euthanasia or assisted suicide when presented with the case of a patient in unremitting pain. When the case is changed to a patient suffering from functional debilitation, or who views life as no longer worth living, one-third no longer supports assisted dying, and one third still does.[9] In Europe, public attitudes differ between countries, with higher rates of acceptance in countries such as The Netherlands, but also Denmark, Sweden, and France, and much lower rates in countries such as Romania, Malta, or Turkey. Factors associated with higher acceptance include weaker religious beliefs, but also younger age, and higher educational level.[10]

Professional attitudes

The American Medical Association, as well as physician associations in countries such as Norway, Germany, and the UK, have opposed euthanasia and assisted suicide, and physician participation specifically, maintaining that assisted dying conflicts with the role of doctors. This opposition, however, is not universal. Physician associations in The Netherlands do not maintain that medical assistance in dying conflicts with the physician's role; the Swiss Academy for Medical Sciences states that assisted suicide is "not a medical act," but nevertheless described circumstances where it finds it to be professionally acceptable for a physician to assist suicide.[11]

Practices

Data from The Netherlands is the most systematically reported, and shows rates of notification increasing from 18% in 1990 to 80% in 2005.[12] In Switzerland, most suicide assistance is performed through right-to-die organizations rather than individual physicians. From 1990 to the mid 2000s, the number of suicide assistance cases has remained stable, with possibly a slight increase in the number of patients suffering from chronic rather than fatal disease.[13]

Serious requests for assisted death are made by only a minority of seriously ill patients. Intractable pain motivates requests infrequently. Psychological, social, or existential suffering, such as loss of community, autonomy, or meaning, seem to motivate euthanasia requests more often.[14] Patients with symptoms of depression have been shown to be four times more likely to request euthanasia than those without such symptoms.[15] Although these results should be taken seriously, they do not signify that all requests for assisted death are associated with depression. Fears that assisted dying would disproportionately affect vulnerable groups have also been voiced, but current data show otherwise.[16]

The link between assisted dying legislation and practices is complex. Up to 3.7% of US physicians reported having – illegally – practiced assisted suicide and up to 9.4% reported having practiced euthanasia.[17] Intensive care unit physicians in France, where euthanasia is illegal, are more likely to report having practiced "deliberate administration of medication to speed death in patients with no chance of recovering a meaningful life" compared with their colleagues from 11 European countries, including The Netherlands.[18] The Dutch Euthanasia Act seems to have been followed by a small decrease in the number of euthanasia and physician-assisted suicide cases.[19] As Belgian doctors have pointed out, more transparent reporting is likely to increase the effectiveness of social control of these practices.[20]

Responding to requests for aid-in-dying

A request for euthanasia or assisted suicide is an emotionally taxing situation, where a thoughtful and respectful response is particularly important. Several elements are crucial. First, some requests are expressions of suffering rather than direct concrete requests for assisted death, but not all of them are. Second, adequate symptom management can significantly decrease the number of such requests. Third, the patient's decision-making capacity is a necessary condition of euthanasia and assisted suicide also where these practices are legal. Fourth, addressing the issue of aid-in-dying explicitly and non judgmentally is preferable to the alternatives. Fifth, even in countries where euthanasia or assisted suicide is legal, there is no entitlement right to obtain it from a physician who disagrees.

Several approaches have been proposed. Two stages in responding to requests for euthanasia or

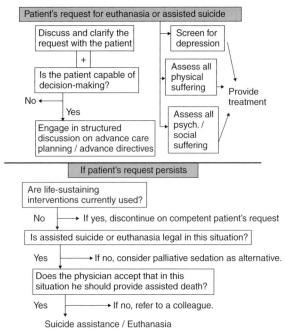

Figure 22.1 Responding to requests for euthanasia or assisted suicide

assisted suicide are outlined in Fig. 22.1. First, these requests should be carefully listened to. Many requests for assisted death are expressions of suffering, and are withdrawn by patients after appropriate symptom management. However, this is not always the case. Although the controversies and emotions surrounding this topic can make these discussions difficult, remaining non-judgmental is important to patient management. The patient's request should be discussed and clarified. If she is truly making a request to die, and is competent to make decisions, a structured discussion about advance care planning should take place, and the possibility of writing advance directives should be offered.

In all circumstances, suffering should be assessed using a holistic "total suffering" palliative care approach. Depression should be screened for and treated if present. Where available, specialized palliative care expertise should be offered. Whenever possible, symptom management should be handled by a team of healthcare providers with complementary expertise. When they are likely to be called upon for specific interventions, such as palliative sedation, anaesthesiologists should be included in discussions

regarding their indication in the patient's specific circumstances. Importantly, palliative sedation does not constitute assisted dying in the sense discussed in this chapter. In some cases, it can be a part of symptom management at this stage.

Many requests will be dropped following these steps. However, some do persist. In such cases, where a competent patient persists in asking to die despite appropriate management of suffering, several situations exist.

One is the situation where a patient is under life-sustaining therapy. Controversies surrounding treatment withdrawal tend to increase as the invasiveness of the intervention decreases: withholding food and water is often more controversial than withholding ventilator support. However, if any life-sustaining intervention is being applied, its refusal by a competent patient is usually considered sufficient grounds to withdraw it.

When no life-sustaining intervention is being used, the next steps will depend on the legal status of euthanasia or assisted suicide, and on the physician's own convictions. Where assisted death is not legal, or in situations that do not fulfill legally described criteria, palliative sedation can again be considered as an alternative at this stage. Indeed, it is sometimes preferred even in areas where assisted death would be legal. Finally, even in situations where euthanasia or assisted suicide would be legally authorised, there is no duty on the part of physicians to perform either intervention. In countries where assisted death is legal, an objecting physician can refer the patient whose request persists to a colleague. Where it is known in advance that a physician would in any case refuse to assist death, this should be made clear to the patient as early as possible. It is of course important to be clear on this point both in countries where assisted death is legal, and in countries where it is not.

Key points

- Palliation with therapeutic intent, including palliative sedation, is not equivalent to assisted death even in cases where the treatment may hasten death.
- Physician assisted suicide and voluntary euthanasia are legal in some jurisdictions.
- Arguments against physician assisted death usually refer to a violation of the physician's

role and/or the potential for coercion of vulnerable patients.

- Arguments for physician-assisted death usually refer to beneficence and patient autonomy.
- Although many patients who request aid-in-dying are depressed, not all requests are associated with depression, nor does the presence of depression necessarily invalidate a request for aid-in-dying.
- Requests for aid-in-dying should be taken seriously and carefully listened to. Screening for and treatment of problematic symptoms and depression may lead to withdrawal of the request.
- When a request for aid-in-dying persists and no life-sustaining treatments are being employed, the response will depend on the legal status of euthanasia or assisted suicide, and on the physician's own convictions.

References

1* Sprung, C.L., S.L. Cohen, P. Sjokvist, M., *et al.* (2003). End-of-life practices in European intensive care units: the Ethicus Study. *JAMA*, **290**(6), 790–7.

2* Sprung, C.L., Maia, P., Bulow, H.H., *et al.* (2007). The importance of religious affiliation and culture on end-of-life decisions in European intensive care units. *Intens Care Med*, **33**, 1732–9.

3 *Schindler v. Schiavo*, 780 So.2d 176 (Fla. 2001).

4 Senate, I. (2009). "Bill no. 1369." Retrieved 5 May, 2009, from http://www.senato.it/service/PDF/PDFServer/BGT/00393277.pdf.

5* Dworkin, G. (2007). Physician-assisted death: the state of the debate. In *The Oxford Handbook of Bioethics*. B. Steinbock, (ed). Oxford and New York: Oxford University Press, pp. 376–92.

6 Emanual, E.J. (2009). Euthanasia and physician-assisted suicide. UpTo Date online. Accessed June 3, 2010.

7* Mauron, A. (2006). La médecine moderne et l'assistance au suicide en Suisse. Synthèse du point de vue de la CNE. *Beihilfe zum Suizid in der Schweiz, Beiträge aus Ethik, Recht, und Medizin*. C. Rehmann-Sutter, A. Bondolfi, J. Fischer, and M. Leuthold (eds.). Nerm: Peter Lang.

8* Hall, M., Trachtenberg, F., and Dugan, E. (2005). The impact on patient trust of legalising physician aid-in-dying. *J Med Ethics*, **31**(12), 693–7.

9 Wolfe, J., Fairclough, D.L., Clarridge, B.R., *et al.* (1999). Stability of attitudes regarding physician-assisted suicide and euthanasia among oncology patients, physicians, and the general public. *J Clin Oncol*, **17**(4), 1274.

10* Cohen, J., Marcoux, I., Bilsen, J., *et al.* (2006). European public acceptance of euthanasia: socio-demographic and cultural factors associated with the acceptance of euthanasia in 33 European countries. *Soc Sci Med*, **63**(3), 743–56.

11 Académie Suisse des Sciences Médicales. (2004). Directives médico-éthiques pour la prise en charge des patientes et patients en fin de vie.

12 Rurup, M.L., Buiting, H.M., Pasman, H.R., *et al.* (2008). The reporting rate of euthanasia and physician-assisted suicide: a study of the trends. *Med Care*, **46**(12), 1198–202.

13 Fischer, S., Huber, C.A., Imhof, L., *et al.* (2008). Suicide assisted by two Swiss right-to-die organisations. *J Med Ethics*, **34**(11), 810–14.

14* Georges, J.J., Onwuteaka-Philipsen, B.D., van der Heide, A., *et al.* (2006). Requests to forgo potentially life-prolonging treatment and to hasten death in terminally ill cancer patients: a prospective study. *J Pain Symptom Manage*, **31**(2), 100–10.

15 van der Lee, M.L., van der Bom, J.G., Swarte, N.B., *et al.* (2005). Euthanasia and depression: a prospective cohort study among terminally ill cancer patients. *J Clin Oncol*, **23**(27), 6607–12.

16* Battin, M.P., van der Heide, A., Ganzini, L., *et al.* (2007). Legal physician-assisted dying in Oregon and the Netherlands: evidence concerning the impact on patients in "vulnerable" groups. *J Med Ethics*, **33**(10), 591–7.

17 Emanuel, E.J. (2002). Euthanasia and physician-assisted suicide: a review of the empirical data from the United States. *Arch Intern Med*, **162**(2), 142.

18 Vincent, J.L. (1999). Forgoing life support in western European intensive care units: the results of an ethical questionnaire. *Crit Care Med*, **27**(8), 1626–33.

19 van der Heide, A., Onwuteaka-Philipsen, B.D., Rurup, M.L., *et al.* (2007). End-of-life practices in the Netherlands under the Euthanasia Act. *N Engl J Med*, **356**(19), 1957–65.

20 Smets, T., Bilsen, J., Cohen, J., *et al.* (2009). The medical practice of euthanasia in Belgium and The Netherlands: legal notification, control and evaluation procedures. *Health Policy*, **90**(2–3), 181–7.

Further reading

Ariès, P. (1974). *Western Attitudes Toward Death: From the Middle Ages to the Present*. Baltimore and London: The Johns Hopkins University Press.

Breitbart, W. (2010). Physician-assisted suicide ruling in Montana: struggling with care of the dying, responsibility, and freedom in big sky country. *Palliat Support Care*, **18**, 1–6.

Emanuel, L. L. (1998). Facing requests for physician-assisted suicide: toward a practical and principled clinical skill set. *JAMA*, **280**(7), 643–7.

Hurst, S. A. and Mauron, A. (2006). The ethics of palliative care and euthanasia: exploring common values. *Palliat Med*, **20**(2), 107–12.

O' Neill, B. and Fallon, M. (1997). ABC of palliative care. Principles of palliative care and pain control. *BMJ*, **315**(7111), 801–4.

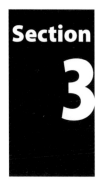

Section 3

Pain management

Ethical considerations in interventional pain management

Andrea Trescot

The Case

Mr. Summers presents to the pain clinic with a several-year history of chronic low back and posterior right leg pain. He describes his pain as 9/10, increased with activity. MRI shows a bulging disc on the right at L45. He has been told that he is not a surgical candidate. He is currently taking six oxycodone tablets per day, noting only temporary relief. He requests larger doses of opioids, but his primary care physician (PCP) has referred him to the clinic with only enough medicines to last until this appointment. The PCP has also indicated that any further pain management, including opioid prescriptions, will have to come from the clinic.

Mr. Summers is agitated and hostile, displaying exaggerated pain behaviors. He has difficulty sitting still during the interview, getting up several times to walk around. Physical examination is difficult to perform because he complains of tenderness with every area palpated, but there appears to be increased right paravertebral tone at the level of the top of the iliac crest. There is pain with extension of the right leg at approximately 70 degrees. Reflexes, strength, and sensory findings are normal other than "break away" weakness. EMG in the past was not completed because he could not tolerate the needle portion of the examination. Careful review of the MRI films shows a high intensity zone on the right at L45, and a mild central bulge at that level.

Evaluation of Mr. Summers suggests a lumbar radiculopathy from a leaking disk or referred pain from internal disc disruption. However, there is also concern that he is a drug-seeker. Management options include injection therapy (lumbar epidural, transforaminal epidural, discogram and possible intradiscal therapy) or more opioids (with or without adjuvant medications). He refuses injections, stating that a friend had injections, and "they didn't help." Furthermore, he states "the pills make the pain go away."

Mr. Summers' insurance will not cover discogram or intradiscal therapies, and requires preauthorization for even office injections. Insurance also covers only short-acting opioids or generic morphine ER, and Mr. Summers states that he has an "allergy" to morphine, which caused nausea. Should the pain specialist give Mr. Summers more opioids, discharge him, or insist on a trial of injections?

> … the profession (of pain medicine) must be informed by scientific knowledge that is contemporary and progressive, but it must also be sensitive to the subjectivity of suffering, … to apply knowledge and skill … that ideally meets each patient's individual medical needs…this is the basis of medicine as tekne … that combines … skill and … art and which is integrative … in the ideal[1]

In 1847, the code of ethics published by the American Medical Association stated "…from the age of Hippocrates to the present time, the annals of every civilized people contain abundant evidences of the devotedness of medical men to the relief of their fellow-creatures from pain and disease …"[2] Despite the intrusion of insurance forms and changing reimbursements, medicine in general and pain medicine specifically continues to be a humanitarian pursuit with goals of relieving suffering and restoring function. Patients rely on physicians to be ethically responsible when recommending care or providing treatment. Pain patients are particularly vulnerable to exploitation, because of a desperation related to unrelieved pain, and the perception that a pill or an injection or a surgery will "fix" the problem. Therefore, each decision in pain medicine needs to be viewed from both a therapeutic and ethical perspective. Pain physicians must define the nature of pain, recognize the variability and subjectivity of its expression in the pain patient, acknowledge the vulnerabilities rendered by pain, describe the inherent characteristics and asymmetry

Clinical Ethics in Anesthesiology: A Case-Based Textbook, ed. Gail A. Van Norman, Stephen Jackson, Stanley H. Rosenbaum and Susan K. Palmer. Published by Cambridge University Press. © Cambridge University Press 2011.

of the patient-clinician relationship, and define the desired pain care end-point.[3]

With multidisciplinary or hospital-based pain clinics, a professional ethicist may be readily available to answer questions, offer advice, or arbitrate difficult decisions, such as whether the physician can ethically demand that a patient be subjected to interventional procedures in order to obtain opioid prescriptions. However, with the proliferation of independent pain physicians and clinics, the availability of multidisciplinary advice, include advice regarding ethics, is diminished. It then becomes incumbent upon the pain provider to resolve the ethical questions that are an inherent part of the care of pain patients.

According to James Giordano, ethicist for the American Society of Interventional Pain Physicians (ASIPP), the ethical crisis in pain care necessitates a three step process: identification of the problems, critical evaluation of various ethical systems, and "a description of how the structure and function of the practice –as a social good – might be enacted within a paradigm of (somewhat) non-hegemonious, integrative pain care."[4] Books such as this one attempt to provide the practical wisdom that is critical to understanding the ethical process. "Because if therapeutic and moral agency are conjoined in the sound practice of pain medicine, then the ethical character of each pain physician becomes instrumental in contributing to and maintaining the overall moral integrity of the profession."[5]

Ethical principles of beneficence and nonmaleficence

An obvious precept of medical care is appropriate diagnosis of problems so that the most effective, and hopefully least harmful, treatment can be offered. One of the greatest limitations of pain management is therefore a lack of objective diagnostic tests. Internal medicine has blood sugar values and blood pressure readings, cardiology has ST depression, and dermatology has pathology results. In pain management, diagnostic testing is of limited utility, because positive findings only indicate the presence of *potential* causes. No test measures pain itself, which is the subjective experience that the patient reports. In the distant past, for example, a myelogram was the standard test to evaluate back pain. Virtually anyone undergoing a myelogram had reported having back pain, and when the test revealed an abnormality, it was assumed to be the cause of the pain, and not merely an incidental finding. MRI studies in asymptomatic patients, however, have now shown "surgically significant"

radiologic findings in as many as 60% of asymptomatic patients.[5] Even more concerning is that up to 40% of completely asymptomatic patients with positive MRIs are offered surgery, one harmful effect of poorly directed MRI over-testing. False positives are not just found in radiologic studies; 15% of asymptomatic patients will have nerve conduction studies that are compatible with the presence of carpal tunnel syndrome.[6] Radiologic and neurodiagnostic studies do not directly demonstrate "pain," so how can the clinician tell if a patient is even really experiencing pain, or is falsely reporting pain for other motives – for example, to obtain narcotics?

The evaluation of pain involves a combination of clues in the history ("pattern recognition"), and a targeted physical exam. It may also require the use of diagnostic injections or other interventional procedures. "The cause of a disorder is hidden in the patient's history and the site of the lesion is detected by physical exam."[7] In this model, diagnostic injections become integral to the evaluation process, much like an Xray to an orthopedic surgeon.

Ethical concerns regarding interventional diagnostic and therapeutic procedures include physician concerns for nonmaleficence, as well as conflicts of interest presented by third-party payers. By their nature, interventional procedures carry risks, both that there can be complications from the procedure and that the results will lead the physician to the wrong diagnostic conclusions and therefore an inappropriate therapeutic path. The subjective nature of pain reporting further complicates evaluation of procedural results. Complications may be mitigated by performing procedures in the safest environment possible, with the most up-to-date equipment, and by an experienced, highly-trained pain specialist. However, multiple factors not under the direct control of the physician or patient, such as third-party reimbursements, may have influence on such important safety factors as where and by whom pain procedures are performed.

Pain procedures can be provided in a variety of physical locations – the office, the hospital outpatient department, or a freestanding ambulatory surgery center. Although "minimally invasive," many of the procedural injections are "maximally dangerous" with the risk of seizures, hypotension, and cardiac arrest. Specialized equipment, such as fluoroscopy and resuscitation equipment, which might mitigate this risk can be quite expensive. In addition, procedures done in the office incur a cost of supplies that, until recently, was not reimbursed. The same procedure done in the hospital or ambulatory surgery center (ASC), in contrast, may be much more expensive for the patient and the insurer. Some insurance programs, including Medicare, in an effort to move procedures out of the more expensive settings, have started to reimburse a "site of service differential" to help cover of the physician cost of providing these services in an office.

Ethical conflicts can arise when deciding where to schedule procedures, particularly if the pain physician involved has a financial interest in an ASC where he or she performs procedures – a situation which is increasingly common. Should the provider perform the procedure in the office (where the cost is low to the patient but the risks of inadequate facilities may be high) or at the ASC (where there would be equipment and personnel to handle emergency issues, but at a higher cost to the patient, and a potential financial conflict of interest for the physician)? Is the procedure being done in the best interest of the patient, or primarily for the financial gain of the provider? The current system of reimbursement in the Unites States, for example, favors serial, potentially ineffective or less effective injections (which keeps the patient coming back) rather than potentially more expensive, but curative treatment.

Insurance companies, in an effort to curb the escalating costs of health care, have at times simply denied a variety of "high tech" procedures because of their cost as a "supply side prudence." But what happens once such technical tools are deemed reasonable and effective? If accessibility to new, more expensive treatments remains restricted, development of new treatments will be of little value.[8] Furthermore, assessment of the clinical effectiveness of the treatment should be as much if not more important than the cost when determining reimbursements and promoting effective pain practice. As new treatments are developed, when the efficacy of interventional procedures is unproven, insurance companies have sometimes cloaked denial of coverage not as "noncovered" service, but rather as "experimental treatment." "Non-covered" is subject to appeal; "experimental" has less recourse. Payers then do not have to claim that the therapy is inappropriate, but merely that it is investigational because its efficacy is unproven.

Assessing efficacy of pain treatment can be difficult. Although there are journals filled with pain studies, studies of pain treatments have been remarkably difficult to do. Unlike blood pressure or HgbA1C, there are

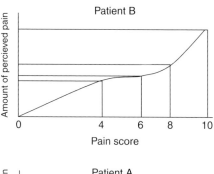

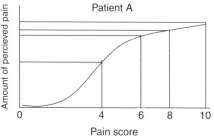

no objective tests for pain, which is by definition a subjective experience. Pain scores, often on a scale of 0 to 10, are useful compare the improvement or lack thereof after an interventional procedure. Although many studies add, subtract and average pain scores, this does not necessarily express the patients' pain experiences, since these numbers do not reflect discrete integers. Pain scores are not strictly linear, and can differ dramatically from patient to patient (Fig. 23.1).

Evidence-based medicine (EBM) is a concept designed to assist the clinician in the decision making process, and can be helpful in determining in general what clinical course to recommend. Studies can be enormously helpful in aiding medical decisions involving choices among competing alternative treatments. Clinical research, especially over the last few decades, as well as a spectacular increase in technological advances, has lead to a huge volume of relevant data and an increase in the complexity of trade-offs among various pain treatments. However, denying a treatment to an *individual* complex pain patient because it has not been shown to be the most effective for a *population* of patients may not be the best approach to an affliction that is highly individual in nature. In the words of Michael Gorback, "We seem to have lost the thread of EBM, which is to use the best evidence available, not deny anything without a positive RCT."[9]

Patient vulnerability

The pain patient is extremely vulnerable in the doctor–patient relationship. He or she is utterly reliant on the provider for continuing treatment of pain. If the patient requires opioid treatment, he or she has few other legal means by which to obtain it. Coercion by the physician is an ever-present possibility. In our case example, the physician may be tempted to threaten to withhold opioid prescriptions if the patient does not agree to undergo interventional pain procedures. Even if the physician does not *intend* to coerce the patient, the patient may nevertheless believe he or she had limited autonomy in deciding what therapeutic options to pursue, and which ones they may refuse.

Not only is the positive outcome of the procedure reliant on the skills and wisdom of the physician, but the negative outcome is as well. The physician has ethical obligations to be extremely vigilant, to confirm that the procedure is within the skill set of the provider, that the technique is the appropriate for this patient at this time, and that the diagnosis and proposed outcomes are as clearly defined as possible.

Professional treatment guidelines – do they help or harm?

Commonly prescribed medical treatments, such as exogenous estrogen to prevent heart disease in postmenopausal women and the efficacy of knee arthroscopies, have, in rigorous testing, not shown to be effective. Professional groups often review relevant clinical studies and physician experience in order to provide general advice about useful and non-useful treatments. It is widely held that adherence to guidelines should improve outcomes overall. However, guidelines do not encourage clinicians to consider and treat each patient as an individual, and do not necessarily stimulate original research. Guidelines are created by a laborious and artificial process, and at times may even be obsolete by the time they are published. They are often published with industry support, and can have a major impact on sales of industry products.[10] Therefore, although well-constructed guidelines generally have positive effects on general patient outcomes, they nevertheless must be interpreted with their shortcomings and conflicts of interest in mind, and in the context of each individual patient's situation.

Prescribing opioids: legal and ethical concerns

The prescribing of opioids is fraught with dangers for physician and patient alike. For patients, the risk of inappropriate use of opioids includes the risks of adverse side effects, ineffective (or less than optimally effective) pain management, problems of opioid tolerance, and in some cases even opioid addiction.

Legal implications in opioid prescribing

Pain management providers must deal with competing problems in pain management: under treatment of pain and opioid abuse. The consequences of over-prescribing as well as under-prescribing opioids can have profound legal implications. Providers who under-prescribe can be accused of abuse, while those who over-prescribe may be subject to charges of drug trafficking.

A number of systems guide and sustain the practice of caring for those who are in pain.[11] The Drug Administration Agency (DEA) has strict penalties for providers prescribing without "a legitimate medical process," who are therefore in violation of the law, and subject to civil and/or criminal penalties.[12] Responsible health-care professionals must expect that they will be held accountable for their actions. Gone are the days when public trust was so complete that healthcare professionals were subject only to a limited sphere of oversight, accompanied by informal and very private sanctions when things had not gone well.[13] In *US vs. Shaygan*,[14] a Mayo Clinic trained internist was charged with 20 counts of prescribing without a legitimate medical purpose. He faced 20 years in prison for writing opioids for pain patients without aggressive treatment or monitoring. In Oregon and California, there have been two cases of physicians sued for under-treating patients. The California case resulted in an initial $1.5 million verdict against the physician (which was subsequently reduced). Another legacy of cases such as this are increasing state regulations of medical practice, such as a new California Law (AB 487) that requires every doctor in California to obtain 12 hours of CME credit in pain management and end-of-life care.[15]

In the US, the Federation of State Medical Boards policies[16] include the following.

- Pain management is important and integral to the practice of medicine.
- Use of opioids may be necessary for pain relief.
- Use of opioids for something other than a legitimate medical purpose poses a threat to the individual and society.
- Physicians have a responsibility to minimize the potential for abuse and diversion.

- A complete patient evaluation should be performed.
- A written treatment plan should be given to the patient.
- Informed patient consent and agreement for treatment should be obtained.
- Periodic review of the course of treatment should take place.
- Physicians should show willingness to refer.
- Physicians should maintain complete and current medical records.
- Physicians may deviate from the recommended treatment steps if there is good cause.

Clinical suggestions

The ethical issues of coercion ("I won't write for pain medications unless you get an injection"), financial gain (injection treatment are much higher reimbursed compared to evaluation and management), opioidophobia (physician concern regarding opioid prescribing), as well as lack of education ("If a patient goes through withdrawal, that means the patient is addicted"), has led to a state of fear as well as greed among some physicians. The patient is caught in the middle, between inappropriate opioid use (both over-prescribing, which leads to iatrogenic addiction, and under-prescribing due to refusal to prescribe) and inappropriate injection therapy (which exposes the patient to multiple expensive but often ineffective treatments, with the concomitant risks of steroid side effects, nerve injuries, potentially increased pain, and possible death). A careful review of the agenda of both the patient and physician should help to clarify the issues of self-interest versus appropriate care.

An approach to the clinical problem

(1) Obtain an appropriate history of prior response to pain interventions.

Getting an accurate history of the initial response to prior injection therapy is critical to interpretating a subsequent negative response. For example, if there was no temporary response the another injection, it may indicate that the local anesthetic wasn't in the right place (failure of accurate diagnosis or failure of accurate placement), or that the patient doesn't respond to that local anesthetic, rather than that injection therapy has failed. A cohort of 1198 consecutive pain patients undergoing interventional procedures were interviewed regarding previous failure of temporary relief from injections or, if no prior injections, a history of difficulty getting numb at the dentist.[17] Of 250 patients with this history were skin tested with lidocaine, bupivicaine, and mepivicaine, 36% (7.5% of the total number of patients) were noted to only be numb to mepivicaine, while another 17% (3.8% of the total) were numb only to lidocaine. Many, if not most, pain procedures are done with bupivicaine, which did not work on 10% of the total population and almost 50% of the patients with a prior failed procedure. In those patients in whom bupivicaine did not work, repeating the same procedure with the appropriate local anesthetic resulted in sustained relief in more than 60% of the patients.

(2) Perform a meticulous physical examination.

A meticulous physical exam, with attention to the most common pain generators, coupled with a recognition of common patterns of pain will help guide to the diagnosis, and from that the appropriate treatment. For example, pain radiating into the groin and the testicles (less commonly described into the vaginal region in women), coupled with the description from the male patient that his testicles "are in a vise" should lead to a directed physical exam of either the ilioinguinal nerve or the iliolumbar ligament.

(3) Use diagnostic procedures appropriately.

Based on the tenderness found on exam, a directed injection (with a peripheral nerve stimulator for the ilioinguinal nerve, or under fluoroscopy for the iliolumbar ligament), using the local anesthetic that works most effectively for this patient and a small dose of depost eroid if appropriate, may establish an accurate diagnosis. Based on the response of those injections, further therapy (cryoneuroablation for the ilioinguinal nerve, radiofrequency lesioning or regenerative injection therapy for the iliolumbar ligament) provides a rational, stepwise approach to the diagnosis and treatment of the presenting pain problem.

Case resolution

The provider discussed with Mr. Summers the inadvisability of long-term opioid therapy in the face of treatable disease, using an analogy of appendicitis ("It would be inappropriate to just give opioids to a patient with appendicitis, though you would be willing to support the patient while you wait for his medical condition to improve or the OR staff to arrive, and you would give opioids postoperatively as the surgical site heals"). After a discussion of the proposed etiology of the pain, and the need for an accurate diagnosis ("you can't treat what you can't diagnose"), and skin testing to identify the most appropriate local anesthetic, the patient agreed to undergo a diagnostic and potentially therapeutic transforaminal epidural. Because of the apparent neuropathic nature of the pain, an anticonvulsant was added to the short acting opioid. Although the desired effect would be improved pain relief and therefore decreased opioid use, the patient and physician also agreed to consider a long-acting opioid such as methadone as an alternative if there was not sustained improvement in the patient's pain with the above interventions. After a detailed informed consent regarding the risks and potential complications of opioid use, and a screening urine drug test, patient was given a prescription for 1 month of opioids and an appointment for the diagnostic injection.

Key points

- A primary goal of medical care is the relief of suffering and restoration of function.
- Pain is a subjective patient experience, and one of the greatest limitations of pain management is a lack of objective diagnostic tests that identify and quantify pain.
- The use of interventional procedures to diagnose and treat pain involves ethical concerns of beneficence and nonmaleficence as well as potential financial conflicts of interest for the physician.
- Third party payers exert additional influence on reimbursements, and the locations where pain procedures can be performed. This in turn can have affects on patient safety, as well as access to new procedures that might be deemed "investigational."
- In pain management, patient vulnerability is a prominent feature of the doctor-patient relationship. Coercion, intentional or otherwise, is an ever-present possibility.
- Opioid prescribing is guided by both legal regulations and professional guidelines. In the US, the Federation of State Medical Boards has express policies on pain management and the obligations of physicians involved in opioid prescribing.

References

1* Giordano, J. and Jonas, W.J. (2007). Asclepius and Hygieia in dialectic: philosophical, ethical and pragmatic bases of an integrative medicine. *Integrative Med Insights*, **2**, 89–101.

2* American Medical Association. (1847) *Code of Medical Ethics of the American Medical Association*. Chicago: American Medical Association Press.

3 Giordano, J. and Schatman, M.E. (2008). An ethical analysis of crisis in chronic pain care: facts, issues, and problems in pain medicine; Part 2. *Pain Physician*, **11**, 589–595.

4* Giordano, J. (2008). Ethics of, and in, pain medicine: constructs, content, and contexts of application. *Pain Physician*, **11**, 391–392

5 Jensen, M.C., Brant-Zawadzki, M.N., Obuchowski, N., *et al.* (1994). Magnetic resonance imaging in the lumbar spine in people without back pain. *NEJM*, **331**, 69–73.

6 Artoshi, I., Gummesson, C., Johnsson, R., *et al.* (1999). Prevalence of carpal tunnel yndrome in a general population. *JAMA*, **282**(2), 152–8.

7 A. Staal, Department of Neurology, Leyden University, Holland.

8 Giordano, J. and Schatman, M.E. (2008). An ethical analysis of crisis in chronic pain care: facts, issues, and problems in pain medicine; Part 3. *Pain Physician*, **11**, 775–84.

9 Michael Gorback, MD, Center for Pain Relief, Houston, TX.

10 Amerlinga, R., Winchester, J.F., and Ronco, C. (2008). Guidelines have done more harm than good. *Blood Purif*, **26**, 73–6.

11 Giordano, J. (2008). Ethic of, and in, pain medicine: constructs, content, and contexts of application. *Pain Physician*, **11**, 391–2.

12 Branding, F.H. (1995). The impact of controlled substance federal aspects of managing regulations on the practice of pharmacy. *J Pharm Pract*, **8**, 130–7.

13 Brushwood, D.B. (2001). From confrontation to collaboration: collegial collaboration and the expanding role of pharmacists in the management of chronic pain. *J Law Med Ethics*, **29**, 69–83.

14 United States v. Shaygan, Case No. 08–20112-CR, 2009.

15 Wilner, A. (2008) Medical-legal aspects of managing chronic pain. AAPM 19th annual meeting. Nashville, TN.

16 Federation of State Medical Boards. www.fsmb.org.

17 Trescot, A. (2003). Local anesthetic "resistance." *Pain Physician*, **6**, 291–3.

Conjoining interventional pain management and palliative care: considerations for practice, ethics and policy

James Giordano and Gerhard Höver

The Case[a]

A 61-year-old woman with metastatic colon cancer presents with intractable abdominal pain. Since her initial diagnosis 13 years ago, she has undergone chemotherapy, multiple colon surgeries, radiofrequency ablation of liver metastases, and excision of a solitary pulmonary metastasis. A CT scan shows enlarging liver metastases involving the capsule and para-aortic lymph nodes.

The patient has been relatively pain-free until 7 months prior to consultation with a local anesthesiologist who specializes in interventional pain managmeent. Prior to consultation, initial treatment of pain consisted of oxycodone and acetaminophen, followed by sustained-release morphine titrated over several months to a total of 1200 mg daily. Sustained release morphine was then supplemented with immediate-release morphine (600 mg) up to four times daily for breakthrough pain. Most recently, she was switched to fentanyl patches plus continued oral morphine. At the time of consultation she was using thirty 100 mcg/h patches every 3 days.

Despite somnolence, she continues to complain of severe constant sharp, aching and "knife-like: upper and lower abdominal pain, with self-rated pain intensity between 7 and 10 on a 0 to 10 scale, with minimal movement bringing pain intensity up to 10.

The anesthesiologist performs a neurolytic celiac plexus block, which decreases her baseline pain from a 7 rating to a 4. A 4 mg intrathecal test dose of morphine reduces her pain rating further to 1–2, with no adverse effects. The anesthesiologist would like to refer her to a multidisciplinary pain clinic for possible implantation of a morphine spinal delivery system, but the patient's insurance company has thus far refused to approve the consultation or implantation, because studies suggest that these devices are cost-effective over continued systemic analgesic management only after 18–30 months of therapy. They point out that she has had significant improvement in her pain after neurolytic block, and is unlikely to survive long enough to make intraspinal therapy cost-effective, even if it provides better quality of pain relief.

A moral obligation to treat pain

Technological advancements within science and medicine have enabled prolongation of the lifespan for those patients with incurable diseases. Yet, at the same time, such relative successes have fostered an increased prevalence of chronic illness and subjective suffering – including intractable pain – due in part to the inability to completely eradicate symptoms, and to the progressive use and sometimes exhaustion of therapeutic and economic resources available to the patient. This has compelled an increased impetus for medicine to develop those dimensions of practice that seek to heal what cannot be cured. To a significant extent, pain medicine and palliative care have arisen from, and seek to meet, this need.

The obligation to treat pain and suffering, while inherent to all of medicine, is by definition most fundamental to the profession of pain medicine and palliative care.[1] Clearly, pain management can be, and often is necessary, albeit not sufficient for rendering sound, palliative care. But technically effective pain care must also be rendered in ways that uphold the moral affirmations of medicine, and while certain ethical (and legal) frameworks exist to guide the tenor, scope and limits of the profession, the actual implementation of care is reliant upon the physician. In this way, the physician is both a therapeutic and moral agent, given that any (if not all) clinical decisions affect the vulnerability of the patient, reflect the asymmetries of knowledge and power between physician and patient, and impact trust within the medical relationship.

The complexity of pain and pain care is such that a simple, "one-size fits all" approach to management is not practical, nor ethically justifiable. An integrative use of interventional, pharmacologic, physiatric, and psychiatric pain management may represent a

Clinical Ethics in Anesthesiology: A Case-Based Textbook, ed. Gail A. Van Norman, Stephen Jackson, Stanley H. Rosenbaum and Susan K. Palmer. Published by Cambridge University Press. © Cambridge University Press 2011.

viable option, both early in and throughout the care of long-term and terminal pain patients. In this context, interventional techniques may be especially useful because of their capacity to effectively reduce pain, make patients more amenable to other therapeutics, and enhance patients' quality of life.

Interventional pain medicine in integrative pain care: practical and ethical claims

If the past 10 years' congressionally declared "decade of pain control and research" in the US has done nothing else, it has certainly instigated: (1) a more internationalized interest in the problem of pain and the difficulties and responsibilities of pain care; and (2) a more well-defined need – and thus goal – for biomedical research to facilitate improved translational applications and models.[2] Despite such progress, interventional management techniques still tend to be under-utilized within palliative care – particularly that which is provided in a paradigm of long-term (i.e., not end-of-life) treatment.

A number of long-held beliefs may contribute to under-utilization. Integrative pain medicine and palliative care may appear to be expensive or not cost-effective from the perspective of hospital operators and insurance companies. The problem chiefly lies in an inability to calculate the cost of pain- and palliative care given the relative uncertainties of matching objective medical treatments to subjectively defined states (i.e., pain and suffering) and ends (e.g., palliation). Long-term pain care can be viewed as cost intensive by insurance providers and hospital operators, with perceived high expenses evoked by the requirements for both medical staff and equipment/facility resource utilization. From a perspective of hospital economics, *prima facie* it might not seem to be "worthwhile" to care for chronic pain patients, given costs incurred relative to payment schedules established according to existing diagnosis-related group (DRG) treatment classification systems. The development and expansion of inpatient and/or outpatient pain- and palliative-care networks are not generally facilitated by current DRG systems. This is because DRGs are not designed to reflect: (1) the wide pathological variance of chronic pain patients; and (2) the finances required to support services necessary to effectively and ethically treat chronic pain conditions.[3] Thus, if the goal of providing high-quality pain medicine and palliative care is to be achieved in light of (1) the noted achievements of technology in medicine and (2) the explicit call to use such advancements to address the increasing incidence and prevalence of chronic pain, then special provisions for adequate funding of both inpatient and outpatient approaches must be developed and implemented.

However, to safely, effectively, and ethically deal with the often complex pathologies of chronic pain patients, it is necessary to maintain multi-disciplinary and integrative treatment provided by professions focal to pain- and palliative care (e.g. specialized physicians, social workers, physiotherapists, psychologists, clergy and secular spiritual counsellors, *et al.*). In this way, treatment would constitute a service of ongoing assessment and interventions that are rendered by a multi-professional, closely-knit team on a regular basis, as appropriate to both the changing status and needs of each specific patient.

It is difficult to categorize chronic pain patients in a homogeneous cost group within current DRG systems, and so an inter-disciplinary pain/palliative care could be seen as impossible to finance because of its requisite utilization of diverse resources. The lack of a more encompassing integrative pain/palliative care paradigm reflects the inchoate nature of the profession of "pain medicine." This has given rise to misconceptions that interventional pain management is a "stand-alone" approach, and led to the opinion that its ongoing, collaborative use with other disciplines (e.g., primary care, physiatry, and psychiatry/psychology) would incur unnecessarily high costs that would be difficult to advocate.

But is this latter opinion correct? Previous studies have shown that the employment of collaborative interventional techniques within an inter-disciplinary pain/palliative care paradigm can be both cost- and time-effective.[4] For example, when compared with long-term use of systemically administered primary and adjunctive/adjuvant analgesics, interventional techniques reveal a very favorable cost: benefit ratio. In the case of the aforementioned patient, the large doses of opioid required to achieve even dissatisfactory pain control were estimated to cost approximately $10 000 per month, while the estimated total combined cost of intrathecal pump placement, intrathecal and oral morphine and the neurolytic block was approximately $5000 per month over the first 3 months.[5] Thus, as this case illustrates, even in those cases in which analgesia is less than complete, but meaningful pain relief is nonetheless achieved, the cost and time savings incurred by reducing the amount of systemic drugs used, and the time needed to obtain stable effects might well balance and justify the initial expenses of interventional procedures. Clearly, however, the use of nerve blocks *and* (rather than "*or*") pharmacological, physical medicine and psychiatric/psychological approaches within a methodologically conjoined treatment protocol affords considerable complementary attributes.

For interventional pain medicine to be truly effective within such a collaborative, integrative system, the interventional pain specialist must realize that the use of techniques and technologies – despite being a significant component of practice – does not in any way lessen the pain physician's practical and moral role and obligations *qua* physician. Interventional pain specialists must assume at least some level of responsibility for the ongoing management of the patients in their charge. The sole provision of interventional techniques without accepting and meeting the broader medical needs of the pain patient, either singularly, or in collaboration with other physicians, might be regarded as a form of abandonment, and in this way rebuts the physician's act of profession. Pharmacologic and psychological management of chronic pain – and the intricacies of dealing with the chronic pain patient in an often litigious environment – can be difficult, but such is the nature of the profession and practice.

Ethically sound practice requires that the physician: (1) use the most current information on pain and pain-related pathologies (e.g., substance abuse, psychopathology); and (2) recognize and understand the medically relevant bio-psychosocial needs a particular patient may have, and how these needs may be served through an integrative, pluralist approach that conjoins other specialties (e.g., psychiatry, etc.).

It is important to remember that from the medical perspective, the "pain patient" is defined by signs and symptoms (i.e., pain and its resultant bio-psychosocial suffering). Assessing and diagnosing pain is often difficult, and establishing precise trajectories and limits of care can be equally troublesome – practically, ethically, and legally. Although interventional pain medicine and palliative care seem to have somewhat different clinical structures, both are focal to apprehending the subjectivity of pain and suffering, and merging patients' subjective experience of pain – and clinicians' personal and professional knowledge and perspectives – to the objectivity of pain assessment and treatment. As

well, both disciplines encounter and must deal with the clinical, economic, moral, and legal problems that are related to medical decisions regarding the nature, scope and extent of such care. Therefore, interventional pain medicine and palliative care could benefit from a shared orientation and inter-disciplinarity, and can be seen as mutual and reciprocal, constituting a larger professional domain that is centered upon the treatment of pain – not merely as an object, but as an existential predicament of the patient who is the moral subject of clinical responsibility.

On the need for policy: bringing stakeholders together

Clinical moral responsibility dictates that when cure is no longer possible, healing care must be maximized. In this way, the collaboration and conjoining of interventional pain management and palliative care may well serve the scope, purposes and obligations of pain treatment. However, facilities committed to this type of inter-disciplinary approach are limited and diminishing, and therefore assembling these resources becomes problematic and non-sustainable. Multi-practitioner pain management practices can be found in most urban areas in the US and throughout western Europe, yet in the US the number of multi-disciplinary pain centers (MPCs) is declining as a result of prior economic concerns, constraints, and misuses. This both reflects the economic turn away from complementarity in pain care, and contributes to it.

This decline has become a quantitative and qualitative barrier to the effective practice of integrative pain/palliative care, and is an intimidating prospect that compels the proposal and ratification of reformed guidelines and policies, both in the US, and on a more global scale. Recent calls for insurance companies, as well as government agencies to establish programs of long-term pain care reflect these concerns and promptings. The primacy of patients' best interests cannot, nor should not be denied, nor subordinated to other, extraneous goals. But medicine does not exist in a socio-economic vacuum, and if these therapeutic and ethical "goods" are to be appropriately rendered to those in pain, the systems utilized toward these ends must be practically enacted, and we must recognize how the relative interests of practitioners, the healthcare and insurance community, and the public at-large affect any realistic dynamic of costs and benefits in the provision of care. In this way, it is important to consider the needs and values of each of these stakeholder groups, not in isolation, but in concert. A strategy of rapprochement is necessary to reconcile the tensions that exist among and between these groups in the best interests of the patient, so as to develop policies that incorporate "… an ethical 'infrastructure and function' that engages ethical systems and approaches in ways that support and sustain the good to be provided on individual and public levels".[6] Physicians should advocate policy development that is directed toward enabling the profession and practice of pain/palliative care to empower the pain patient.

It is important to see the patient not only as a victim of her disorder, despite the reality that medical treatment is, in the first place, based upon the presence of identifiable and categorical symptoms and distress. It is also important to see that the pain patient has fears and hopes. Reflection upon her existential problems is not only a personal challenge for the patient, as well as her family, friends, and others, but can also pose professional challenges and opportunities to the clinician.

Unavoidably, life entails some measure of pain and suffering. This should not foster a sense of existential nihilism. To the contrary, it serves as a motivation to move away from any passive consideration or experience of pain and suffering, and assume a more active, anticipatory and therefore authentic approach to care. In this sense, "care" may be translated from its Latin origin, *cura*, as "concern" or "regard," and this is philosophically consistent with the goals, ends, and "promise" of pain/palliative medicine.[7]

It has been said that philosophy teaches humanity how to suffer. In light of this, the authors propose that a philosophical, and practical conjoinment of pain/palliative care affords purchase to learn not only how we suffer (i.e.- a focus upon pain and its meanings), but how we can – and should – concern, regard, and treat those in pain.

Key points

- As prolonged survival of previously terminal medical conditions has increased, so has the prevalence of chronic and/or intractable pain and suffering.
- A "one-size-fits-all" approach to pain management is not practical, nor ethically justifiable.

- Interventional pain management techniques and integrative pain medicine are under-utilized, due to misperceptions by hospital operators and insurance companies about cost effectiveness.
- Employment of collaborative interventional techniques, however, has been shown to be both cost and time effective.
- Even in cases of incomplete pain relief, *meaningful* pain relief may nevertheless be achieved by use of a multi-disciplinary approach.
- Physicians should advocate policy development that is directed toward developing and enabling the profession and practice of pain/palliative care.

Acknowledgments

This work was supported, in part, by funding from the Nour Foundation, and an American Academy of Pain Medicine-Pfizer National Visiting Professorship at Texas Tech University Health Sciences Center (JG). This work was completed as part of the N3P3 Project (Neuroscience, Neurophilosophy and Neuroethics of Pain, Pain Care, and Pain Policy) that conjoins the authors and their respective institutions. Thanks to Drs. Mark V. Boswell, Carlos Gomez and James Harrison for intellectual collaboration on prior work regarding the role of interventional pain medicine in palliative care.

Notes

[a] Although this is a fictional case, some facts and cost analysis are based on an actual case reported in the literature: (Seamans, D.P., Wong, G.Y., and Wilson, J.L. (2000). *J Clin Oncol*, **28**(7), 1598–1600.)

References

1* Giordano, J. (2006). Hospice, palliative care, and pain medicine: meeting the obligations of non-abandonment and preserving the diginity of terminally ill patients. *Del Med J*, **78**(11), 419–22.

2 Boswell, M.V. and Giordano, J. (2009). Reflection, analysis and change: the decade of pain control and research and its lessons for the future of pain management. *Pain Physician*, **12**, 1–7.

3* Ewald, H. (2004). *Stationäre Palliativmedizin. Finanzierung und Qualitätskriterien unter DRG-Bedingungen*, 3. Petersberger Gesundheitssymposium; Palliativmedizin: Herausforderung für das Gesundheitssystem. 1 July.

4 Manchikanti, L., Singh, V., Kloth, D. *et al.* Interventional techniques in the management of chronic pain. *Pain Physician* 2001; 4(1): 24–98.

5 Seamans, D.P., Wong, G.Y., and Wilson, J.L. (2000). Interventional pain therapy for interactable abdominal cancer pain. *J Clin Oncol*, **18**(7), 1598–600.

6 Giordano, J., Schatman, M.E., and Höver, G. (2009). A crisis in chronic pain care – an ethical analysis, Part I. Facts, issues, and problems. *Pain Physician*, **12**, 803–13.

7* Graf, G. and Höver, G. (2006). *Hospiz als Versprechen: Zur ethischen Grundlegung der der Hospizidee*. Der Hospizverlag.

Further reading

Giordano, J. (2006). Pain, the patient and the physician: philosophy and virtue ethics in pain medicine. In *Ethical Issues in Chronic Pain Management*, Schatman, M.E. (ed.) NY: Informa, pp. 1–18.

Giordano, J. (2009). *Pain: Mind, Meaning and Medicine*. Glen Falls, PA: PPM Communications.

Giordano, J., Benedikter, R. and Schatman, M.E. (2009). In: Giordano J, Boswell MV (eds.) *Pain Medicine: Philosophy, Ethics and Policy*. Oxon, UK: Linton Atlantic, pp. 39–50.

Höver G (2001/2) „Qualität" Bedeutung und ethische Dimensionen einer Schlüsselkategorie hospizlicher Arbeit. *Rheinisches Jahrbuch für Volkskunde*, **34**, 205–12.

Maricich, Y. and Giordano, J. (2009) Chronic pain, subjectivity, and the ethics of pain medicine: A deontic structure and the importance of moral agency. In: Giordano J, Boswell MV . (eds.) *Pain Medicine: Philosophy, Ethics and Policy*. Oxon, UK: Linton Atlantic, pp. 85–94.

Pain management

Opioid therapy in addicted patients: background and perspective from the UK

William Notcutt

Three Cases[a]

Case 1

Alesha, age 35, has chronic leg pain secondary to vascular damage from previous recurrent groin infections associated with intravenous opioid use. Having a baby was the stimulus to come off her drugs but she has struggled to maintain this state because of her pain and her impoverished living conditions. She sometimes smokes cannabis to relax and help her sleep. She uses codeine, which is of minimal help for the pain. She is supported by a psychiatric social worker who attends the clinic with her and she has never missed an appointment. These are now at 3-month intervals. She does not get on with her GP who she describes as an "Arse."

Should she be prescribed a long-acting opioid, such as slow release morphine, in a dose that will give her reasonable control?

Case 2

Ian, age 54, has been admitted to hospital with acute alcohol poisoning. He drinks two to three bottles of spirits a day. He also takes morphine for chronic back pain due to two wedge fractures of lumbar vertebra. He has been with the addiction services in the past, but has a chaotic lifestyle. His GP provides him with oral morphine for his pain. He only likes immediate release opiates, but has remained on a stable dose for some months. On the acute medical ward he is suffering severe withdrawal symptoms and has been given chlordiazepoxide. He has not had morphine for 2–3 days.

Should he have his morphine restarted at the previous dose?

Case 3

Peter, age 40, has had three prison terms for violence. He has a significant history of drug misuse. He has chronic low back pain for 12 years and has been through a full range

of investigation and therapy. He is using slow release morphine, diazepam, and amitriptyline. When he can get cannabis, he finds this is very effective for symptom control. He says that his back is much worse now and asks for an increase in opiate. He indicates that he might go back to buying on the street.

Should the physician increase his morphine dose, or prescribe him a synthetic cannabis analogue?

Most, if not all, doctors and nurses in the UK are now educated in the basics of ethics and are familiar with the common four principles of autonomy, beneficence, nonmaleficence, and justice/fairness. They are easy to understand and to apply to clinical practice as a source of guidance. Further, there is a perception in the UK that a court would look favorably on a doctor who has acted using reasonable and demonstrable ethical process in decision-making, whatever the outcome (based on the UK tradition of the Bolam Test[1] and later, the Bolitho judgment,[2] in determining negligence).[3]

Ethical principles

Autonomy

Just because a patient has a dependency problem, this is no justification for denying their right to have their pain managed in an appropriate fashion and to being involved in decisions about treatment. Pain control may be difficult to achieve but clinicians have a duty of care to attempt this. The patient should have some autonomy to determine, within reason, his or her preferred approach. In cancer care we allow the patient to decide on treatment, from a range of drug and procedure options that may all be potentially toxic and harmful. Equally, we don't agree to harmful therapeutic options. Doctors and nurses also have the right to not being abused, either by the patient, relatives, friends, or by the state authorities.

Clinical Ethics in Anesthesiology: A Case-Based Textbook, ed. Gail A. Van Norman, Stephen Jackson, Stanley H. Rosenbaum and Susan K. Palmer. Published by Cambridge University Press. © Cambridge University Press 2011.

Beneficence

There is a widely held acceptance that pain control has benefits for both the individual and those around him/her. Therefore, beneficence is achieved by working towards this goal. However, determining the balance between analgesia and feel-good/pleasure effects in a patient with a significant dependency potential is difficult. A patient is likely to derive health benefits from having a prescribed, standardized, and uncontaminated source of their drug rather than being tempted to purchase on the street. Working with others to control abnormal behaviors associated with pain and to reduce chaotic lifestyles will be helpful, although for some patients this may become mere containment of the situation rather than progressive improvement. Containment, however, is better than deterioration.

Nonmaleficence

Providing a legitimate source of a drug for pain has its risks. A patient may see this as a way to support a drug dependency habit if the doctor can be convinced that the pain is the dominant problem. However, failing to help a patient with chronic pain may have a major impact on the rest of the family and local society. A similar situation occurs when such a patient is admitted to a ward with an acute pain problem. They can be disruptive when they cannot get their usual level of drug intake, or the extra medication, or alternatives needed to control the additional pain. One common reason for failure to manage this situation is that the doctors lack knowledge in prescribing appropriate amounts of medication. For example, finding patients prescribed a mere 10 mg of oral morphine for breakthrough pain, when their normal daily baseline intake is 500 mg of morphine, is a common occurrence. Similarly, wholly inadequate bolus doses of opioid are often programmed into PCA devices for post-operative pain in these patients, because doctors are terrified of causing an overdose by giving more than the standard dose used for an opioid naïve patient. Lack of adequate education in pain management for all clinicians is a serious systemic ethical failure.

Inevitably there are the occasional tragedies, as opioids are dangerous in the wrong hands. A patient of the author's, who had proved very difficult to manage, went for a night out with a friend. While away, the troubled adolescent daughter broke into her mother's apartment with some friends and decided to have a party. She searched out her mother's slow-release morphine for a "trip," vomited while unconscious, and died. While these occurrences should lead to a search for safeguards, they are not an adequate excuse for not providing, or attempting to provide, appropriate analgesia for pain.

Justice

Perhaps the most common ethical principle that is flouted is that of justice and fairness. Patients with dependency problems are often given a low priority for pain therapy due to their drug habit, lifestyle, attitudes to staff, and other personal issues. We easily lose impartiality, objectivity, compassion, interest, and patience. Interventional treatments are refused on "psychological" grounds. However, we have a "duty of care" and if we will not deliver it, then we should find others who will (perhaps comparable to the duty of a physician-conscientious objector to abortion to nevertheless find other caregivers for the patient). Overcoming the negativity can be very difficult when addressing the pain problems of the addicted patients who, for example, usually do not have interesting problems, are often not "nice" patients to treat, may be difficult to trust, and often waste clinical time and appointments, among other issues.

The principle of double effect

In the past, doctors have extensively debated the ethics of a principle of "double effect" of opiate use in palliative care, although the evidence that this is a problem is almost nonexistent.[4] (For further discussion of "double effect" see Chapter 15). In the UK it does not seem to be considered as a significant concern. However, the doctrine of "double effect" is broader, explaining the permissibility of an action that may have some benefit but might also cause harm as a side effect. A judgment has to be made between the potential benefits and the harms. Therefore, perhaps we should redefine the use of the term and apply it to the use of opioids (and other drugs) in relieving pain in the potentially dependent patient.

Opiate prescribing in the UK

As in the US, the UK has seen a substantial increase in the prescribing of opiates for non-malignant pain. There are perhaps two major causes. First, since the early 1980s, doctors have become confident in the management of the use of opiates in malignancy and this experience has been translated to non-malignant pain. Second, with the exception of gabapentinoids, there have been no significant pharmacological advances in

Table 25.1. Often misunderstood or misused terms in opioid dependency

Term	
Tolerance	A pharmacologic property defined as the need for increasing doses to maintain therapeutic effects.
Physical dependence	A physiologic phenomenon defined solely by the development of an abstinence (withdrawal) syndrome following discontinuation of therapy, substantial dose reduction, or administration of an antagonist drug
Psychological dependence	A desire to continue a medication because it produces a sense of well-being; abstinence leads to anxiety, but not withdrawal syndrome.
Withdrawal syndrome	A clinical syndrome of physiologic manifestations after acute removal of a particular medication or substance. In the case of opioid withdrawal, symptoms and signs can include flu-like symptoms, yawning, agitation, restlessness, anxiety, insomnia, dilated pupils, piloerection, nausea and vomiting, abdominal pain, tachycardia, and hypertension.
Pseudo-addiction	The development of aberrant behavior in cancer patients who are experiencing unrelieved pain. With improved analgesia, the behaviors cease.
Chemical coping	A syndrome described in some pain patients who periodically display aberrant behaviors or have a mixed response to opioid therapy. Described by some as a "middle ground" between compliant opioid use and addiction.
Substance misuse or abuse	Excessive or inappropriate use of a chemical substance.
Addiction	A psychological and behavioral syndrome characterized by: (1) loss of control over drug use; (2) compulsive drug use; and (3) continued use despite harm.

pain treatment except in modes of drug delivery. The desire for simple techniques for relieving pain has led doctors, particularly pain clinicians, to see opioids as a useful and valuable option and so there has been a drift to expand their use.

In the author's own experience, in general, prescribing habits by pain specialists have had an "educational role" and are taken up by general practitioners, albeit a year or two later. However, in general, training in the management of chronic pain is still woefully inadequate.[5–7] Furthermore, few doctors, including pain clinicians, develop a comprehensive practice in the area of chronic pain in the opioid-dependent patient, because they often find the legal, ethical, and practical problems overwhelming.

Opioid dependency – a misunderstood problem

Despite the increasing recognition of chronic pain and opioid use, there is still much misunderstanding in the minds of doctors and nurses over the terminology associated with opioid dependency. Doctors still often describe patients as being addicted to their analgesics when in reality they may have some degree of dependency, but are not engaged in patterns of behavior associated with addiction (Table 25.1). Conversely, people with dependency problems may develop acute

or chronic pain, acute flare-ups of chronic pain, or pain associated with malignancy, AIDS or other life-limiting diseases. Furthermore, such patients may be taking their drugs for a variety of reasons (euphoria, escapism, relief of withdrawal symptoms, medicinal purposes, or a combination). The need for training in this area has been recognized and this is incorporated into the International Association for the Study of Pain (IASP) Curriculum.[8] The reality is that there are large numbers of clinicians that are highly skilled in interventional pain practice, but the same is not true for treating pain in patients with dependency.

Key differences between the UK and the US

The organization of the Health Service is a major difference between the UK and the US. All patients have a general practitioner who is the key both to ongoing prescribing and to the access to secondary care. There is a very limited role for the hospital emergency department to act as a primary health clinic and the access to a supply of opioids at this point is minimal. In hospital practice there is usually good, regular communication with the general practitioner. The normal practice would be to agree that there should only be one prescribing point for the patient. Initially, the pain clinic may manage prescribing until optimum dosing is achieved before returning this to the general practitioner. Some pain services have also developed strong links with the local addiction services to manage the addict with pain problems by running joint clinics.

Hence, in the UK, there is very little ability to go from doctor to doctor to obtain more and more prescription drugs. In practice, patients occasionally "lose" their drugs or use an excess, although they quickly learn that their requests for replacement are rarely accepted. The ability for the well off and well connected to access such drugs from private practitioners is limited. Close oversight by regulators identifies aberrant and/or high cost prescribing of opioids prescribed in primary care in locality. Prescribing opiates for registered addicts is managed through the addiction services, in general. Therefore, the access to opiates is reasonably well controlled and GPs take part in the long-term management of patients using opiates for pain, often sharing care with the pain clinics and palliative care services.

Diversion of prescribed opioids does not appear to be a great problem in the UK. In the past, problems of diversion were well recognized with short-acting opioids such as Dipipanone (Diconal), Dextromoride (Palfium) and Pethidine (Meperidine). This was resolved by either the agreed local banning of the drugs, or by agreed tight restriction in prescribing. Furthermore, it is well recognized in primary care now through education that these drugs have no use for managing chronic pain. It is notable that, in the UK, the use of diamorphine (heroin) has never been discontinued, unlike most other countries. Its use is principally within hospital practice and in palliative care. There has neither been any evidence of a significant problem with diversion nor any contribution to the widespread problems of recreational heroin use. Some addicts have been prescribed pharmaceutical grade heroin regularly to manage their addiction and there is also open debate about the possibilities of this approach to reduce their health problems. For the addict then there would be little incentive to exchange a quality product for other street drugs.

In contrast, the mild opioid, Dextropropoxyphene, combined with Paracetamol is widely used and well tolerated by many patients. It has been withdrawn recently because of concerns over its potential lethal effect when taken in deliberate overdose. The withdrawal of the drug led to many patients suffering increased pain when they were unable to find a suitable alternative.

The regulatory authorities however, did not appear to engage in any debate on the ethics of this with pain clinicians. There are many other aspects of modern life that are useful and safe, but dangerous in the hands of the irresponsible. The drug alcohol and the automobile are two good examples.

Professional guidelines

The clinician trying to treat the problem patient with opioid dependency will find little evidence from clinical trials to guide pain management. What information there is has been extensively reviewed but the advice and guidance available are based on opinion and consensus.[9, 10] We are left in a situation where we are often faced with complex patients with complex problems and with limited resources and abilities to manage them. Trying to do the best for these patients is not determined by long-established medical and scientific principles. The American and British Pain Societies have however, produced guidelines giving practical advice.[11, 12]

The British Guidelines also give examples of specific patient problems and how to deal with them. However, most patients present with a number of interconnected issues that are not easily resolvable, as in our case examples. The objective of achieving good pain control, good coping skills, and compliant, limited drug use is usually unattainable. Therefore, compromise and pragmatism are often needed to contain unsolvable problems. If this is supported by the explicit use of ethical principles, it may be possible to find the optimum way forward.

In the UK, Clinical Ethics Committees are still emerging and evolving. They have commonly provided an advisory service to the clinician to help with decision-making but in general, do not hand down formal judgments. Unfortunately, most public debate of ethical issues seems to revolve around exotic problems at the extremes of life rather than the everyday problems of clinical practice. Occasionally, clinicians refer complex cases to the courts for a decision, thereby obtaining the protection of the law, but in reality, handing over medical problems to nonclinicians.

Case resolution – UK perspective

Case 1

After getting to know Alesha, we discussed the use of strong opioids, recognizing the risks. She opted for transdermal fentanyl and settled at a stable dose.

Unfortunately she developed skin problems and had to discontinue the drug. She used oral ketamine for a short period but disliked its effect on her. She moved to slow release morphine twice a day, having originally been reluctant to have access to a quantity of tablets. In this way her autonomy was respected in her participation in the management of her care.

Her general practitioner prescribed the medication under the pain clinic's instruction, and was the only source of supply thereby reducing harm. Having originally been seen at 4-weekly periods, she is now seen in the pain clinic every 3 months. She is happy and confident with her current progress and pain control, as is her social worker and she has had fairness in her treatment. This approach has also helped improve her relationship with her general practitioner.

Case 2

Ian had a chaotic lifestyle. The opioid helped his back pain as did his alcohol. There was no other treatment that would be of help to his back in these circumstances as he was not suitable for vertebroplasty. On the ward he was accurate in his description of his opioid usage (confirmed by his general practitioner). He was also clearly suffering severe alcohol withdrawal symptoms.

We restarted his regular morphine dose (to treat pain and prevent opioid withdrawal), and quickly controlled his alcohol withdrawal symptoms (with chlordiazepoxide and other supportive measures). His symptoms and his abusive behavior settled. His general physical condition improved and he was discharged home. He was lost to follow-up in primary care.

Normally, opiate prescription for primary opioid addiction would be in the hands of addiction services and not the general practitioner. Here, the opioid was used for pain. It can be considered that controlling some of his pain with morphine was better for him than his using alcohol for the same purpose therefore being beneficent. Two risks of harm are possible: diversion to pay for alcohol, and overdose. His right to use a medicine that helped his pain was negotiated and managed by his general practitioner. Restarting his morphine on the ward was beneficial to him (and to those around) and it was helpful to have recognized and treated his dependency. The duty of care was met. The general practitioner will continue the long-term care as best he can.

Case 3

Perhaps the most important ethical principle in managing Peter is fairness in management, however limited, within the medical services. He was not a friendly individual. He had been offered and had tried other treatments thereby fulfilling his right to appropriate management of his problem. Dose escalation was not an option, as it was very unlikely to provide any improvement in pain control. His threat to obtain street opioids was unlikely to be carried through as his mobility and finances were limited.

In the UK, admitting cannabis use to a medical practitioner is not uncommon and, in some communities, its use is so widespread, it would be reasonable to include it in a review of a patient's pharmacological pain management. Its use here is probably recreational/euphoric as much as therapeutic. This then can be seen as beneficial for him in helping him cope. However, prescribing a substitute would likely be ineffective through his need to get some form of "high." The likelihood of harm from this is minimal (nonmaleficence). Therefore, accepting its use and the overall safety of the drug in comparison to most others in routine use for pain, is the current management approach. He will continue to be seen regularly to support the general practitioner in his management (duty of care).

Key points

- Ethical problems presented by opioid-dependent patients who are suffering pain are challenging, but can be guided by simple principles of ethical medical practice.
- A patient's dependency problem is not a justification for denying appropriate pain management. Clinicians have a "duty of care" to try to achieve pain control.
- Appropriate pain control benefits both the patient and those surrounding them. Containment of aberrant behaviors may be the best that can be achieved; however, containment is better than deterioration
- A major problem with pain management in the patient with opioid dependency is lack of physician knowledge about appropriate prescribing; education of physicians is key to developing reasonable prescribing practices.

- A principle like that of "double effect" might be useful in defining appropriate physician behavior in relieving pain in the potentially dependent patient.

Notes

a These are real examples from a single UK clinic. In this chapter, Dr. Notcutt discusses management of the cases from a UK perspective incorporating basic clinical ethics. In the following chapter, the same cases will be discussed by Dr. Ballantyne from a US perspective. The UK perspective presents what actually happened, while the US perspective presents how the cases may be handled differently by a physician in the US, understanding that opinion and practice vary considerably even within a single practice, and certainly across any single nation.

References

1 Bolam v. Friern Hospital Management Committee [1957] 1 WLR 583. The Bolam test states that if a doctor reaches the standard of a responsible body of medical opinion, he is not negligent.

2 Bolitho v. City and Hackney Heath Authority [1998] 9 MLR 26 (HL). In this judgment, it was determined that a judge must be satisfied that the body of expert opinion relied upon must have some demonstrable logical basis, and is not accepted solely because it comes from an expert body.

3 Hurwitz, B. (2004). How does evidence based guidance influence determinations of medical negligence? *BMJ*, **329**, 1024–8.

4 Fohr, S.A. (1998). The double effect of pain medication. *J Palliat Med*, **1**, 315–28.

5* The Pain Education Special Interest Group of the British Pain Society. (2009). Survey of undergraduate pain curricula for healthcare professionals in the United Kingdom. The British Pain Society, London UK.

6* Annual Report of the Chief Medical Officer on the State of Public Health 2008. Department of Health Publications (2009) pp. 33–39 [www.dh.gov.uk].

7 Notcutt, W. and Gibbs, G. (2010). Inadequate pain management: myth, stigma and professional fear. *Postgrad Med J* (accepted for publication).

8 Charlton, J.E. (ed). (2005). *Core Curriculum for Professional Education in Pain*, Seattle: WA, IASP Press.

9 AAPM Clinical Guidelines for the Use of Chronic Opioid Therapy in Chronic Noncancer Pain. APS Evidence Review American Pain Society. opioid/pub/pdf/org. ampainsoc.WWW_final_evidence_pdf.report.

10 Ballantyne, J. and LaForge, S. (2007). Opioid dependence and addiction during opioid treatment of chronic pain. *Pain*, **129**, 235–55.

11 Clinical Guidelines for the Use of Chronic Opioid Therapy in Chronic Noncancer Pain. (2009). American Pain Society – American Academy of Pain Medicine Opioids Guidelines. *J Pain*, **10**(2), 113–30.

12 Pain and substance misuse: improving the patient experience. (2006). London UK: British Pain Society.

Further reading

AAPM Council on Ethics. (2005). Ethics charter from American Academy of Pain Medicine. *Pain Medicine*, **6**(3), 203–12.

American Pain Society. (2009). Clinical guidelines for the use of chronic opioid therapy in chronic noncancer pain. American Academy of Pain Medicine Opioids Guidelines. *J Pain*, **10**(2), 113–30.

American Pain Society. Evidence Review: APS-AAPM Clinical Guidelines for the Use of Chronic Opioid Therapy in Chronic Noncancer Pain. www.ampainsoc.org/pub/pdf/opioid_final_evidence_report.pdf.

Bannister, J. (2005). Running a pain and dependency clinic. In *Managing Pain and Addiction – Opening Pandora's Box*. University of Dundee. Conference communication.

British Pain Society. (2006). Improving the Patient Experience: Pain and Substance Misuse. London, UK.

Fishbain, D. (2003). Chronic opioid treatment, addiction and pseudo-addiction in patients with chronic pain. *Psychiatric Times Newsletter*, **20**, 2.

Littlejohn, C., Baldacchino, A., and Bannister, J. (2004). Chronic non-cancer pain and opioid dependence. *J Roy Soc Med*, **97**, 62–5.

Portenoy, R.K. (2006). Opioid therapy for chronic non-malignant pain: clinicians' perspective. *J Law Med Ethics*, **24**(4), 296–309.

26 Opioid therapy in addicted patients: background and perspective from the US

Jane C. Ballantyne and Joseph Klein

The three cases

Please refer to the previous chapter's cases for discussion.

Opium addiction as a social problem

Although opium derivatives have been used since antiquity for medicinal and recreational purposes, recognition of opioid addiction as a significant social problem emerged only relatively recently. The opium eaters of the eighteenth and nineteenth centuries consumed fairly low doses of active drug. Intoxication and addiction certainly existed, but the lack of widespread availability prevented broad societal ramifications. Nonetheless, a stigma was attached to opium consumption by a largely religious society that valued suffering as a moral good. The Quakers, for example, likened the soul to a physical entity; intoxicating substances impaired self-restraint, leading to lapses in moral judgment and consequent damage to the soul. Despite these views, few restrictions on opium existed.

With the emergence of purified morphine and later heroin, the deleterious effects of opioids on individuals and society came into focus. In the US, the number of narcotic addicts exploded, crime rose, and worker productivity declined. Legislation soon followed. The Harrison Act of 1914 restricted opioid and cocaine distribution to registered physicians and pharmacies. By the 1920s, authorities jailed physicians for distributing opioids outside their professional "course of conduct," thus setting a precedent that would affect opioid prescribing for decades. Britain soon followed with its own legislation, the Dangerous Drugs Act, in 1920.

Regulatory influence

In the US, after *Webb versus the United States*[1] and provisions of the 1914 Harrison Narcotic Drug Act made it illegal for physicians to prescribe opioids for the treatment of opioid addiction, opioid treatment of pain practically ceased. Not knowing which of their patients might be addicted, doctors in the US were intimidated lest they lose their medical license, or worse still, suffer criminal prosecution. The laws in other Western countries were less constraining. In the UK, guided by the Rolleston Committee (1924–1965), physicians were allowed to give their addicted patients diamorphine (heroin), syringes, and needles. At the time, heroin proliferation was less of a problem in the UK than in the US: in 1958 there were only 62 known heroin users in the UK, a number that would soon increase severalfold. In *The (London) Times* in 1955 it was argued:

> 'Heroin addiction in Great Britain is practically unknown and it is difficult to see why administrative action ... should be allowed to hinder the relief of suffering.'[2] "Do not let us follow along the path of prohibition – a bad and dangerous way'.[3]

In a description of the London drug scene in the 1960s, the preacher Kenneth Leech wrote:

> 'To cut off the supply by prescription would be easy; it has been done in the United States where doctors are not allowed to prescribe for addicts, with the result that the provision of drugs has become a flourishing industry and drug addiction increases there yearly.'[4]

The differences between the US and other Western countries persisted into the late 1960s when US President Richard Nixon's "War on Drugs" led to even stricter regulations. The effect on the medical use of opioids in the US was disastrous. By the second half of the twentieth century, both addiction and pain were undertreated, with baleful consequences. When the iniquities of undertreatment were recognized, opioid advocacy was born. In the US, addiction advocacy brought about the re-establishment of opioid (methadone) treatment for addiction in 1974 (Narcotic Addict Treatment Act); pain advocacy during the 1970s and

Clinical Ethics in Anesthesiology: A Case-Based Textbook, ed. Gail A. Van Norman, Stephen Jackson, Stanley H. Rosenbaum and Susan K. Palmer. Published by Cambridge University Press. © Cambridge University Press 2011.

1980s brought about the re-establishment of opioids for the treatment of acute and cancer pain, principles that were later extended to chronic pain.

Prevalence of prescription opioid abuse

Historically, under-treatment of pain as a consequence of draconian anti-drug laws occurred mainly in the US. The swing of the pendulum towards over-use, or at least careless use, of opioids for pain seems also a uniquely American problem,[5] reflected in alarming statistics that demonstrate precipitous increases in prescription opioid abuse over the past decade, to the extent that prescription opioid abuse is now more prevalent in the US than is illicit heroin abuse.[6] (Figure 26.1) Successful marketing of "designer" opioids increased prescribing of opioids for chronic pain.[7] Increased prescribing for pain resulted in increased opioid analgesics in homes, pharmacies, and on the streets, and has likely contributed to the disturbing increases in prescription drug abuse and related deaths seen in the US.[8] Surveys such as the National Household Survey do not exist in the UK, and it may be that, without an effective early warning system, the extent of the problem of prescription opioid abuse is unknown in UK.[9] Whatever the benefits of the UK's relatively forgiving approach to controlling addiction in terms of not having inhibited opioid prescribing for pain to the same extent as in the US, UK policies seem to be failing to control problematic illicit drug use when compared to other European countries. The UK now has the worst illicit drug problem in Europe, a situation that is bound to impact UK general practitioners at the intersection of pain and addiction. Effective confinement of prescription opioid use to medical use, as appears to have been achieved in the UK, seems ideal, yet the balance between prescription and illicit opioid abuse will always be precarious.

Enactment of laws and their effect on opioid prescribing for pain

In the US, the Controlled Substances Act of 1970 unified many previous laws under a single framework regulating the manufacture, distribution, prescription, and dispensing of opioids and other substances with abuse potential. Controlled substances were assigned to one of five schedules based on their medical utility and abuse potential. The Controlled Substance Act defines neither legitimate medical purpose nor standards of professional practice: this falls to the state medical boards, professional societies, the Department of Justice, or even lay juries in criminal trials. Criminal charges against physicians generally arise only when both bad practice and bad intention by the practitioner are established.

Because of legal constraints placed on opioid prescribing in the US, gross negligence (bad practice) may lead to criminal prosecution even when there is good intention. For example, a physician is more likely to be accused of involuntary manslaughter if the drug chosen for overdose by a suicidal patient is an opioid rather than a noncontrolled drug such as a tricyclic antidepressant. In *People v Schade*, a physician was convicted of involuntary manslaughter when a patient with known addiction and suicidal ideation killed himself with an opioid that had been prescribed within days of a previous suicide attempt. The jury deemed this to be reckless facilitation of a suicide. Had the medication not been a controlled substance, the physician more likely would

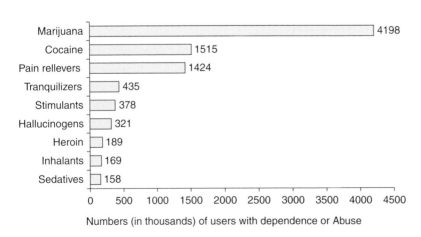

Figure 26.1. Dependence or Abuse of Specific Illicit Drugs among Persons Aged 12 or Older: 2003

have faced malpractice (a civil action not subject to incarceration), rather than criminal charges.[10]

The perception of risk of even being investigated, let alone being tried and convicted on criminal charges, has deterred many physicians from aggressively treating pain with controlled substances. In the US there is a risk also of being charged with undertreatment of pain. In 2001 a California physician was convicted of elder abuse for underprescribing pain medications in a malpractice suit. The jury awarded the family $1.5 million.[11] Cases such as these have raised significant societal debate on the role of the courts in dictating what constitutes a "legitimate medical purpose," a role historically the purview of state medical boards and professional societies. Contradictory legal precedent places physicians in a quandary: prescribe liberally and risk possible criminal investigation or prescribe sparingly and risk civil proceedings for the undertreatment of pain. The war on drugs collides with another American phenomenon, patient advocacy for the right to pain control. Physicians are left caught in the middle.

Because UK drug regulations are less restrictive than those in the US, criminal prosecution of physicians on charges related to opioids were virtually unheard of until the notorious case of Harold Shipman in 1998. Harold Shipman was a general practitioner who was tried and convicted of the murders of 15 elderly patients. He had administered diamorphine (a legal drug in the UK for clinical use). After his trial, a special inquiry (the Shipman Inquiry) found evidence to suggest that he had, in fact, killed as many as 250 people. The press coverage of the case was such that Harold Shipman's activities became well known in the UK. Unlike the US, where criminal prosecution of physicians had occurred relatively frequently with an insidious effect on opioid prescribing for pain, the Shipman case had an immediate and profound effect on opioid prescribing in the UK. The Shipman Inquiry was damning in its criticism of the General Medical Council (the body that accredits British doctors) saying that the body had protected doctors at the expense of protecting patients.[12] The inquiry suggested two ways in which risk might be reduced, which had been recognized in earlier legislation but never implemented: they found that doctors should not be allowed to prescribe controlled substances: (1) for their own use; or (2) when not in "actual practice" (with an active medical license). Another provision that had been suggested in earlier regulations, but never implemented, was that all private prescriptions should be written on special

forms. In 2006, the Misuse of Drugs Regulations were changed, and new arrangements made for prescribing controlled substances on special forms.[13]

Demanding opioids: the impact of cultural and healthcare system differences

At the end of the twentieth century, doctors stopped worrying that opioid treatment of chronic pain was neither effective nor safe, and caution turned to confidence. It was believed that treatment could relieve people of the burden of chronic pain and improve their lives. This philosophical shift was important for persuading the medical community that opioids should be widely used for the treatment of chronic pain. But what if, after all, opioids are not so effective for relieving pain and improving lives, as has been suggested by several recently published epidemiological studies?[14] Is patient *desire* for opioid treatment of their pain enough?

Studies are beginning to show that pain treatment, any pain treatment, can produce positive patient satisfaction ratings even if that treatment fails to produce the results treating clinicians want to see (improvement in pain, function, and quality of life).[15] Simply validating a pain complaint by continuing treatment may be enough to satisfy patients. But if that treatment is an opioid, then there are several reasons why the treatment could produce good satisfaction ratings despite failing to achieve the primary goals of treatment. Only a few patients will develop true addiction, but many if not all patients receiving continuous opioid treatment will develop dependence (physical and psychological).[16] They may therefore give up opioids only with difficulty, even when such drugs are not working well. By the definition of addiction, those patients that do develop iatrogenic addiction will desire opioids beyond their ability to improve quality of life. Many patients will rely on opioids to treat symptoms other than pain ("chemical copers"). The addictive properties of opioids introduce complications such as deliberate or careless diversion. There is also a sense that there is nowhere to go beyond opioid treatment – that there is nothing better, so it must be good.

The issue of patients desiring opioid treatment, even when the treatment fails to achieve conventional treatment goals, exposes some important differences between the US and the UK. Consider first the profound cultural differences that drive ethical and moral arguments in these two countries. Liberty and the right to pursue happiness were fundamental to the constitution of the New World – values that have remained central to the American character ever since. In the US, the rights of the individual are of primary importance. In healthcare, this means that patients dominate in healthcare decisions, provided they or their insurance can pay. Statutes are written to ensure that patients have a right to determine their own treatment, including Intractable Pain Statutes that establish the right of patients to receive opioids for the treatment of intractable pain.[17] Physicians are supposed to help inform patients about the capability of a treatment to achieve its goals, and to steer the patient's decision within a guidance-co-operation model, as distinct from the paternalistic model of care seen more often in government run healthcare systems. This forms the basis of the shared decision-making that is prevalent in US healthcare.

Medical ethics: the role of patient choice

The most difficult ethical arguments arise when there is this difference of opinion between the patient and physician, especially when the argument pitches the individual patient against the needs of society.[18] In the US, there is cultural bias to allow patient choices, while in the UK healthcare system and culture, a more socialist approach is encouraged. This difference becomes important when considering the role of patient satisfaction as an "outcome" of opioid treatment. Addiction risk aside, if opioid treatment of chronic pain effectively achieves any of the conventional goals of treatment (e.g., sustained pain relief), most people would agree that there is a strong argument for providing it. If the treatment is desired but not effective, or even harmful, then differences in the value placed on patient satisfaction will be starkly exposed.

The US healthcare system is unique in that it is the only system in the world that relies on employers, through insurance agencies, to fund healthcare. Medicare and Medicaid fund healthcare for the elderly and the impoverished, respectively. The truly uninsured are a small minority of the population. Healthcare in the US is therefore driven by marketing – not by welfare – politics, and the model of American healthcare is a business model.

Attention to pain, and successful treatment of pain, have become important markers of quality of care. Measures of patient satisfaction are now included in most hospital outcome metrics, and are used for accreditation of US hospitals, as well as to assess the performance of individual clinics and clinicians. Failure to compete in terms of patient satisfaction could mean institutional failure, loss of institutional support, or loss of livelihood for clinicians. Patient satisfaction with opioid treatment without any other demonstrable benefit presents a dilemma for some clinicians, who may feel pressured to prescribe against their better judgment. The conflicts that can arise in discussing withdrawal of opioid treatment in patients who have not demonstrated traditional signs of clinical efficacy may deter many clinicians, since it is much easier to simply prescribe the opioids the patient is seeking. A business model of healthcare may thus promote a tendency to overprescribe.

Case resolutions

Case 1

The best way to keep Alesha's addiction under control is to formalize her addiction treatment, ideally in recognition that she needs both *pain* and *addiction* treatment. Opioid maintenance or analgesic treatment alone will not be enough to control either her pain or her addiction, and counseling and other nonmedical interventions should be an integral part of treatment. In the US, a patient like this may fall through the cracks if she doesn't have some sort of healthcare coverage (e.g. Medicaid). It is highly likely that this patient will suffer a relapse if she does not receive appropriate treatment. The ethical issues that arise here are: (1) that the stigma of addiction affects physicians' prejudices and their willingness to treat pain with opioids; and (2) she may be denied appropriate medical care because of lack of, or limited, benefits – a reason some may argue at the broad political level that it is unethical to continue with the current healthcare system and its disparities.

Case 2

Ian is in a high-risk, low-benefit category for opioid pain treatment. He presents a high risk of misuse due to his alcoholism and chaotic lifestyle, and he has a pain condition that can be effectively treated using non-opioid approaches. Ideally, he should be offered both addiction and chronic pain treatment, the latter being with nonopioid approaches. The ethical issue here is whether physicians can and should withhold opioids if they believe that in prescribing, they could do harm. In the US, the physician risks losing DEA certification or medical license if prescribing to a patient who subsequently harms him/herself. Fear of liability thus becomes a significant factor in clinical decision making.

Case 3

Evidence and expert opinion strongly suggests that open-ended dose escalation doesn't work, and eventually leads to opioid refractoriness. Peter should be advised that, if the opioid is no longer working well, his choices include opioid holiday or opioid switch, but not dose increase. Peter's concomitant marijuana issue is always tough. Since marijuana use is illegal in the US, the physician can either take the hard line of not prescribing opioids to patients who use marijuana (which may be revealed on the urine toxicology screen even if the patient doesn't admit to use) or deal with it in a "don't ask, don't tell" manner. He would probably not be prescribed a synthetic cannabis analogue because it doesn't work well for pain. This author would not be threatened by the patient's statement about going back to buying on the street, since she cannot prevent that. Ethically, the physician is bound to treat pain to the best of their ability according to their knowledge. In this case, that would be with a rational and stable does of opioid, with the usual safeguards. Although for a patient who has already threatened to "buy on the street," there will always be a risk of him selling his prescribed opioid, on balance this tendency may be better controlled if he is provided with a stable dose of opioid in a medical setting. Some American physicians may fear regulatory scrutiny in this situation, with appropriate documentation of this rationale for the treatment decision, they would be unlikely to be faulted by the authorities.

treatment has long been maintained as being humane, ethical, and necessary.

- Physician choices in the US are influenced by legal issues; US physicians can be held liable for both over-treatment and under-treatment of pain, while in the UK such cases are rare.
- Fears of civil or criminal prosecution may unduly influence physicians in the US, placing self-interest ahead of the traditional prioritization of beneficence and respect for patient autonomy.
- Differences between the US and UK in healthcare provision additionally influence opioid prescribing.
- Lack of universal healthcare coverage in the US means that, at one end of the spectrum, for the uninsured, it may not be possible to offer appropriate care for pain and addiction.
- At the other end of the spectrum, strong patient advocacy and the established rights of the insured, mean that patients dominate in healthcare decisions, including the right to receive opioids. The paternalistic approach more predominant in universal healthcare systems is not appropriate in the US. This produces ethical dilemmas for the US physician whose concept of risk versus benefit may differ from that of the patient, and who additionally may be driven to produce good patient satisfaction ratings in a market-driven healthcare system.

Key points

- Differences in history, culture, healthcare systems, laws, and attitudes have significantly affected perspectives on the ethical management of opioid use between the US and the UK.
- Use of illicit opioids in the US has lead to reactionary legislation with harsh penalties.

  The present state of affairs is that abuse of prescription opioids is more prevalent in the US than abuse of "street" heroin.
- Opioid treatment of pain has periodically come under intense scrutiny in the US, resulting in fluctuations between under- and overtreatment of pain. In the UK, opioid

References

1 Webb *et al.* v United States, 249 US 96 (1919).

2 Horder, T.J. (1955). Manufacture of Heroin. *The Times*, London. 26th May;11e.

3 Webb-Johnson, A.E. House of Lords debates, 13th December 1955, vol 195, columns 45–6

4 Leech, K. (1991). The London Drug Scene in the 1960s. Policing and Prescribing, eds. Whynes D and Bean P. McMillan, London UK, pp. 43–4.

5* Zacny, J., Bigelow, G., Compton, P., *et al.* (2003). College on Problems of Drug Dependence taskforce on prescription opioid non-medical use and abuse: position statement. *Drug Alcohol Depend*, **69**(3), 215–32.

6 Office of Applied Studies (2008). Results from the 2007 National Survey on Drug Use and

Health: National findings (DHHS Publication No. SMA 08–4343, NSDUH Series H-34. Rockville, MD: Substance Abuse and Mental Health Services Administration.

7* Van Zee A. (2009). The promotion and marketing of oxycontin: commercial triumph, public health tragedy. *Am J Public Health*, **99**(2), 221–7.

8* Kuehn, B.M. (2007). Opioid prescriptions soar: increase in legitimate use as well as abuse. *JAMA*, **17**(3), 249.

9* Spence, D. (2010) Bad medicine: pain. *Br Med J*, **340**, b5683.

10 Romanow, K. (2003). Criminal law: physician convicted for recklessly prescribing OxyContin. *J Law Med Ethics*, **31**(1), 154–5.

11 Bergman v. Eden Medical Center, No. H205732–1 (Cal. Super. Ct. Aug. 20, 2001).

12 The Shipman Inquiry. http://www.the-shipman-inquiry.org.uk/home.asp.

13 Department of Health (2006). Safer Management of Controlled Drugs (CDs): Private CD prescriptions and other changes to the prescribing and dispensing of controlled drugs (CDs). Guidance for Implementations. Gateway Reference: 6820.

14 Eriksen, J., Sjogren, P., Bruera, E., *et al.* (2006). Critical issues on opioids in chronic non-cancer pain. An epidemiological study. *Pain*, **125**, 172–9.

15* Ballantyne, J.C. and Fleisher, L.A. (2010). Ethical issues in opioid prescribing for chronic pain. *Pain*, **148**(3), 365–7.

16* Ballantyne, J.C. and LaForge, S.L. (2007). Opioid dependence and addiction in opioid treated pain patients. *Pain*, **129**, 235–55.

17 Dubois, M.Y. (2005). The birth of an ethics charter for pain medicine. *Pain Med*, **6**(3), 201–2.

18* Rubin, S.B. (2007). If we think it's futile, can't we just say no? *HEC Forum*, **19**(1), 45–65.

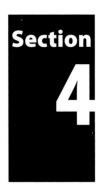

Section 4

Research and publication

Ethics in anesthesiology research using human subjects

A.M. Viens

The Case

A group of anesthesia researchers undertook a research project to determine if injection of a sedative drug into the subarachnoid space would improve effectiveness of pain control post-operatively for labor and delivery. The literature at the time had scant information about toxicity of the drug in question when administered in this way, although some anesthesiologists had been doing so anyway. While a handful of studies had demonstrated no obvious adverse outcomes in animal models, several studies suggested dramatically otherwise, including one study in which rabbits demonstrated serious spinal cord histological changes. No study had examined the use of the drug in the dosage and mode of administration proposed by the investigators. The investigators obtained institutional ethics review board approval and the study was carried out. No human subjects appeared to suffer an adverse effect. A modest improvement in analgesia was seen in some, but not all, patients. The project was written up and submitted to a journal for publication.

All anesthesiologists will encounter ethical issues related to research. It may be through engaging in their own primary or clinical research projects, in their practice treating a patient who is a research participant in a project from another treating speciality, applying for research funding and ethics approval, publishing research results, or even through determining departmental/divisional funding priorities. The focus of this chapter will be solely on the ethics of conducting research involving human subjects – in particular, some of the main ethical issues that arise with the kind of research conducted by anesthesiologists in clinical settings.

The history of anesthesiology research on human subjects, while at times undertaken in varying degrees of ethically permissible ways, has produced many techniques that are the mainstay of modern surgical, perioperative and intensive care. It should be recognized by anesthesiologists that both clinical research and

research ethics share a common reason for undertaking such activities: to improve clinical practice and care. Research constructed, conducted, and disseminated in an ethical fashion will likely lead to quality improvement, improved outcomes, shared knowledge and best practices, amongst other considerations.

Research ethics in general, and the ethical conduct of clinical research in particular, are concerned with ensuring research participants and their interests are protected, and that the clinical research they are involved in serves the interests of science and the community in which it is conducted.

Most anesthesiologists will split their time working in the operating room, intensive care unit, or pain clinic and divide the rest of their time in administrative, teaching, and research roles. Each of these positions and environments will have their own obligations associated with them; and it is often the case that many of the obligations and issues that arise in the clinical setting will have some overlap with research activities.

Anesthesiologists conducting research have obligations to patients, colleagues, and society that should be adhered to. Some of the main research-based obligations include the following.

- Study design and performance should be based on a thorough knowledge of the scientific literature and other relevant sources of information.
- Studies should address a research question of sufficient value to participants to justify risk exposure.
- There should be clear research question(s) that can be answered reliably and efficiently.
- Sufficient number of participants should be enrolled in a reasonable period.
- All research projects should be reviewed by relevant research ethics committee(s) for consideration, comment, guidance, and approval before the study begins (even studies that are

Clinical Ethics in Anesthesiology: A Case-Based Textbook, ed. Gail A. Van Norman, Stephen Jackson, Stanley H. Rosenbaum and Susan K. Palmer. Published by Cambridge University Press. © Cambridge University Press 2011.

noninvasive or involve accepted therapies need approval both for regulatory reasons and to consider issues of confidentiality, cost and voluntariness).

- Informed consent should be obtained for all parts of the project, including any resulting adverse effects that may require modification of protocols or care.
- Undue inducements, duress, or coercion should not be used in recruiting or retaining participants.
- Research should be conducted only by individuals with the appropriate medical qualifications and scientific training.
- Findings should be valid and reproducible.
- Research design should be preceded by careful assessment of predictable risks and burdens to the individuals and communities, and participation should be dependent upon confidence that the risks involved can be satisfactorily managed.
- Research protocols, and information given to participants, should have clear provisions for treating and/or compensating subjects who are harmed as a consequence of participation in the research study.
- Participant privacy and confidentiality in the collection, analysis, storage and/or reuse of identifiable and anonymized data should be ensured.
- Positive and negative research findings should be disseminated.

To some, these may seem like scientific or legal considerations, and not ethical considerations. However, these considerations are ethical in that designing and executing a study that is not scientifically rigorous or exhibits scientific misconduct puts participants at risk of burden, loss, or harm.

Why anesthesiology research is special

The kind of research conducted by anesthesiologists deserves special attention by virtue of the fact that a good deal of the human subject research conducted will be with participants who are potentially themselves vulnerable – children, women in labor, critically ill patients – or in temporary vulnerable states – individuals who are sedated, unconscious, about to undergo surgery, in pain, or being resuscitated. This is not to say that vulnerability is not found in other areas of research, merely that it is an acute and central concern in anesthesiology and peri-operative clinical research. Moreover, the unique environment in which clinical anesthesiology research is conducted and consent is

obtained, also presents specific challenges. As a result of this, this chapter will focus on three areas where these issues are especially important for the ethical conduct of clinical anesthesiology research: enrollment and consent, potential conflicts of interest, and the balance of risk and benefit.

Enrollment and consent in clinical research

Free and informed consent to participate in a research project must be obtained from the participant or from an appropriate legally designated representative for participants who do not possess the capacity to consent. Participants incapable of providing consent for research participation require special protection.

The consent process should involve providing the participant with sufficient information – in lay language – that includes the aims of the research and potential outcomes, inclusion and exclusion criteria, what happens if the participant agrees to take part, what methods, techniques, or devices will be used, any risks or benefits to participating, what will happen to specimens or data obtained from research, arrangements for ensuring anonymity or confidentiality, and how results will be disseminated, amongst other relevant considerations.

It should be made clear that the primary purpose for medical research is to understand the nature of disease and/or improve preventive, diagnostic, and therapeutic interventions. As such, the decision to participate in research need not result in any direct personal benefit – even if there are associated indirect benefits. It should also be made clear that a decision not to participate will have absolutely no effect on their clinical care.

Research participants need to be given sufficient time to reflect on the information contained within the project description and consent form, and to consult with friends or family members (should they wish). The unique environment in which most clinical anesthesiology research takes place will make this a challenge that must still be accommodated.

It must be made unambiguous that research participants and their data (assuming it is not anonymised) can be withdrawn from a study at any time without explanation and that this withdrawal will also have absolutely no effect on the quality or level of their clinical care. Research involving general anesthetics or other potent central nervous system depressant medications will constrain a participant's ability to exercise their right to withdraw from a study and this factor must also be taken into account and accommodated within the design and conduct of a study. Due attention must also be paid to the fact that approaching patients in a clinical setting for research purposes will raise questions about a patient's privacy and the confidentiality of medical information and research data.

The Canadian Anesthesiologists' Society[1] suggests that pre-operative consent for clinical anesthesiology research may be obtained either before admission or on the day of the scheduled surgery provided that:

(1) Patients are not under the influence of premedication.

(2) Risk to the patient and time commitment to the study are not significantly different from routine clinical care (e.g., during drug trials in which a patient may be randomly assigned to receive one of several anesthetic regimens, using approved medications).

(3) After verbal explanation from the investigator or research assistant, and in the absence of the investigator or research assistant, patients are given time to read the information sheet and consider the risks and benefits. Patients should have an opportunity to raise any further questions or seek clarification on any points concerning the nature of the study, alternatives, risks, benefits, etc.

(4) Patients who feel they are under duress, or require more time to make a decision, should be advised to decline participation in the study.

(5) Investigators document in the healthcare chart the nature of their consent process for patients who agree to participate in a research protocol.

Dual role of anesthesiologist and clinical researcher

When anesthesiologists who treat patients also engage in clinical research, they take on dual roles that have important differences that may give rise to potential conflicts or obligations that come into tension with an anesthesiologist's duty of care.[2]

One area of potential concern is financial conflicts of interest.[3] While the vast majority of clinical research is undertaken for scientific reasons, it is undeniable that there are a number of positive upshots that can result, including promotion, tenure, funding, prestige, etc. As a result, the existence and even appearance of conflicts

of interest must be mitigated or removed. Other financial conflicts of interest may include finder's fees, institutional funding and sponsorship, owning stock in a company whose product you are researching, or being involved in a spin-off company that may commercialize the results of the study. Research protocols, participant information sheets, the consent process, and publication/presentation of the resulting research findings should include information regarding all potential conflicts of interest, including funding, sponsors, affiliations, and positions.

Another area of concern is that potential research participants may be in a dependent relationship with anesthesiologists – either as the direct treating physician or by being a patient who is treated by a colleague on the same service. Many patients will find an approach to participate in a research project by their treating anesthesiologists or a project being conducted at the institution in which they are receiving treatment more difficult to turn down than they might otherwise have in a different setting. Anesthesiologists need to be careful in their approach of potential participants for enrollment that the attitude, situation, or environment is not in any way coercive or involves an unnecessary pressure. If possible, it may be advisable to have an appropriately qualified individual who is completely independent of the physician or research relationship conduct the participant enrollment and/or consent process.

According to King and Churchill,[2] physician-researchers should:

- Discuss the differences between research and medical practice with patients.
- Disclose both physician and researcher roles to patients, and distinguish them ("switch hats") as needed.
- Consistently use "research" terminology, not "treatment" language, when referring to investigators, subjects, and experimental interventions.
- Present benefit to society as the sole or primary goal of research.
- Explain that benefit to research participants, while often hoped for, is always uncertain and may be unlikely or impossible, depending on the design and phase of the trial.
- State when clinical benefit from the experimental intervention in a study is not possible or not likely.

- When clinical benefit from the experimental intervention in a study is reasonably possible, describe it clearly, including its nature, magnitude, duration, likelihood, and limits.
- Remember that, even though clinical research is not medical practice, researchers can, do, and should care about and for their research subjects.

The Helsinki Declaration[4] maintains that, "The physician may combine medical research with medical care only to the extent that the research is justified by its potential preventive, diagnostic or therapeutic value and if the physician has good reason to believe that participation in the research study will not adversely affect the health of the patients who serve as research subjects." When holding the dual role of clinician and researcher, in circumstances where the two come into conflict (or the potential exists to give rise to the appearance of conflict), the role of clinician must take priority over the role of researcher.

Risk, benefit, and clinical trials

Many of the risks and benefits associated with participation in clinical anesthesiology research are based on the use of the anesthetic itself and not participation in the research project.[1] However, this is not always the case. The case study at the beginning of the chapter, which is based on an actual research study, contains a number of ethical issues of concern that could arise in other clinical anesthesiology research.

The investigators conducted their research project when there was inadequate information at the time the study was performed, regarding the safety of the proposed procedure. The benefits arising from the study were questionable – very effective labor analgesia already existed at the time and, as such, the research outcome did not appear to warrant the risks. The quality of the informed consent obtained could also be called into question, since the investigators very probably did not disclose the results of some animal model experiments, which affects the accuracy of communicating the full risks and benefits of participation. It is difficult to imagine that many patients would have agreed to the experiment if they knew what happened to the rabbits. The fact that these issues were not flagged by the research ethics committee leads one to believe that either there was a failure to adequately screen the study or the investigators did not provide

all of the scientific information available on safety and efficacy – or both.

Moreover, even with such issues, the journal in which the research was published could not resist the desire to publish the findings given the lack of negative outcomes and the parallel publication from an unconnected source of a well-designed animal model that, in some aspects, paralleled the experiment involving human subjects. While the journal did include an editorial accompanying publication of the article that outlined the ethical dilemmas in which the editors found themselves in, it does raise the question of whether publishing the results will have the effect of making it easier to justify other cases of publishing unethical research results. The Helsinki Declaration[4] requires that medical research must conform to prior "… adequate laboratory and animal experimentation…" and that "[r]eports of research not in accordance with the principles of this Declaration should not be accepted for publication". (For more on publication ethics, see Chapter 35.)

This example is also illustrative of an issue that frequently occurs in clinical anesthesiology research directed at symptom management (e.g., pain, anxiety, nausea), for which adequate, if not perfect, treatments already exist. That is, that this study exposed its subjects to potential adverse neurologic consequences for minimal gain in an area that already has significant proven treatments. When undertaking this kind of research, investigators should be able to demonstrate that there is no reasonable alternative therapy or methodology that would eliminate or mitigate the risks associated with participating in the research study. (See also Chapter 32.) While we must be vigilant against the increased risk of harm associated with participating in research, it must also be recognized that such risks include being exposed to untested or unevaluated medical interventions.[5]

While research ethics is a large area with many interesting and complex issues, this chapter has only been able to touch on some of the main ethical concerns associated with clinical anesthesiology research. Researchers are encouraged to apply, and interpret, existing ethical guidance to research design and conduct, as well as to do further research and reading on issues in which they want more in-depth information and analysis. In addition to the ethical issues discussed here, it is very important that professional, institutional and legal requirements concerning research with human subjects within your jurisdiction are adhered to, and respected.

Key points

- Research studies involving human subjects should be based on a thorough knowledge of the scientific literature, and should address questions of sufficient importance to warrant the risks.
- All research should be reviewed by relevant research committees for guidance and approval.
- Informed consent should be obtained from subjects, without undue inducements, duress or coercion.
- Subjects should be given sufficient time to reflect on the information they are given about the research study.
- Decisions not to participate or to withdraw from a study should never affect the quality or level of a patient's care.
- Conflicts of interest on the part of the researcher should be avoided or mitigated, and where they exist be disclosed to subjects.
- Both positive and negative results of the research should be disseminated.
- Particular care should be given when research is directed at conditions for which adequate, if imperfect, treatments already exist.

References

1* Committee on Bioethics (1999). *Guidelines on the Ethics of Clinical Research in Anesthesia*. Toronto: Canadian Anesthesiologists' Society.

2* King, N.M.P. and Churchill, L. (2008). Clinical research and the physician-patient relationship: the dual roles of physician and researcher. In *The Cambridge Textbook of Bioethics*. Singer, P.A. and Viens, A.M., eds. Cambridge, UK: Cambridge University Press, pp. 214–21.

3* Lemmens, T. and Luther, L. (2008). Financial conflicts of interest in medical research. In *The Cambridge Textbook of Bioethics*. Singer, P.A. and Viens, A.M., eds. Cambridge, UK: Cambridge University Press, pp. 222–30.

4* World Medical Association. (2008) *Declaration of Helsinki: Ethical Principles for Medical Research Involving Human Subjects*. Washington: World Medical Association.

5* Ashcroft, R.A. and Viens, A.M. Clinical Trials. In *The Cambridge Textbook of Bioethics*. Singer, P.A. and Viens, A.M., eds. Cambridge, UK: Cambridge University Press, pp. 201–6.

Further reading

Beauhamp, T.L. and Childress, J.F. (2001). *Principles of Biomedical Ethics*, 5th edn. New York, NY: Oxford University Press

CIOMS (2002). *International Ethical Guidelines for Biomedical Research Involving Human Subjects*. Geneva: Council for International Organisations of Medical Sciences.

Faden, R. and Beachamp, T.L. (1986). *A History and Theory of Informed Consent*. New York, NY: Oxford University Press.

Freedman, B. (1987). Scientific value and validity as ethical requirements for research: a proposed explanation. *IRB, Rev Hum Subj Res* **17**, 7–10.

Maltby, J.R. and Eagle, C. J. (1993). Informed consent for clinical anaesthesia research. *Can J Anaesth*, **40**, 891–6.

Levine, R.J. (1988). *Ethics and Regulation of Clinical Research*. New Haven, CT: Yale University Press.

Slowther, A. and Kleinman, I. (2008). Confidentiality. In: Singer P.A. and Viens, A.M., eds. *The Cambridge Textbook of Bioethics*. Cambridge, UK: Cambridge University Press. pp. 43–8.

Sykes, K. and Bunker, J., eds. (2007). *Anaesthesia and the Practice of Medicine: Historical Perspectives*. London: Royal Society of Medicine Press.

28

Animal subjects research Part I: Do animals have rights?

Nancy S. Jecker

The Case of Laika

In 1957, a stray dog from Moscow named Laika, described by her keepers as "quiet and charming," became the first animal to orbit the planet, and the first death in orbit. Training for her mission included subjection to confinement in progressively smaller cages for up to 20 consecutive days, during which she was whining and restless and would stop urinating or defecating for prolonged periods of time. She was placed in centrifuges simulating rocket acceleration and the noises of the spacecraft, causing extreme changes in her blood pressure and pulse. On the day before her mission, Dr. Vladimir Yazdovsky took her home to play with his children. He later said, "I wanted to do something nice for her: she had so little time left to live."[1]

In the capsule, she was confined by a harness that allowed her only to sit, stand and lie down in one place. A launch pad malfunction kept her waiting for 3 days in freezing temperatures inside a capsule the size of a washing machine before she was launched into orbit. Although it was reported at the time that Laika lived for 7 days in space and was then was mercifully euthanized with a pre-programmed portion of poisoned food, in 2002 it was revealed that she had, in fact, died only a few hours into orbit as a result of broiling heat due to a thermo-regulator failure.[2] In 1998, Oleg Gazenko, one of the scientists involved, expressed his regret:

> "Work with animals is a source of suffering to all of us … The more time passes, the more I'm sorry about it. We shouldn't have done it. We did not learn enough from this mission to justify the death of the dog."[3]

The case of Laika, and other cases involving the use of animals to serve human ends, raise moral questions such as the following. Is there something distinctive about humanity? Do humans have a special moral status that nonhumans lack? Is there a quality that human beings alone possess that qualifies them for higher moral standing? If not, should we broaden our conception of who is a member of our moral community? If it is sometimes acceptable to use animals in research, when it would not be acceptable to use human beings, and what accounts for this difference?

In this chapter we consider what it means to say that a being deserves moral consideration. We ask what it means to say that a being has a right to life. We then consider the claim that, even if a being *lacks* a right to life, it deserves to have its interests taken into account. Finally, we consider the application of these ideas to research with animals.

Human beings, animals, and persons

Throughout this discussion the term, "person," refers to *any living being of any species* whose characteristics entitle it to a right to life. Thus the term "person," as defined here, is a moral or ethical term, not a biological one, and quite distinct from the term "human being."

The term, "human being," refers to anything that is biologically alive and belongs to the species, *Homo sapiens*. In this definition, the term "human being" obviously includes normal human children and adults, but also includes prenatal human life, human beings with physical or mental abnormalities, and humans in a persistent vegetative state who will never regain consciousness.

To assume that only instances of human life could count as persons in a moral sense, and so possess a right to life, would be a moral error analogous to claiming that only members of favored racial groups possess certain rights or are persons. The latter mistake is called racism; the former might thus be called speciesism. To avoid this mistake, we cannot assume membership in a species represents a necessary or sufficient condition for personhood, but must instead identify a quality independent of species that establishes personhood.

In many cases most agree about who is and is not a person. For example, normal adult human beings

Clinical Ethics in Anesthesiology: A Case-Based Textbook, ed. Gail A. Van Norman, Stephen Jackson, Stanley H. Rosenbaum and Susan K. Palmer. Published by Cambridge University Press. © Cambridge University Press 2011.

are considered to be the sort of beings of whom personhood can be predicated. Many will also agree that certain living things are not persons. For instance, there is not widespread belief that trees are persons. That is not to say that we ought not to take good care of trees. Saying that trees are not persons is merely saying that trees do not have a right to life, nor are trees entitled for their own sake to have their lives preserved.

In-between the cases of trees and normal human beings, is a spectrum of less obvious cases. Do permanently unconscious human beings, human fetuses, human beings who will live in the distant future, or intelligent life that we might encounter on other planets qualify as persons? What about members of other terrestrial species? Are nonhumans animals, such as dogs, chimpanzees, or dolphins, persons?

To focus on the specific question of whether personhood applies to nonhuman animals (henceforth referred to simply as "animals") here on earth, let us consider three distinct views one might hold. First, what we shall call a *conservative* position claims that no animals are persons with a right to life. A second, *moderate* position asserts that at least some animals deserve moral consideration for their own sake, but no animals have a right to life. A third view, which we shall call a *liberal* view, holds that at least some animals are persons with a right to life.

Are animals "persons"?

The "conservative" view

Perhaps the best known proponent of the conservative position is Immanuel Kant. Kant believed that human beings alone qualify as persons by virtue of their rational capacities. He wrote:

> … every rational being, exists as an end in himself and not merely as a means to be arbitrarily used by this or that will…Beings whose existence depends not on our will but on nature have, nevertheless, if they are not rational beings, only a relative value as means and are therefore called things.[4]

For Kant, humanity had an intrinsic and unconditional value. By contrast, animals had only a relative or instrumental value. Elaborating this position in "Duties to Animals and Spirits," Kant stated:

> … if a man shoots his dog because the animal is no longer capable of service, he does not fail in his duty to the dog,…but his act is inhuman and damages in himself that humanity which it is his duty to show towards mankind."[4]

Kant understood our duties to human beings as *direct duties*, but regarded our duties to animals as *indirect duties*. *Direct duties* are duties we owe someone for their own sake. Indirect duties are duties we owe to someone for the sake of someone else. For instance, if a child is cruel to animals by pinching a cat's tail, Kant's worry was that the child may go on to develop a corresponding sentiment of cruelty to humans, and may treat humans cruelly too. The reason that it is wrong for a child to pinch the tail of an animal, according to Kant, is that doing so will ultimately harm human beings, who matter morally for their own sake. Thus, the child has a duty to the cat for the sake of her fellow human beings.

The philosophical basis for the above distinction is Kant's idea that human beings, by virtue of their rational agency, are persons and possess intrinsic moral worth. Kant's position is not speciesist, because the ultimate basis for the dignity of human beings is not species membership, *per se*, but rational nature. As Wood notes, "Kant thought it quite likely that there are rational beings on other planets; they would be ends in themselves every bit as much as human beings …"[5]

It follows from Kant's philosophy that we should not cause suffering to animals, for example, by performing painful experiments "for the sake of mere speculation, when the end could also be achieved without these."[6] However, Kant thought that we do have a right to kill animals, provided we do not cause pain and suffering or kill merely for sport. Kant encouraged the humane treatment of animals who work for us, as well as gratitude. In his lectures, he told a story about the philosopher, Leibniz, who reportedly returns a worm to its leaf when done examining it.[7] For Kant, this exemplified the attitude humans should cultivate toward animals.

Despite the fact that Kant's philosophy encourages the humane treatment of animals, critics charge that it gives insufficient regard to animals. Allen Wood maintains that, by virtue of the fact that animals are not persons in Kant's approach, we are permitted to treat animals solely as instruments or objects of human goals. To illustrate this, he asks us to imagine the following possibility:

> If it happened to be a quirk of human psychology that torturing animals would make us that much kinder toward humans (perhaps by venting our aggressive impulses on helpless victims), then Kant's argument

would apparently make it a duty to inflict gratuitous cruelty on puppies and kittens so as to make us that much kinder to people.[8]

If Wood's reasoning is correct, then even though Kant himself rejects cruelty to animals, his philosophy still allows this possibility.

In response, defenders of Kant's approach can argue that it is inconsistent with Kantian ethics to treat animals as mere things for our use or enjoyment. Kantian philosophy, as they interpret it, emphasizes our positive duties *with regard* to animals, even if we have no duties *toward* them. O'Neill, for example, argues that the fact that Kant's allowance for indirect duties to animals is not trivial, because "Kant endorses more or less the range of ethical concern for non-human animals that more traditional utilitarians allowed: welfare, but not rights."[9]

Contemporary Kantian scholars further develop Kant's conservative position in a variety of ways. Christine Korsgaard proposes that what distinguishes humans is their capacity for a special sort of rationality. Humans alone use reason to reflect about *morality*, to be what Korsgaard calls "sources of normativity."[10] Humans alone face the *problem* of normativity: the problem of considering the morality of their reasons for acting and deciding what they ought to do. According to Korsgaard,

> We human animals turn our attention on to our perceptions and desires themselves, on to our own mental activities, and we are conscious *of* them. That is why we can think *about* them … And this sets us a problem that no other animal has. It is the problem of the normative… The reflective mind cannot settle for perception and desire, not just as such. It needs a reason.[7]

While some animals act on reasons, Korsgaard insists that only humans act on *normative* reasons. Korsgaard believes a capacity to consider the moral basis for action is a necessary feature of moral personhood that humans have and that animals lack. She concludes that animals on earth are not the kind of beings for whom personhood is possible.

The "liberal" view

In contrast to conservatives, both moderates and liberals argue that animals deserve moral consideration in their own right. They claim that many morally important qualities, such as rationality, exist in some intelligent animals. Singer and Cavalieri hold that apes display many fragments of the forms of

rationality that we find in humans.[11] Moreover, some human beings *lack* rationality and the corresponding ability to morally evaluate their reasons for acting. Human infants are potentially, but not actually, rational; permanently unconscious human beings lack rationality altogether; and humans with certain forms of dementia or mental retardation may possess only fragments of rationality. In all of these cases, human beings cannot be what Korsgaard calls "sources of normativity." Many moderates and liberals conclude that, if rationality in some form is a necessary and sufficient condition for personhood, then at least some humans are not persons, and at least some animals are persons.

If personhood and humanity are not coextensive, this creates an opportunity to explore the possibility that animals possess a right to life – the position favored by liberals. One way this position is defended is to underscore the idea that there is no criterion that all humans *possess* and all animals *lack* that is a necessary requirement for personhood. Tom Regan, for example, states the general argument in support of a conservative stance looks like this:

The conservative argument

(1) For X to be a person, X must have A.
(2) Humans have A.
(3) Animals do not have A.
(4) Therefore, humans are persons and animals are not.[12]

Regan rebuts the conservative argument by showing that there is no quality, A, that can be used in the premises of this argument to establish the argument's conclusion. For example, suppose the conservative proposes that the quality most essential for personhood is sentience. Regan's reply would be that some humans, such as those in a persistent vegetative state, lack sentience, while many animals have it. Or, suppose a conservative proposes instead that possessing a concept of self is essential for personhood. Regan's reply would be to call attention to the fact that this quality is inadequate, since some human beings, such as infants and those with profound mental retardation, lack a concept of self. Likewise, if the quality considered fundamental to personhood is possession of positive interests, such as desires, goals, hopes, and preferences, Regan would point out that there are humans who lack these qualities and animals who have them.

Regan concludes that at least some animals *satisfy* whatever criterion one might advance as a necessary condition for personhood, and at least some human beings *fail to satisfy* it. In other words, there is no A which is non-arbitrary and such that all humans possess A and no animals possess A. Therefore, it is inconsistent to believe that all and only humans possess a right to life. Regan says we must therefore choose between two options:

(1) Deny a right to life to both animals and defective humans, or

(2) Grant a right to life to both animals and defective humans.

Regan himself endorses the latter option, granting a right to life to *both* animals and impaired human beings. However, it would seem that to ethically justify current practices, such as using animals in biomedical research or consuming meat, we would be forced to choose the former option: deny both animals and impaired human beings a right to life. Yet, if we choose this option, we are left with the question of how we can ethically justify a requirement to treat impaired humans better than animals. The conclusion Regan and other liberals draw is that, to avoid this consequence, we should predicate personhood of impaired human beings, and also acknowledge that at least some animals are persons as well.

Both the conservative and liberal positions represent a "deontological" approach to ethics. Deontological approaches hold that there are certain overriding moral principles or duties that apply irrespective of whether fulfilling their requirements is burdensome or produces the best consequences overall. If the basis of our duties to humans or animals is *rights*, then we must discharge our duties regardless of whether doing so is convenient or promotes the general happiness. According to a rights-based liberal view, any practice that fails to respect the rights of those animals who possess them is wrong. So if we eat, hunt, experiment on, or use animals for entertainment, this is wrong if the animals in question have a right to life, even if it produces a tremendous amount of benefit for others. Likewise, if all human beings are persons with a right to life, as conservatives claim, then there is no condition where we would be justified in sacrificing a human life in order to bring about the greater good for society at large.

The "moderate" view

Let us set aside the question of whether animals are persons with a right to life, and turn to consider a different question, namely: is it wrong to cause animals to suffer? Peter Singer thinks that, regardless of where one comes down on the question of whether animals have rights, they have *interests*,[13] specifically, an interest in avoiding suffering. According to Singer, it is wrong to eat meat given modern methods of meat production or to use animals in scientific research for trivial purposes, because of the interest animals have in avoiding suffering. Thus, according to Singer, the *moderate position* is sufficient to establish that we must bring animals into our sphere of moral concern. Even if it is sometimes acceptable to use animals or to end their lives painlessly, many of our current practices would have to change if the moderate position is correct.

In support of this approach, Singer advances the following *Principle of Equal Consideration*:

> The interests of every being must be given equal consideration, in proportion to their degree of seriousness for the being in question.

This principle begins with the idea of having an *interest*. According to Singer, the capacity for suffering or enjoyment is sufficient to establish that a being has an interest. A cat or dog, for example, suffers terribly if it is picked up by its tail and thrown across the room, and so it has a clear interest in avoiding this. Similarly, some experiments subject animals to pain, stress, anxiety, illness, and other forms of suffering. Without a doubt, animals have an interest in avoiding suffering produced in this way.

But there is a difference between *equal consideration* and *equal treatment*. In fact, equal consideration for the interests of humans and animals might require very different treatment. Consideration for the interests of a pig might require no more than that we leave a pig with other pigs in a place where there is adequate food and room to run freely, whereas concern for the interests of a child growing up in America might require that we teach the child to read.

In some cases, the greater mental power of normal adults will mean that they will suffer more. They will anticipate suffering, remember it, and have a fuller idea of their predicament. In other cases, the greater mental powers of normal adults will mean that they suffer less. As Singer notes, prisoners during wartime are able to understand that:

> although they must submit to capture, search, and confinement, they will not otherwise be harmed and will be set free at the conclusion of hostilities. If we capture wild animals, however, we cannot explain that we are not threatening their lives.[10]

Singer draws on these ideas to develop the following argument against certain forms of animal experimentation.

(1) The interests of every being must be given equal consideration, in proportion to their degree of seriousness for the being in question.

(2) Animals have a very serious interest in avoiding suffering and in being able to live in a way that allows their instinctive desires and drives to be satisfied.

(3) Animal research causes serious suffering and does not permit animals to satisfy instinctive desires and drives.

(4) A great deal of animal research satisfies no direct or urgent purpose, or satisfies only relatively minor human interests.

(5) Therefore, continuing with a great deal of animal research involves weighting relatively minor human interests above very serious interests of the animals in question, and hence is morally unacceptable.

(6) In many cases, it is not possible to conduct these experiments without using the sorts of methods which are objectionable.

(7) Therefore, *in many cases*, we should end current animal research.

Note that Singer's argument does not conclude with an absolute probation against inflicting pain and suffering on animals. Nor does it ban experiments that result in the painless death of animals. Singer is not saying that all experimenting on animals ought to stop immediately. Instead, the argument establishes that the suffering of animals must be taken seriously and justified by the positive benefits it helps to bring about. It is consistent with this argument to allow experimenting on animals in situations where the trade-offs justify the pain and suffering inflicted. As Singer notes, "We have still not answered the question of when an experiment might be justifiable. It will not do to say 'Never!' Putting morality in such black and white terms is appealing, because it eliminates the need to think about particular cases; but in extreme circumstances, such absolutist answers always break down." Singer proposes that a good test of whether an experiment is ethically justified is to consider whether or not we would consider conducting it on humans who are impaired and have a mental life similar to the animal we are proposing to use. For Singer, the ethically crucial requirement is that

our actions produce as much pleasure and happiness and as little pain and misery as possible for all beings that have the capacity to experience happiness and misery.

The general structure of Singer's argument can be applied in many other areas. For example, Singer advances a similar argument in support of taking seriously the suffering of animals used in modern methods of meat production. As in the argument about using animals in experiments, Singer is not putting forth an absolutist conclusion. Rather than supporting strict vegetarianism, he allows for the possibility that eating meat is sometimes morally acceptable. For example, it is permissible to consume meat when a wild animal that is painlessly killed is eaten by people who would otherwise suffer hunger.

Opponents of Singer's moderate position argue that the position entails consequences we are not willing to accept. One such consequence is that, just as we are sometimes ethically allowed to eat animals, or to end the lives of animals painlessly in a medical experiment, so too we would sometimes be ethically allowed to eat humans for meat or to end their lives painlessly in a medical experiment. This objection to Singer holds that by failing to recognize the inviolability of the moral claims of all morally considerable beings, "utilitarianism cannot accommodate one of our most basic prima facie principles, namely that killing a morally considerable being is wrong."[14]

In contrast to a conservative or liberal position, a moderate position is vulnerable to such an objection precisely because it does not ascribe a right to life to humans or animals. Thus, for a moderate, such as Singer, our duties to other beings, whether human beings or animals, depend on what competing interests happen to be at stake in any given situation.

In contrast to the deontological approaches of Kant and Regan, Singer's approach is an example of a consequentialist view. Consequentialist arguments hold that the moral worth of our actions is measured solely by the consequences they produce, not by their conformity to an overarching principle or duty. For this reason, Singer can say, for example, that:

> Torturing a human being is almost always wrong, but it is not absolutely wrong. If torture were the only way in which we could discover the location of a nuclear bomb hidden in a New York City basement and timed to go off within the hour, then torture would be justifiable.[13]

Likewise, experimenting on brain-damaged human beings will almost never be justified, but under rare circumstances could be.

Key points

- There are three distinct answers one might give to the question, is there anything morally distinctive about humanity?
- The "conservative" answer: humans alone have moral standing and a right to life.
- The "liberal" approach: some animals possess qualities that conservatives equate with moral standing and "personhood," and some human beings lack those qualities.
- The "moderate" view: what is morally important about humans and animals is their capacity to suffer; both humans and animals have an interest in avoiding suffering.
- For moderates, the moral acceptability of animal research depends on the balance of the suffering produced weighed against the importance of the interests the research serves: when animal research serves relatively minor, indirect, or nonurgent interests, but causes serious suffering, it is morally unacceptable.
- Both liberals and conservatives hold that there are absolute prohibitions against harming "persons" or treating them as a means only; these apply regardless of whether abiding by such prohibitions produces the best consequences overall.
- For both liberals and conservatives the moral acceptability of research with animals or human beings depends on whether or not the subjects of research are persons with a right to life.

References

1   Isachenkov, V. Space Dog Monument Opens in Russia. AP Moscow. Friday April 11, 2008 http://www.msnbc.msn.com/id/24069819/.

2   Whitehouse, D. First Dog in Space Died Within Hours. BBC News, World Edition. Monday 28 October 2002, 10:34 GMT. http://news.bbc.co.uk/.

3   Oleg Gazenko, speaking at a Moscow news conference in 1998.

4   Kant, I. (1998). *The Groundwork for the Metaphysics of Morals*, Mary J. Gregor (trans.), Cambridge, UK: Cambridge University Press, p. 428

5   Wood, A. (1998). Kant on duties regarding nonrational nature I. *Proceedings of the Aristotelian Society Suppl.* **72**, 189–210 at 189.

6   Kant, I. (1996). *Metaphysics of Morals*, Gregor, M., ed., transl. Cambridge, UK: Cambridge University Press, p. 193.

7* Kant, I. (1997). *Lectures on Ethics*, transl. by P. Health; Health, P. and Schneewind, J., eds. New York: Cambridge University Press, pp. 212–13.

8   Wood, A. (1998). Kant on duties regarding nonrational nature I. *Proceedings of the Aristotelian Society Suppl*, **72** (sup plement), 189–210 at 194–5.

9   O'Neill and Kant O. on duties regarding nonrational nature II. *Proceedings of the Aristotelian Society Suppl*, **72**, 211–228, at 223.

10* Korsgaard, C. (2005). Fellow creatures: Kantian ethics and our duties to animals. *The Tanner Lectures on Human Values*, **25**, 77–110.

11 Singer, P. and Cavalieri, P. (1993). *The Great Ape Project*. Fourth Estate, London, discussed in O'Neill O. Kant on Duties Regarding Nonrational Nature II. *Proceedings of the Aristotelian Society*, **72 (suppl)**, 211–228 at 224.

12* Regan, T. (1976). Do animals have a right to life? In *Animal Rights and Human Obligations*. Regan, T. and Singer, P., eds. New Jersey: Englewood Cliffs, pp. 197–204.

13* Singer, P. (2009). *Animal Liberation, updated edition*. New York: Harper Collins.

14 The moral status of animals. *Stanford Encyclopedia of Philosophy*. Accessed http://plato.stanford.edu/entries/moral-animal/ (Accessed March 8, 2009).

Further reading

Kant, I. (1963) Duties to animals and spirits. In Kant I, *Lectures on Ehics,* transl. by L. Infield. New York: Hackett Publishing Company, p. 240.

Research and publication

Animal subjects research Part II: Ethics of animal experimentation

Gail A. Van Norman

The Case

Fifty hemophilic mice are anesthetized with an intraperitoneal injection of ketamine (which kills six mice), followed by blunt force trauma to a knee joint in half of the survivors. Post-trauma analgesics are administered only on day 0 and 1 following knee trauma. Two days later, and every 2–4 days thereafter, all mice are placed on a rotating rod and forced to ambulate until they fall off. Blunt trauma is administered in the test group weekly, and the process repeated. After 4 weeks, all mice are killed to examine their joints. The authors conclude that joint trauma and hemarthrosis leads to problems with ambulation and hemophilic synovitis – "consistent with clinical experience."[1]

The editors of the journal in which this experiment appeared commented that the manuscript "proved challenging on review," citing obligations of journal editors to assure that investigators minimize animal pain and suffering. One reviewer points out that progressive joint functional limitation is well known in human patients with hemophilia, particularly following trauma associated with hemarthrosis. He also raises concerns about animal suffering, pointing out that, although they were given analgesia for a brief period following acute trauma, the mice were forced thereafter to ambulate on traumatized joints without analgesia.[2] Mice in the test group lost weight, limped, and fell off the rotating rod more quickly, all of which might be signs of pain and suffering that went untreated.

Nonhuman animals are used as subjects in research experiments, as test subjects for industries, and as objects for dissection and instruction in science classrooms – a subject of intense moral dispute. Most reviews addressing the ethics of animal research describe this debate as a war of wills between scientists and animal rights activists. Extremism on both fronts garners media attention. Leading scientists, and even some ethicists to insist that there is "no consensus" about the appropriate use of, and treatment of animals in testing, education, and research. But this is a distorted and misleading perspective. Specific moral

frameworks regarding the use of animals by humans are evolving; nevertheless, there *is* moral, scientific, and public consensus about animals in research. It is likely that this consensus will evolve as our understanding of nonhuman animals deepens – their experiences, intelligence, and capacities for suffering, pain, and enjoyment. But it is imperative that every physician and researcher who uses animals in teaching, testing, and/ or experimentation understands that they have explicit ethical obligations to their animal subjects.

Moral justifications of animal research

At its heart, the debate over the use of animals in research is centered on a single moral question: are humans *morally justified* in using animals in this way? Ethical arguments favoring animal experimentation generally fall into two categories: (1) humans have higher moral standing than animals and have a right to use animals in experiments that better human lives, and (2) the benefits of animal experimentation outweigh the harms, and that animal experimentation is sometimes the only way in which science can answer important questions necessary to human well-being.

The moral standing of humans versus animals

Western culture is heavily imbued with Judeo-Christian traditions, in which animal interests are subordinate to those of humans. Earth and its contents were bequeathed by a Creator to humankind to benefit humans. This view is still prominent among conservative Judeo-Christian leaders:

> "The animal rights movement can best be understood by viewing it as an attempt to undo the opening chapters of the biblical Book of Genesis." [3]

In the last 50 years, detrimental effects of human populations on the environment have begun to threaten global repercussions. The views of conservative

---

Clinical Ethics in Anesthesiology: A Case-Based Textbook, ed. Gail A. Van Norman, Stephen Jackson, Stanley H. Rosenbaum and Susan K. Palmer. Published by Cambridge University Press. © Cambridge University Press 2011.

Judeo-Christian philosophers toward man's relationship with the planet and nonhuman animals have begun to shift in response, but still describe the ethical obligations of humans in the utilitarian framework of serving the ultimate interests of mankind – i.e., we should take care of the environment and animals because, if we don't, it will lead to depletion of resources and jeopardize the future of human existence.

Many twentieth-century religious scholars were challenged to reconcile new scientific theories and evidence (e.g., the theory of evolution and the fossil record supporting it) with mainstream theology. Pierre Teilhard de Chardin, a Jesuit priest and paleontologist, argued that, in parallel with biological evolution, humans are a part of a continuum in a "spiritual evolution" that also includes plants and animals.[4] Breaking down bright theological lines between animals and humans begs the question of whether our relationship with animals should really be viewed only through a utilitarian glass. Are we allowed to treat animals in ways that only promote human interests? Or do they have legitimate "interests" of their own? (For more discussion of ethical arguments regarding animal interests and rights, see Chapter 28.)

Are humans and nonhuman animals fundamentally different?

Up until the mid-to-late twentieth century, Western biologists operated under a "Cartesian" paradigm that attributed minimal, if any, intelligence to nonhuman species. Reasoning, emotions, and suffering were believed to be uniquely human attributes – animals were merely pre-programmed, instinct-driven robots that did not have moral standing.

> "They eat without pleasure, cry without pain, grow without knowing it; they desire nothing, fear nothing, know nothing."[5]

Current research demonstrates unequivocally that, far from being simple bundles of instinctual programming, the intellectual abilities of animals parallel that of humans in many startling ways. The manufacture and use of tools, long held to be a uniquely human ability, is now well described in nonprimate and even non-mammalian species.[6] Animals demonstrate "culture," in which uniquely individual and adaptive behaviors are passed within social groups by observation and mimicry, and not by instinct or genetic programming.[7] The great apes appear to be capable of learning and using symbolic language, an important marker of abstract thinking.[8] Meadow voles demonstrate

"episodic recall," believed to be an important marker of sentience.[9] Whales and dolphins understand symbolic representations and have self-awareness,[10] which has also been demonstrated in primates, elephants,[11] and magpies.[12]

Why have animal researchers been slow to acknowledge these critical similarities with humans? Zoologist Frans de Waal proposes that "Our culture and dominant religion have tied human dignity and self-worth to our separation from nature and distinctness from other animals." This cultural bias, he argues, keeps scientists from recognizing how similar humans and other animals really are, and thereby weakening arguments of human moral superiority.[13]

Bioethicist Bernard Rollin suggests that scientists now have an "ideology" of their own, in which they assert that science is "objective" and not burdened by moral values. "The bottom line," he says, is the belief that "science might provide society with the facts relevant to making moral decisions, but it steers clear of any ethical debate."[14] But if it were true that there is no moral dimension to scientific endeavor, then there would be no need to argue that animal experimentation is permissible, nor that cruel experimentation on human subjects must be disallowed because it violates moral principles. Almost any experiment that simply produced new information would be allowed under such an ideology, without regard for treatment of any of its subjects, human or animal. The idea that medical research is immune from moral consideration has long been discredited, as exemplified in the Doctor's Trial at Nuremberg after World War II.

Most bioethicists concede that many animals have at least some moral standing, although *which* animals and *how much* moral standing are unclear. Deliberately causing an animal to suffer due to pain, fear, starvation, illness, or poor conditions of care constitutes a moral harm to be prevented or mitigated, and considered carefully against the benefits such conditions might produce. Apart from any consideration of animal "rights," many ethicists propose that cruelty to animals should still be discouraged, because it is likely that those who are cruel to animals will be cruel to humans as well.

Assessing the benefits of animal research

There is no doubt that animal experimentation has contributed to advances in anesthesia, cardiovascular and orthopedic surgery, treatment of such diseases as diabetes and hemophilia, vaccines, antimicrobial agents, cancer therapy, treatment protocols for trauma and shock, and many other areas. Yet is it simply not sensible to assert that medical science would have come to a complete halt without animal experimentation. As Harold Hewitt, himself an animal researcher, points out:

> 'It underrates the ingenuity of researchers to assert that medical progress would have been seriously impeded had animal experiments been illegal, although a different strategy would have been required. It is the skill of the scientist to find a way around the intellectual, technical and ethical limits to investigation. No one complains, surely that we have been denied the benefit of potential advances by prohibiting experiments on unsuspecting patients, criminals or idiots.[15]

The contributions of animal experimentation to human medicine may also be greatly over-estimated. Critical analysis of the quality of animal experimentation leads to disturbing conclusions. A systematic review of animal experiments in fluid resuscitation, for example, found that many studies were fraught with poor design, were statistically underpowered, showed evidence of publication bias, and were seldom subjected to cross-species analysis or meta-analysis to determine if the results were even applicable to humans.[16] Animal trials have been frequently conducted simultaneously with human trials, and were thus superfluous. They often set out to answer questions that had already been answered or could have been answered by a systematic review of existing studies.[17] Historically, animal experimentation has, at times, been frankly misleading. It probably actually impeded such endeavors as developing the polio vaccine; understanding the role of asbestos exposure and lung disease; understanding the connections between tobacco smoke and lung cancer; and in developing other cancer treatments.[18]

An analysis of 76 animal studies cited in seven prominent scientific journals found that almost half were never subsequently tested in human trials. Of those that had been tested in humans, 18% were contradicted in the humans. Only 37% were eventually confirmed in human studies. Almost two-thirds of animal studies were *not* confirmed by testing in humans, and did not result in any human benefit.[19] Another review of 221 experiments involving over 7000 animals found that results were in agreement with human studies in only 50% of cases. The authors found that basic methodological errors, such as lack of randomization and blinding, poor sample size, and publication bias probably contributed to poor concordance with human studies.[20] In the words of physician R. Burns, "As

physicians, researchers, and educators, we must take a long-overdue objective look at how and why we use animals in research and education. A great deal of animal-based research adds very little to our understanding of the diagnosis and treatment of our patients."[21]

How many animals are used in research and testing laboratories? According to the United States Department of Agriculture (USDA), the use of "reportable" animals in research has declined steadily, from over 2 million animals in 1992, to just over 1 million in 2007.[22] Because a 2002 amendment to the Animal Welfare Act (AWA) exempted laboratories from reporting research on birds, rats, and mice, USDA statistics only reflect the use of cats, dogs, hamsters, rabbits, guinea pigs, primates, and farm animals. Rats and mice are estimated to comprise approximately 95% of laboratory animals in research, and it is estimated that over 20 million animals are actually experimented on every year in the US.[23] In 2007, about half of the *reported* experiments produced pain in the subjects, and almost 80 000 animals were subjected to pain without analgesia. An accurate number regarding how many "exempted" animals are subjected to untreated pain during research protocols is unavailable, but presumed to be in the millions.

According to the Home Office of Great Britain, approximately 3.7 million procedures were done on animals – including all vertebrates and one species of octopus – in research in the UK in 2008 that was deemed "likely to cause pain, suffering, distress, or lasting harm." In only about 35% of procedures was some form of anesthesia or analgesia used.[24]

Public perceptions and public consensus

Scientists rightfully point out that research based solely on tissue cultures and cell lines may not accurately mimic conditions found in a human being. Many tests felt to be essential to human health, such as testing drugs and chemicals for teratogenic potential, do not currently have reasonable alternatives to animal testing and pose too high a risk for human testing. Would we be willing to give up important health protections for human beings in order to eliminate animal research entirely?

A 2008 US poll found that public concern about treatment of animals is significant; all but 3% believe that animals require protection, and a startling 25% believed that animals should have the *exact same rights as humans* to be free from harm and exploitation. A significant portion of respondents (35%) would ban all medical research on animals, and 39% would ban all product testing on animals.[25] In a 2007 poll, 37% rated medical testing on animals as "morally wrong."[26] A 1994 comparison of public opinion regarding animal research across 15 nations indicates that opposition to any research that causes pain or injury to animal subjects is common globally – ranging from about 35% in Portugal to almost 70% in France.[27]

The three Rs

In 1954 William Russell, a zoologist and classical scholar, and Rex Burch, a microbiologist, were appointed by the Universities Federation for Animal Welfare in the UK to systematically study the ethical aspects of laboratory research. The result was the seminal publication of *The Principles of Humane Experimental Technique* in 1959.[28] They stated that "the humanest possible treatment of experimental animals, far from being an obstacle, is actually a prerequisite for successful animal experimentation." In fact, as J. Edward Gates from the University of Maryland observes, "Pain and stress adds an uncontrollable variable into an experiment, and so it is in the interest of good science to control pain and distress whenever possible."[29]

Russell and Burch introduced the "3 Rs" of humane experimentation. These principles were: (1) *replacement* of animal subjects whenever possible with other methodologies, human volunteers, or computer modeling; (2) *reduction* of animal use by using fewer animals or obtaining more information from the same number of animals; and (3) *refinement* by improving scientific procedures and husbandry to minimize actual or potential pain, suffering, distress, or lasting harm, and increase animal welfare when animal use is unavoidable. These principles now form the bedrock of ethical animal use in laboratory research.

Current issues

Most Western nations now have laws regulating the treatment of animals in research and industry testing. In the US, federal legislation includes the AWA, initially passed in 1966. The Health Extension Act in 1985 and amendments to the AWA required the establishment of Institutional Animal Care and Use Committees (IACUCs), to oversee conditions of laboratory animals, review and approve animal research protocols, and educate and train investigators in ethical issues and aspects of animal handling such as anesthesia, analgesia, and euthanasia. In Great Britain, the Animals (Scientific

Procedures) Act of 1986 (ASPA) regulates experimentation that might cause "pain, distress, suffering or lasting harm" to any vertebrate animal (and one species of octopus).[30] In 1999, the UK introduced ethical review of scientific research involving living animals through local ethical review committees. In the European Union (EU), agreement on the protection of animals in research was codified in the 1986 European convention for the Protection of Animals used for Experimental and Other Scientific Purposes.[31] Laws and regulations of the US, UK, EU, and others have recognized the "3Rs" as foundational to ethical animal experimentation, and explicitly call for the replacement of animals in scientific research whenever possible.

> 'A research institution that receives money and support from the public is responsible for conducting research according to the limits set by society…the use of animals in research is a *privilege*, and not a *right*. The consensus at this time in the United States is that animals should be treated humanely and that pain and distress should be minimized when animals are used for research or teaching purposes.'[29]

A number of national and international scientific organizations provide information for researchers seeking alternatives to animal experimentation and testing, as well as the use of live animals in education. Several resources may be found in "Further reading" at the end of this chapter.

IACUCs in the US, and ethical review committees in the UK can play a significant role in enforcing the 3Rs, by refusing to approve studies that are poorly designed; are not anticipated to significantly alter existing knowledge; could have been conducted in humans or alternative models; do not use the bare minimum number of animals; and do not provide adequate management of pain and distress. However, there is considerable resistance among IACUC's to becoming reviewers of "scientific merit" rather than simply overseeing animal care.[32] In addition, it is clear that many IACUC members do not have adequate education in ethical issues in animal research and ethical decision-making to perform well as ethics reviewers.[33]

Because publication is an important determinant of research funding, professional promotion, and academic prestige, peer-review journal editors and reviewers have significant power to impact researcher behavior. Yet evidence points to a systematic lack of competent peer-review in animal studies. In an analysis of 271 published animal research studies,[34] only 59% stated the hypothesis they were testing, over 85% did not use randomization or blinding to reduce bias, and 30% did not identify the statistical methods used in analysis. In many, basic information was omitted, such as the total number of animals, and the strain, sex, age, and weights of the animals used – all factors that clearly can affect experimental results.

A study of journal editorial policies among 236 randomly selected English language peer-review journals that publish animal research found that 53% did not have a relevant editorial policy. Of 111 journals that did have policies, only one explicitly mentioned adherence to the 3Rs, and only one had a statement that adherence to their policy was a prerequisite for publication.[35]

Subjecting animal studies to the same strict level of review afforded human subjects studies, and requiring adherence to ethical guidelines as a prerequisite for publication may be important ways to encourage more rigorous research design, and conformation to the principles of replace, reduce, and refine.

Key points

- Mainstream scientific study has now challenged long-held beliefs that animals are fundamentally different than humans in many morally relevant ways.
- Public opinion, scientific communities, and biomedical ethicists agree that researchers have moral obligations to reduce or eliminate animal suffering in research, and to strive to eliminate animal experimentation altogether.
- The 3Rs of animal research ethics: replace, reduce, and refine have been adopted internationally in legislation and regulations regarding animal research.
- Animal researchers have ethical obligations to seek alternative models whenever possible, to design research protocols that use the fewest numbers of animals for meaningful results, and to offer humane care that reduces pain, distress and harm when using animals in research.
- IACUCs have regulatory obligations to review research protocols to assure that redundant, insignificant, or poorly designed research is not allowed.
- Biomedical journals should have established policies regarding publication of animal research, including emphasis on the 3Rs, and pledges not to publish studies that do not meet editorial or humane guidelines.

References

1 Mejia-Carvajal, C., Hakobyan, N., Enockson, C., and Valentino, L.A. (2008). The impact of joint bleeding and synovitis on physical ability and joint function in a murine model of haemophilic synovitis. *Haemophilia*, **15**, 119–26.

2 Berntorp, E. (2008). Protecting the joints of mice and men. *Haemophilia*, **14**, 117–18.

3 Environmental stewardship in the Judeo-Christian tradition: Jewish, Catholic, and Protestant Wisdom on the Environment. Barkey MB, edit. (2009). The Interfaith Council on Environmental Stewardship. Action Institute, Grand Rapids MI. http://www.acton.org/ppolicy/environment/ppolicy_environment_theology_monograph.php.

4* Teilhard De Chardin, P. (1959). *The Human Phenomenon*. New York, NY: Harper and Row

5 Philosopher Nichoas Malebranche, 1638–1715.

6 Taylor, A.H., Hunt, G. R., Holtzhalder, C., and Gray, R.D. (2007). Spontaneous metatool use by New Caledonian crows. *Curr Biol* **17**(17), 1504–7.

7 Byrne, R.W., Barnard, P.J., Davidson, I., *et al.* (2004). Understanding culture across species. *Trends in Cognitive Sciences*, **8**(8), 341–6; Madden, J.R. (2008). Do bowerbirds exhibit culture? *Anim Cogn*, **11**(1), 1–12.

8 Tanner, J.E., Patterson, F.G., and Byrne, R.W. (2006). The development of spontaneous gestures in zoo-living gorillas and sign-taught gorillas: from action and location to object representation. *J Devel Process*, **1**, 69–102.

9 Ferkin, M.H., Combs, A., delBarco-Trillo, J., *et al.* (2007). Meadow voles, *microtus pennsylvaicus*, have the capacity to recall the "what", "where", and "when" of a past single event. *Anim Cogn*, **11**(1), 147–59.

10 Marino, L., Connor, R.C., Fordyce, E., *et al.* (2007). Cetaceans have complex brains for complex cognition. *PLoS Biol*, **5**(5), e139.

11 Plotnik, J.M., de Waal, F.B., and Reiss, D. (2006). Self-recognition in an Asian elephant. *Proc Natl Acad Sci USA*, **103**(45), 17053–7.

12 Prior, H., Schwarz, A., and Gunturkun, O. (2008). Mirror-induced behavior in the magpie (Pica pica): evidence of self-recognition. *PLoS Biol*, **6**(8), e202.

13* De Waal, F. (2001). *The Ape and the Sushi Master; Reflections of a Primatologist*. New York, NY: Basic Books.

14 Rollin, B.E. (2007). Animal research: a moral science. *EMBO Rep*, **8**(6), 521–5.

15 Hewitt, H. (1990). Benefits of animal research and the doctor's responsibility. *BMJ*, **300**, 811.

16 Roberts, I., Kwan, I., Evans, P., *et al.* (2002). Does animal experimentation inform human healthcare? Observations from a systematic review of international

animal experiematns on fluid resuscitation. *BMJ*, **324**, 474.

17* Pound, P., Ebrahim, S., Sandercock, P., *et al.* (2004). Where is the evidence that animal research benefits humans? *BMJ*, **328**, 514–17.

18 Dennis, C. (2006). Cancer: Off by a whisker. *Nature*, **442**, 739–41.

19 Hackam, D.G. and Redelmeier, D.A. (2006). Translation of research evidence from animals to humans. *JAMA*, **296**, 1731–2.

20 Perel, P., Roberts, I., Sena, E., *et al.* (2007). Comparison of treatment effects between animal experiments and clinical trials: systematic review. *BMJ*, **334**, 197–203.

21 Burns, R. (1989). Animals in research. *Acad Med*, **62**, 780.

22 Animal care annual report of activities, fiscal year 2007. United States Department of Agriculture, August 2008. http://www.aphis.usda.gov/publications/animal_welfare/content/printable_version/2007_AC_Report.pdf

23 Trull, F.L. and Rich, B.A. (1999). More regulation of rodents. *Science*, **284**, 1463.

24 Statistics of scientific procedures on living animals: Great Britain 2008. Home Office. Ordered by the House of Commons to be printed. London. July, 2009. http://www.homeoffice.gov.uk/rds/pdfs09/spanimals08.pdf.

25 Post Derby tragedy, 38% support banning animal racing. The Gallup Organization. May 15, 2008. http://www.gallup.com/poll/107293/PostDerby-Tragedy-38-Support-Banning-Animal-Racing.aspx.

26 Americans rate the morality of 16 social issues. The Gallup Organization. June 4, 2007. http://www.gallup.com/poll/27757/Americans-Rate-Morality-Social-Issues.aspx.

27* Pifer, L., Shimizu, K., and Pifer, R. (1994). Public attitudes toward animal research: some international comparisons. *Soc Animals*, **2**(2), 95–113.

28* Russell, W. and Burch, R. (1959). *The Principles of Humane Experimental Technique*. London: Methuen and Co. Ltd.

29 Gates, J.E. Committee Chair, Appalachian Laboratory, University of Maryland Center for Environmental Science (Lecture: Insitutional Animal Care and Use Committee, General Information).

30 Animal (Scientific Proceures) Act 1986. Great Britain. http://www.archive.official-documents.co.uk/document/hoc/321/321.htm

31* European Convention for the Protection of Vertebrate Animals used for Experimental and Other Scientific Purposes. Strasbourg, 18.III.1986 (amended Dec 2, 2005 to reflect formation of the European Union).

http://conventions.coe.int/treaty/en/treaties/html/123.htm

32 Rowan, A.N. (1990). Animals, science, and ethics – section IV. Ethical review and the animal care and use committee. *Hastings Cent Rep*, **20**(3), s19–24.

33 Houde, L., Dumas, C. and Leroux, T. (2009). Ethics: views from IACUC members. *Altern Lab Anim*, **37**(3), 291–6.

34* Kilkenny, C., Parsons, N., Kadyszewski, E., *et al.* (2009). Survey of the quality of experimental design, statistical analysis and reporting of research using animals. *PLoS One*, **4**(11), e7824.

35* Osborne, N.J., Payne, D., and Newman, M.L. (2009). Journal editoral policies, animal welfare, and the 3Rs. *Am J Bioeth*, **9**(12), 55–9.

Further reading

Cavalieri, P. (2009). The ruses of reason strategies of exclusion. *Logos*, **8**(1).

Fund for the Replacement of Animals in Medical Experiments (FRAME). http://www.frame.org.uk/page.php?pg_id=152.

Gaul, G.M. (2008). In US, few alternatives to testing on animals. *The Washington Post*. April 12.

Harrison, P. (1992). Descartes on animals. *Philos Quart*, **42**(167), 219–27.

Hastings Center Report Special Supplement. (1990). *Animals, Science and Ethics*. Donnelley, S., and Nolan, K. eds. **20**(3), s1–32.

Hobson-West, P. (2010). The role of 'public opinion' in the UK animal research debate. *J Med Ethics*, **36**, 46–9.

The Humane Society of the United States. Biomedical Research. http://www.humanesociety.org/issues/biomedical_research/Accessed March 1, 2010.

The Johns Hopkins Center for Alternatives to Animal Testing. http://caat.jhsph.edu/contact/index.htm.

Kilkenny, C., Parsons, N., Kadyszewski, E., *et al.* (2009). Survey of the quality of experimental design, statistical analysis and reporting of research using animals. *PLoS One*, **4**(11), e7824.

Langley, G. (2009). The validity of animal experiments in medical research. *Revue Semestrielle de Droit Animalier*, **1**, 161–8.

NC3Rs. National Center for Replacement, Refinement, and Reduction. http://www.nc3rs.org.uk/.

The Royal Society for Prevention of Cruelty to Animals. Research Animal Science. http://www.rspca.org.uk/sciencegroup/researchanimals Accessed March 1, 2010.

Universities Federation for Animal Welfare. http://www.ufaw.org.uk/.

30 Ethical function of human subjects review boards: a US perspective

Jeffrey H. Silverstein

The Case

An investigator submits a project that proposes to use an antibiotic for treatment of an unusual infection that afflicts as small number of patients following colonic interposition following esophagectomy. Although the number of cases of this type of postoperative esophagitis are small, the suffering of the patients with this complication is severe. The proposed antibiotic is approved for clinical treatment of anaerobic infections but is a second line drug and is not frequently used for this purpose in clinical practice. A related drug is one of the most commonly used therapies for treatment and prophylaxis of anaerobic infections, being administered to thousands of patients every day in the US.

The application is extensive and includes a number of case reports of successful treatment of post esophagectomy colonic interposition inflammation and a small animal study that also suggests the treatment will be effective. The side effect profile of the medication is similar to many antibiotics – including gastric distress, possible allergy and the risk of subsequent resistant infection.

The project accrues a small number of patients and is reviewed annually for two subsequent years. Few adverse or unanticipated events are reported. During the third annual evaluation, one of the IRB reviewers notes that there is a specific warning from the Food and Drug Administration (FDA) indicating that a similar drug (not the one in use, but the more common one that is administered regularly) has been shown to cause cancer in a small number of mice when administered for prolonged periods of time. The drug proposed for this project has never been reported to cause cancer in either animals or humans and the related drug has never been reported to cause cancer in humans. In reviewing the literature and documentation, it is clear that this warning was known when the project was initially reviewed, but was not included in the presentation from the investigator, nor was it noted by the IRB reviewers during the initial review or the first two annual reviews of the project.

Was it ethical to approve the study initially? Did the IRB do its job in reviewing this project? What is the nature of the lapse in initial reporting by the investigator? Should the participants be notified of a failure to inform them of this risk of malignancy?

In a previous chapter, Dr. Viens describes the ethical basis for the conduct of research on human subjects. All researcher who have participated in these activities rapidly learn that adherence to the ethical principles outlined are not left up to the individual investigator, but require a formal review process by independent individuals. This review process is the basis of extensive regulatory statues.

What is the purpose of an IRB and how did they evolve?

The history of protecting human subjects in research goes back into antiquity. While it might be thought that societies would proactively define norms and mores regarding how one can experiment on fellow humans, in practice, our regulatory structure has evolved almost exclusively in the wake of scandal and disaster. Indeed, the history of human subjects protections and the initial creation of formalized institutional review boards followed a specific series of incidents that were both unacceptable and well publicized.

Most treatises on human subjects protection begin their discussion with the effort at codifying research ethics undertaken by the Judges for the Nazi Doctors Trial following World War II. In this case, experiments were conducted, some with little legitimate scientific intent, which caused extreme suffering and frequent deaths. Many were specifically designed to understand the limitations of human tolerance to hypothermia, low oxygen tension high altitude situations and immersion in salt water, all problems suffered by combatants on both sides of the conflict. These experiments were intended to assist scientists in developing means to support soldiers and sailors engaged in the war effort.

Clinical Ethics in Anesthesiology: A Case-Based Textbook, ed. Gail A. Van Norman, Stephen Jackson, Stanley H. Rosenbaum and Susan K. Palmer. Published by Cambridge University Press. © Cambridge University Press 2011.

Some were published in reputable scientific journals. Nonetheless, these experiments were widely considered unethical and the war crimes tribunal following the war prosecuted the doctors involved in these experiments. The judges assigned to the trial found that there were essentially no coherent codes of conduct regarding human experimentation for reference. Therefore, in 1947, they elaborated what has become known as the Nuremberg Code (Table 30.1) as a guide document for understanding what should have happened in the wake of tragedy.

On the basis of this construct, many of the doctors and participants in those experiments were convicted. Many of the concepts were elaborated upon in a subsequent document created by the World Health Organization, which is called the Declaration of Helsinki. The Declaration is an ethics document, as opposed to a regulatory or legal document. Its continued evolution has created controversy in the last few years.[1]

A key moment in the evolution of American research oversight was the seminal publication in 1966 of an article in the *New England Journal of Medicine* entitled "Chronicle of 22 unethical studies."[2] The author Henry Knowles Beecher was one of the most famous anesthesiologists of his day and the anesthesia laboratories at Harvard still bear his name. This article delineated a large series of published studies that Dr. Beecher contended had failed to follow the ethical principles of the day.

The Tuskeegee experiment and the Belmont Report

The first set of human subjects regulations were elaborated by the then nascent National Institutes of Health. However, the true watershed event in US research ethics was the description of the Tuskeegee experiment. Officially titled " Tuskeegee syphilis study or Public Health Service syphilis study," the Tuskeegee experiment, at least in its initial conception, was a scientifically valid observational study of the natural history of syphilis. When this started in 1932, syphilis was a major health problem with no cure and which created a hugely varied pantheon of symptoms. A similar study was under way in Sweden at the time. Unfortunately, when it became known that syphilis could be cured with penicillin in the mid 1940s, the scientists involved did not stop or redesign the study. The subjects were all male African-American prisoners in southern jails who had no idea that they were part of a research study. The national scandal that

Table 30.1. The Nuremberg Code

Nuremberg Code
• Voluntary informed consent
• Anticipate scientific benefit
• Benefit outweighs risk
• Animal experimentation first
• Avoid suffering
• No intentional death or disability
• Protection from harm
• Subject free to stop
• Qualified investigators
• Investigator will stop if harm occurs

erupted led to the formation of the National Bioethics Commission and the elaboration of what became known as the Belmont Report.

The Belmont Report elaborated three basic principles: autonomy, beneficence, and justice, which remain the ethical underpinnings of American human research protections.[3] This was soon followed by federal regulations that created a standard for evaluation, review and consenting for humans participating in research subjects. The role of Institutional Review Boards (IRBs) was carefully described "The IRB shall be sufficiently qualified through the experience and expertise of its members and the diversity of the members, including consideration of race, gender, and cultural backgrounds and sensitivity to such issues as community attitudes, to promote respect for its advice and counsel in *safeguarding the rights and welfare of human subjects*…the IRB shall be able to ascertain the acceptability of proposed research in terms of institutional commitments and regulations, applicable law, and standards of professional conduct…The IRB shall therefore include persons knowledgeable in these areas."[4]

Of note, there are two separate, related, but distinct sets of regulations in the USs. Most research undertaken at medical schools with funding from the NIH are governed by the Department of Health and Human Services Protection of Human Subjects found at 45 CFR 46 (CFR = Code of Federal Regulations). However, there is a separate, similar, but not identical set of regulations that govern the Food and Drug Administration. Anyone proposing to submit a drug for FDA approval must follow those regulations.[5] In many cases, both sets of regulations apply simultaneously.

Even with this set of regulations in place, IRBs remained somewhat sleepy backwaters of compliance in major medical schools. Following another series of scandals, federal authorities removed the authorization to use federal monies for research from a number of major educational institutions in the late 1980s and early 1990s. This resulted in a major overhaul and significant augmentation of the human subjects protections programs in all major schools and the rapid evolution of independent institutional review boards. Since that time, there has been an appreciation that human subjects protections is a profession, which has evolved it's own certification process for individuals (CIP – certified IRB professional) and an accreditation process for programs (AAHRPP – Association for the Accreditation of Human Research Protection Programs).

IRBs have frequently been referred to as ethics boards and indeed the charge includes the assessment of the ethics of a proposed study. However, in practice modern IRBs are responsible for assuring that investigators are in compliance with the regulations regarding human subjects research. Thus, the content of informed consent documents, which is delineated in US federal regulations and compliance with specific protections afforded to special groups of potential participants are required activities that IRBs must document. This compliance function frequently appears to take precedence over the pure ethics of a clinical trial. Whether this type of review is more or less beneficial to the goal of protecting human subjects is an interesting ethical question in its own right, but one beyond the scope of this chapter.

In the index case presented above, both the IRB and the investigator apparently failed to properly identify a specific risk. This failure could be described as a failure of the principle of beneficence, and nonmaleficenc (the principle to do no harm). It can also be seen as having severely limited the autonomy of the participants, whom, in the absence of a potentially critical piece of information, might not have been able to make an informed decision regarding their participation. Appropriate actions following the identification of such risks should include the notification of participants.

Determination of risk, risk/benefit ratio, and risk management

One of the principal obligations of IRBs is the determination of the level of risk posed to a participant and assuring that the risks are both acceptable and minimized by appropriate research design risk. This idea is frequently couched in the phrase risk/benefit ratio, which makes this determination sound like a

calculation with a definable answer. Risk involves the expected value and likelihood of one or more future events. Unfortunately, the concept of risk is not defined in federal regulations and remains a particularly difficult concept to apply in the setting of human experimentation. Bioethicists, such a Ezekiel Emmanuel from the National Institutes of Health have argued for an actuarial definition of risk, based on the statistical likelihood of a an untoward occurrence. In this construct, human research is, for the most part, much safer than many daily human activities such a driving a car or participating in a contact sport such as football. On a practical basis, IRBs find themselves considering risk in a relation to a relative level of tolerance or acceptability. So, while the risk of driving a car is well understood, it is also generally acceptable in that very few individuals would consider not using an automobile based on the risk of death or injury, while a much lower absolute likelihood of injury or death in a biomedical research is not so well accepted.

The index case provides an interesting example. The cancer warning for the drug was established based on animal experiments of a related drug. There was no indication that the related drug actually did produce cancer in any humans and the actual drug in use was never tested for chronic use in animals, so the actual drug proposed for the study had never been reported to cause cancer. The warning was based on very little information and could arguably be dismissed from a scientific basis; however, failing to note the warning was clearly an error on the part of both the investigator and the review board. Any risk of cancer, no matter how small or theoretical, might be legitimately considered to be significant.

What is the IRB's role in scientific review?

A frequent complaint leveled against current IRBs is the tendency to review the scientific design of a research proposal. Investigators argue, with some justification that scientific review occurs at other venues. Particularly for major grants, such as those funded by the National Institutes of Health, extensive review by panels of experts have critiqued the scientific content of the proposal. One could legitimately argue that IRBs, even with some direct expertise, are not as well equipped and provide little added value to previous professional scientific review. Even in the absence of this highly sophisticated professional review process, many institutions have internal scientific review bodies that can provide high quality review of the science underlying a proposal. These groups should be at least as good at evaluating the current standard of care and determining whether an experiment is justified and well designed.

High-quality scientific review should be extremely helpful to an IRB reviewing a project. A human subjects' reviewer should be able to have confidence that a project reviewed and funded by an auspicious national body represents quality science. One might argue that a project prepared by a major pharmaceutical manufacturer who employs skilled personnel with extensive experience in research design is equally well designed. It is beneficial for these projects to have previous focused scientific review prior to submission to the IRB.

IRBs are supposed to minimize risk by ensuring appropriate research design. This is the standard justification used by most IRBs to question a study design. A number of circumstances arise. For major projects that have been reviewed, it may be that the contingencies of human subjects protections were not considered during the design or review of the project. For projects reviewed by the National Institutes of Health, this changed a few years ago, so that all projects including human subjects must now have a section describing human subjects protections. This change in the scientific review process has been a major improvement in scientific review that should minimize discrepancies seen in the past.

Even with this process, there may remain legitimate differences in the evaluation of a design. A poignant example has arisen in the latest rendition of the Declaration of Helsinki, which seeks to minimize the use of placebo controls. The supporters of this document contend that the use of placebos in rarely justified. For example, if a new analgesic was to be tested, one could argue that we don't need one that is better than nothing, but rather one that is as good as or better than current therapy. Therefore, one should not design a trial that compares such a drug to placebo, but rather to an active standard of care control drug. Interestingly, the US FDA has rejected the current Declaration of Helsinki over this issue (among others) and continues to support and sometimes require placebo-controlled studies prior to approval of a new drug. IRBs frequently have a difficult time reconciling these different positions.

Furthermore, much research that is reviewed by IRBs has not undergone such extensive, if any peer review and might have been written by individuals with little experience is writing research proposals.

These projects probably benefit from the expert reviews provided by an IRB. Much current science could be argued to be repetitive with little to be offered in terms of significant scientific progress. While major funding agencies require a project to be innovative and significant, the tremendous expansion of the medical literature has resulted in large numbers of scientific reports that do not have a major impact. Pharmaceutical companies are particularly interested in maintaining drugs on patent and are frequently accused of testing new articles with limited advantages over existing medications. For the most part, IRBs have been reluctant to take issue with well-designed research which promises minor scientific or medical value. Most IRB members would find that role unappealing and difficult to fulfill.

A difficult problem arises when poorly designed research poses minimal or no risk, but is unlikely to answer the proposed questions, due, for example, to a lack of proper controls or the inclusion of too few patients to achieve statistical significance. Some IRBs would argue that poor science represents an unacceptable risk, even if the primary "risk" involved is wasting the time of a participant. Others would argue that, in the absence of any definable risk of injury, for example, in an innocuous anonymous survey, the IRB is not justified in suggesting alterations to a project. Because the primary model ensconced in the regulations is based on significant clinical trials, it can be argued that applying these principles to minimal risk types of projects is either inappropriate or a waste of resources.[6] Although an ongoing problem, there is little appearance that this issue will be resolved at a federal level any time soon.

In the index case, there was no concern regarding the design. Had the information regarding the risk of the test substance been discussed at the initial review, the project most likely would still have been approved, although the information regarding this risk would have been discussed and included in the information provided to potential participants. In the age of the internet, where information is easily accessible, it is reasonable to question whether it is the responsibility of IRB reviewers to "go beyond" what the researcher supplies in order to do a thorough review. In the index case, this did not happen during the initial review, but did occur during subsequent review. It is hard to argue that IRBs should not be looking for this additional information, but it is also difficult to set standards for what should be reviewed.

New issues facing IRBs

IRB review is a continually evolving process. In recent years, issues of privacy and confidentiality have become major focuses of human subjects protections under the guise of the Health Insurance Portability and Accountability Act of 1996. Initially designed to avoid loss of insurance based on violations of privacy, the rules regarding privacy and confidentiality have proven daunting to review and enforce. Consent documents have expanded greatly to accommodate required language. Investigators have legitimately complained that the requirements are excessive and impair research activities. Balancing these concerns are the very real problems associated with identity loss and the concerns that private health information could be used to discriminate against individuals. IRBs have also become embroiled in the desire to minimize conflicts of interest in research. All of this activity has created an increasing burden for investigators, IRB members and human subjects protection program staff members. Fortunately, there seems to be a movement to simplify and streamline some of these review processes. One can only hope that we will achieve a balance of appropriate review and adequate protections which can be accomplished in an efficient and professional manner.

Key points

- Regulation of human subjects research has evolved in the wake of scandals involving mistreatment of human research subjects.
- Modern human subjects protections had their roots in the war crimes trials of German physicians who experimented on prisoners during World War II.
- Important early declarations regarding the ethical treatment of human research subjects include the Nuremberg Code, and the WMA Declaration of Helsinki.
- The description of the Tuskeegee Experiment was a watershed event in the history of US human research ethics, leading to the publication of the Belmont report elaborating the ethical principles in treatment of human subjects research.
- US IRBs have largely functioned as regulatory bodies assuring compliance with federal regulations.

- Determination of risks and assuring that risks are both acceptable and minimized is an important part of IRB review. Minimization of risk includes assurance of appropriate research design.
- Additional new issues facing IRBs include protection of the identities of human subjects, and the minimization of conflicts of interest in research.

References

1* The World Medical Association Declaration of Helsinki. Ethical Principles for Medical Research Involving Human Subjects. Adopted by the WMA General Assembly, Helsinki, Finland, June 1964. Last amended by the WMA General Assembly, Seoul, October 2008. http://www.wma.net/en/30publications/10policies/b3/index.html.

2* Beecher, H.K. (1966). Ethics and clinical research. *N Eng J Med*, **274**(24), 1354–60.

3 The National Commission for the Protection of Human Subjects of Biomedical and Behavioral Research. (1979). The Belmont Report: Ethical Principles and Guidelines for the Protection of Human Subjects of Research. Dept of Health, Education and Welfare.

4 21CFR56.107. Code of Federal Regulations. Title 21, volume 1. Part 56: Insitutional Review Boards. Subpart B: Organization and Personnel. Revised April 1, 2009.

5 Informed consent: 21 CFR 50, Institutional Review Boards: 21 CFR 56.

6* Gawande, A. (2009). *The Checklist Manifesto, How to Get Things Right*. New York: Henry Holt.

Further reading

Annas, G.J. and Gordon, M.A., eds (1992). *The Nazi Doctors and the Nuremberg Code. Human Rights in Human Experimentation*. New York: Oxford University Press.

Code of Federal Regulations. TITLE 45:Public Welfare Department of Health and Human Services, Part 46. Protection of Human Subjects http://www.hhs.gov/ohrp/humansubjects/guidance/45cfr46.htmP.

Jones, J.H. (1983). *Bad Blood: The Tuskeegee Syphilis Experiment*. New York: The Free Press

Wendler, D., Belsky, L., Thompson, K.M., and Emanuel, E.J. (2005). Quantifying the federal minimal risk standard: implications for pediatric research without a prospect of direct benefit. *JAMA*, **294**, 826–32.

31

Research with vulnerable persons such as children and prisoners

Samia Hurst and Bernice Elger

The Case

Complex regional pain syndromes (CRPS) are increasingly recognized in children, and treatment is unsatisfactory in many cases. An anesthesiologist designs a clinical research project to study the efficacy of lumbar sympathetic blockade (LSB) with lidocaine compared to intravenous (IV) lidocaine in pediatric patients with CRPS who have not responded to traditional therapy. The study is a double-blind placebo-controlled study, involving 40 children between the ages of 7 and 12. All will receive general anesthesia and placement of a lumbar sympathetic catheter. Patients will then be randomized to receive either IV lidocaine plus saline via lumbar sympathetic catheter, or LSB with lidocaine plus IV saline. In obtaining informed consent, the researcher explains to parents and children (to the degree that the children can understand) the risks of general anesthesia and lumbar sympathetic catheter placement.

In answer to the expressed desires and expectations from patients and parents of pain relief, the researcher informs them that the "real" drug may be effective (in fact, he thinks it will be), but that it is equally important that researchers determine if LSB lidocaine is ineffective in relieving the pain. Several parents express concerns that their children may be subjected to the risks of general anesthesia and of lumbar catheter placement, but not receive the benefit of pain relief. They want assurances that their children will receive lidocaine and not placebo.

What are the ethical considerations in human subjects research when the patients who are being studied belong to vulnerable groups, such as children? Should human subjects research be conducted in vulnerable populations?

Vulnerable persons enrolled as research participants require special protection. This is recognized in a number of international and national regulations, including the US federal regulations on research with human subjects (see Table 31.1). When designing and conducting a research study, it is important to know which potential participants are vulnerable, which studies do or do not justify their inclusion, and what protections are necessary when they do participate in research.

This does not mean that vulnerable persons should never be enrolled in research. Historically, scandals have involved abusive studies where vulnerable persons were included because they were less able to resist. Excluding vulnerable persons from research entirely, however, can lead to their exclusion from: (1) research with potential benefit; and (2) the more general benefits of the research endeavor: knowledge about conditions relevant to them, their sometimes specific needs and risks, and the possibility to generalize available data to the situations they present with.

Who is vulnerable?

Attempts to define vulnerability have differed in their scope.[1] A European "principle of vulnerability" presents it as a universal expression of the human condition.[2] Such broad definitions, encompassing humanity in its entirety,[3,4] are unhelpful in protecting human subjects as they cannot provide reasons for *special* protection. In a more restricted definition, "vulnerability" in research on human subjects is often applied to individuals who are unable to give informed consent or more likely to be exploited.[5] National and international regulations are based on this sort of definition: vulnerability is usually linked either to consent or to the risk of harm.

One way to synthesize these different definitions is to consider that vulnerability as a claim to special protection is an *identifiably increased likelihood of being wronged*.[6] It encompasses any wrongs, including those we incur when something to which we have a valid claim is denied us. Defining vulnerability in this way means that we start by identifying the sorts of wrongs likely to occur in the conduct of research, then identify those more likely to suffer these wrongs. Many individuals are vulnerable in this way; but this definition makes the identification of different kinds of vulnerability, and the development of targeted protections, easier.

Clinical Ethics in Anesthesiology: A Case-Based Textbook, ed. Gail A. Van Norman, Stephen Jackson, Stanley H. Rosenbaum and Susan K. Palmer. Published by Cambridge University Press. © Cambridge University Press 2011.

Table 31.1. Vulnerability in research according to international guidelines

Belmont report	• Racial minorities • The economically disadvantaged • The very sick • The institutionalized
U.S. – Department of Health and Human Services (DHHS) 45 CFR 46	• Children • Prisoners • Pregnant women and foetuses
Declaration of Helsinki	• Incompetent persons • Persons susceptible to coercion • Persons who will not derive direct benefits from participation • Persons for whom research is mixed with clinical care
CIOMS	• Those with limited capacity or freedom to consent or to decline to consent… [including] children, and persons who because of mental or behavioural disorders are incapable of giving informed consent, • Junior or subordinate members of a hierarchical group…[such as] medical and nursing students, subordinate hospital and laboratory personnel, employees of pharmaceutical companies, and members of the armed forces or police, • Elderly persons, • Residents of nursing homes, • People receiving welfare benefits or social assistance and other poor people, • The unemployed, • Patients in emergency rooms, • Some ethnic and racial minority groups, • Homeless persons, • Nomads, • Refugees or displaced persons • Prisoners • Patients with incurable disease • Individuals who are politically powerless • Members of communities unfamiliar with modern medical concepts
ICH tripartite guidelines	• Members of a group with a hierarchical structure such as medical, pharmacy, dental, and nursing students, subordinate hospital and laboratory personnel, employees in the pharmaceutical industry, members of the armed forces, and persons kept in detention • Patients with incurable diseases • Persons in nursing homes • Unemployed or impoverished persons • Patients in emergency situations, • Ethnic minority groups, • Homeless persons • Nomads, • Refugees, • Minors, • Those incapable of giving consent

DISCOVERY LIBRARY
LEVEL 5 SWCC
DERRIFORD HOSPITAL
DERRIFORD ROAD
PLYMOUTH
PL6 8DH

Protecting vulnerable persons in research

Necessary protections have two components: fair subject selection, and the specific care required to minimize wrongs to vulnerable persons once they are enrolled in research. Recruitment of research subjects should respect fairness in the distribution of research-related risks and benefits. It is not justifiable to conduct research on an "easily available" population – for example, the rural poor in developing countries – simply because the study will be easier to conduct with them than with persons living in better circumstances. Neither is it defensible to reserve access to potentially beneficial research to the socially privileged. The rationale for the planned recruitment strategy must be based on the balance of potential harms and benefits and the need to obtain generalisable results, and discussed in the protocol.

Specific care requires that the risks and needs of those more likely to suffer wrongs in the conduct of research be identified, and targeted special protections outlined. Protecting vulnerability in clinical research starts with a good grasp of criteria for ethical research, in general. Investigators designing research with vulnerable subjects, and ERCs reviewing such research, should ask themselves the following questions:

(1) In which ways are potential research subjects at risk of being wronged in this research?

(2) Are some potential subjects identifiably more likely than other persons to incur this wrong, or likely to incur it to a greater degree?

(3) Am I/are we among those who share in the duty to minimize, or avoid, this wrong?

(4) If yes, what should we do to avoid this wrong or minimize its increased likelihood or degree, or ensure it is compensated in ethically justifiable ways?

Based on the sorts of wrongs that can occur in clinical research, examples of vulnerability are outlined in Table 31.2; examples of protections tailored to the wrongs involved are outlined in the Table 31.3. In some cases, excluding vulnerable persons from participation in a research project will be an appropriate way to minimize the risk of harm or other wrongs. Sometimes, however, it won't be. A study designed to address health problems specific to a vulnerable population, such as research on advanced dementia, could benefit the same population of vulnerable persons from which subjects are recruited, and cannot be conducted on nonvulnerable subjects: a condition

known as the *subsidiarity principle*. A study that, although it could be conducted enrolling only non-vulnerable subjects, could be designed in a way to give sufficient extra protection for vulnerable subjects. When such studies offer prospective benefit to research subjects, excluding vulnerable populations rather than providing protections to allow their recruitment can itself be harmful. If a subject in a research protocol with prospective benefit is imprisoned during the study, for example, terminating his participation may not be in his interest. In the rest of this chapter, we focus on two specific populations of individuals often vulnerable in the conduct of research: children and prisoners.

Research involving children

Why are children vulnerable?

Going from the state of being a child to that of being an adult is a continuous process, during which societies identify varying points as the threshold marking the passage from one state to the other. Children are considered vulnerable because, during much of their development, they are incapable of decision-making regarding medical intervention. Even when they are capable of decision-making for clinical care, consent for research requires something more: research-related risks are born for the benefits of others, a fact potential subjects are at risk of misunderstanding even in the best of cases. Although minors who are mature adolescents can often understand the consequences of their choice regarding medical interventions and then provide informed consent for clinical care, this is not considered sufficient in the case of research. Additionally, we are more reluctant to expose children to research-related harms, in part again because the risks undergone in this context cannot be consented to by the child herself, but also because we recognize a general responsibility of protection towards children beyond that which their parents endorse.

What follows from the vulnerability of children for research ethics?

Fair subject selection requires that children be enrolled only when the research question cannot be answered by conducting the study with adults – for example, because the targeted condition is specific to children or because the research question regards the situation of children specifically. When children *are* recruited in research, protections are required to circumscribe

Table 31.2. Vulnerability as a greater likelihood of being wronged

Requirements*	Examples of vulnerability
Social or scientific value	• Lack of access to either benefit or knowledge derived from research
Scientific validity	• Rare disease, leading to difficulties in reaching statistical power to demonstrate therapeutic effectiveness
Fair subjects selection	• All persons likely to be victims of discrimination
Favorable risk-benefit ratio	• Potentially higher risks: unstable patients, emergency research, foetuses, pregnant women • Potentially lower benefits: subjects in phase I studies, terminally ill patients • Subjects whose risk-benefit ratio might sometimes be the object of lesser concern to those responsible for protection: terminally ill patients, disenfranchised persons, poor subjects in developing countries, subjects without access to health care outside of research.
Independent review	• All persons likely to be victims of discrimination, if those responsible for review share discriminatory views.
Informed consent	• Difficulties in receiving or understanding the relevant information: not knowing the language used, or how to read • Lack of decision-making capacity: some children, some patients with mental disorders, comatose patients. • Lack of freedom to make a voluntary choice • Through limited freedom: prisoners • Through social weakness: minorities, refugees, sometimes women • Through hierarchical weakness: lab employees, students
Respect for potential and enrolled subjects	• Health care providers, researchers and students close to the study team who are at increased risk of faulty confidentiality • Groups and communities at risk of stigmatisation in the interpretation of study results

*With permission from Emanuel, E. J., Wendler, D. and Grady, C. (2000). What makes clinical research ethical? *JAMA*, **283**(20), 2701–11.

acceptable risks and to compensate the lack of consent by the children.

Limiting risks to children has implications for the timing of a protocol. Interventions relevant to both children and adults should undergo at least initial testing on adults in order to minimize unknown risks at the time when children will be recruited to assess questions more specific to them. Other implications regard the design of a protocol. Under US regulations, ERCs may approve research involving children under three sets of circumstances: "minimal risk," "prospect of direct benefit," and "minor increase over minimal risk." A prospect of direct benefit is defined as a research situation where risks are justified by the anticipated benefit to the subjects and where the relation of the anticipated benefit to the risk is at least as favourable as that of alternatives available to potential subjects.

Linking the acceptable risk threshold to the prospect of direct benefit in this manner has come under criticism for conflating risks acceptable in therapy and in research, and allowing healthy children to undergo greater research-related risk than those accepted in the case of sick children. An alternative proposed by Wendler is based on the "net risks test."[7] As any assessment of risk in research, it should focus on the *research-related risk*: risks that potential research subjects would not run outside the protocol. Sick children enrolled in research will often undergo standard therapy as well as experimental interventions, and risks inherent to the standard therapy are not research-related. The assessment should further focus on the *net risk*: risks that are not balanced by the prospect of direct benefit to the child. Paediatric pharmacokinetic studies, for example, hold no prospect of direct benefit: their entire risk is a net risk. A phase III study of a novel therapy proven effective in adults, however, does hold a prospect of direct benefit for sick children. Such a study can still have a net risk, however, especially if the expected

Table 31.3. Protection of vulnerable subjects by Ethics Review Committees*

Are potential research subjects at risk of being wronged by this research project?	Example 1: breach of confidentiality	• Health care providers are at greater risk. • IRBs share in the duty of protection • Minimization: could require specific anonymisation of data to limit colleagues' access to their personal information
Are some potential subject identifiably more likely than other persons to incur this wrong, or likely to incur it to a greater degree?	Example 2: unfavourable risk/benefit ratio	• If they stand to benefit less, terminally ill patients may be at greater risk. • IRBs share in the duty of protection. • Their risk/benefit ratio should be specifically examined by researchers and IRBs rather than assumed to be the same as for other potential subjects.
Is our IRB among those who share in the duty to minimize, or avoid, this wrong?	Example 3: being enrolled without valid consent	• Subjects of emergency research lack time to think through the options. • IRBs share in the duty of protection. • This can be minimized if consent is asked at that time only for those parts of the protocol that are truly urgent. • The remaining problems with consent at that time can be compensated by including a requirement that an independent clinician confirm that enrolment is not contrary to the potential subject's interest.
If yes, what should we do to avoid this wrong, or minimize this increased likelihood or degree, or ensure it is compensated in ethically justifiable ways?	Example 4: being denied the benefit of research	• Patients in developing countries who lack access to care are excluded from an important part of the social benefits of research. • Although IRBs are not alone in bearing some responsibility for this, it is among the points they should examine in general, and thus also for the purposes of protecting the vulnerable • Minimization: reasonable availability (World Medical Association 2008) aims to minimize this problem • Compensation: fair benefits (Participants in the 2001 Conference 2002) aim to compensate it.

*With permission from Hurst 2008.

benefit is modest. Finally, ERCs should assess this *net research-related risk* and accept it if it is no greater than "those associated with routine medical and psychological examination"[8] or "those ordinarily encountered in daily life."[9] US regulations combine these two thresholds. Comparison of the net research-related risks posed by a study should be with "the level of risk average children face in daily life (or during routine examinations),"[10] or the level "normally encountered in the daily lives of people in a stable society"[11,12] in order to avoid placing an excessive burden on children suffering from diseases requiring invasive treatment or living in circumstances such as war-torn countries, whose risks in daily life far exceed what is acceptable in research.

Because children are unable to provide consent for their own participation in research, permission must be sought from their parents or other legal guardians. US regulations specify that the permission of both parents is required unless: (1) the investigational procedure involves no more than minimal risk; (2) there is a prospect of direct benefit to the child; or (3) "one parent is deceased, unknown, incompetent, or not reasonably available" or "only one parent has legal responsibility for the care and custody of the child." EU directive 2001/20/EC specifies that research can only be conducted on minors if "the informed consent of the parents or legal representative has been obtained,"[13] apparently requiring the agreement of both parents.

Regulations also require that older children and adolescents should be informed to the level they can understand, and that they should provide *assent* – defined as "affirmative agreement" in US regulations and provided in writing – when they are capable of doing so.[14] Determining when assent should be sought is delicate as children's ability to understand research participation varies across, but also within, age groups. While it is usually found that children under 7 years of age are not capable of giving assent, and those over 14 years often are, this requires specific assessment, especially in the intermediate age group. Letting families decide when children are old enough to be involved in a decision to enroll in research is one possibility, but it should be applied with caution; data suggest that considerable disagreements can arise within families on this point, including reluctance on the part of the parents of capable children to involve them.[15] Children sometimes wish their parents to decide for them, and this, of course, should be respected.

Protections provided by parental permission and children's assent are further complemented by requirements that explicit refusal by children be respected.[8] EU directive 2001/20/EC further specifies that "parental consent must represent the minor's presumed will,"[13] and that no financial incentive may be offered. Children who are unable to assent to research may become able to do so, especially in long-term studies. In such cases, their assent (or consent as the case may be), must be sought at that time.

With such protections in place, a (small) net risk in research involving children is acceptable. Allowing such studies is not only necessary to allow the conduct of research needed by children themselves, it is also compatible with motivations of altruism for research participation, a reason accepted by many parents as well as children.

Research involving prisoners

Why are prisoners[a] vulnerable?

Prisoners are not a homogenous group. Statistically, they include a higher percentage of members from other vulnerable groups, such as the poor, illiterate, mentally ill, and – in many countries – foreigners who do not understand or speak the local language sufficiently to understand explanations regarding research.

As a group, prisoners are vulnerable due to their particular situation: being detained and therefore being deprived of the freedom to move freely, which implies that they are, possibly, under the influence of different kinds of pressures. Several prison-related factors are relevant for ethical considerations about research involving prisoners.

First, prisoners are vulnerable because they have limited choices: they cannot freely choose and consult their own physician. Their access to healthcare depends on the available health structures. Prisoners might not have access to alternative healthcare or adequate and independent clinical advice when a research study is carried out in a prison.

Second, prisoners are vulnerable because the pressures from prison officers and co-detainees, as well as pressures resulting from their living conditions, could interfere with free informed consent. Prisoners might accept participation in research because they fear punishment if they do not participate. Hierarchical structures are strong among prison inmates and leaders might force others to participate or, on the contrary, could force inmates not to participate. Prisoners are also vulnerable to real or perceived incentives to become a research subject, especially if they think that participation could be advantageous because research subjects obtain better living conditions or shorter prison terms than other prisoners.

Among ethics scholars and researchers, controversy exists as to whether prisoners should be considered competent to give informed consent. At one extreme are those who, based on the principle of beneficence, claim that, since studies are lacking which prove prisoners' capacity to give truly informed consent, one should not let them decide on their own. At the other extreme is the opinion that prisoners should not be treated differently from other potential research subjects, since their mental faculties are not fundamentally changed by detention. A part of this question is empirical: there has been insufficient exploration of whether prisoners have a tendency to make different decisions while in prison from those they would make if they were not detained. A second argument refers to the right to respect autonomy: being deprived of liberty does not include deprivation of the autonomy to decide about one's body and healthcare-related issues.

Treating prisoners, by definition, as incompetent concerning health-related matters is a violation of their human rights.

What follows from the vulnerability of prisoners for research ethics?

The vulnerability of prisoners has triggered various strategies for their protection against research risks and abuse.[16,17] Strategies are used either alone or cumulatively by different guidelines and legislations.

The first is characterized by different forms of restrictions. The most extreme form is general prohibition of all forms of research with prisoners as is the case in some of the US. Others, such as US federal regulations, allow only certain categories of research to be carried out with prisoners. Categories are allowed either because they imply only minimal risk or because their benefits are particularly important and outweigh the (limited) risks.[18] The Council of Europe varies restrictions according to the type of benefit. It restricts only research that does not promise *direct* benefit to prisoners. If research is expected to produce indirect benefit, i.e., benefit only to prisoners as a group, it is allowed only if three conditions are fulfilled: "(i) Research of comparable effectiveness cannot be carried out without the participation of persons deprived of liberty; (ii) The research has the aim of contributing to the ultimate attainment of results capable of conferring benefit to persons deprived of liberty; (iii) The research entails only minimal risk and minimal burden". Research without at least indirect benefit is prohibited.[16,17]

A second strategy is to require higher efforts than with nonprisoners to assure informed consent and freedom of choice. This could imply that prisoners should be informed several times and particular tests could be indicated to ensure that they have understood the information. It could also mean to provide prisoners with more time than nonprisoners to consider their decisions. Most regulations prohibit incentives in the form of money or better living conditions or influence on prison terms. Other means to ensure that prisoners' choices are in line with their best medical interest is to grant them access to an independent and qualified doctor who is not part of the research team who could advise prisoner patients impartially.

A third strategy is to increase oversight mechanisms by research ethics committees (RECs) or ERCs.[b] In the US, for example, ERCs that approve research with prisoners need to have a particular composition including a prisoner representative who has experience with prison healthcare. RECs should receive clear indications how to evaluate specific ethical issues concerning research with prisoners such as the principle of subsidiarity and issues of distributive justice: prisoners should not bear a disproportionate burden of research risks, and research should be carried out inside prisons only if results of comparable efficiency and meaning cannot be obtained with nonprisoners. Stricter oversight mechanisms might include the obligation to visit the prison before, during, and after the study to control whether confidentiality, informed consent, and other ethical requirements are respected.

A fourth strategy is to require special ethical training for researchers carrying out research with prisoners to assure that they are aware of ethical issues and specific risks related to research with prisoners, and engage themselves in the protection of prisoners from abuse through research.

Such strategies are important to protect prisoners from the risk of abuse, and preferable to their exclusion from research entirely. Empirical studies inside prisons can be beneficial and are necessary to obtain evidence-based answers to some research questions that need to be addressed in order to improve prisoners' healthcare.

Key points

- With children, prisoners, and other vulnerable populations, the challenge is to find the right balance between protection from abuse and the need to grant vulnerable populations access to participation in research.
- Although the exclusion of vulnerable subjects from a specific study will sometimes be an appropriate way to minimize their risk of being wronged in the conduct of research, this will not always be true.
- Studies designed to address health problems specific to a vulnerable population are needed to improve care for this very population, and often cannot be conducted on others.
- Participation in research can hold a prospect of benefit from which it is sometimes wrong to exclude vulnerable persons. In such cases, enrollment with special protections tailored to the sort of wrong to be avoided is ethically preferable to exclusion.

Notes

a In this text, the term "prisoner" is meant to include any kind of detained person, in any kind of detention facility. The term prison is used in its British meaning all kinds of detention facilities, such as jails, federal prisons or other places of detention.

b Institutional review boards (terminology used in the US). In this chapter we do not make any difference between the terminology: both REC and IRB refers to the competent body of research oversight in a given country.

References

1* Ruof, M. C. (2004). Vulnerability, vulnerable populations, and policy. *Kennedy Inst Ethics J*, **14**(4), 411–25.

2* Rendtorff, J. D. (2002). Basic ethical principles in European bioethics and biolaw: autonomy, dignity, integrity and vulnerability – towards a foundation of bioethics and biolaw. *Med Health Care Philos*, **5**(3), 235–44.

3* Callahan, D. (2000). The Vulnerability of the Human Condition. *Bioethics and Biolaw, Volume II: Four Ethical Principles*. P. Kemp, J. Rendtorff and N. Mattsson Johansen. Copenhagen, Rhodos International Science and Art Publishers; and Centre for Ethics and Law in Nature and Society.

4* Kottow, M. H. (2004). Vulnerability: what kind of principle is it? *Med Health Care Philos*, 7(3), 281–7.

5* Lott, J. P. (2005). Module three: vulnerable/special participant populations. *Dev World Bioeth*, **5**(1), 30–54.

6 Hurst, S. A. (2008). Vulnerability in research and health care: describing the elephant in the room? *Bioethics*, **22**(4), 191–202.

7 Wendler, D. (2008). Is it possible to protect pediatric research subjects without blocking appropriate research? *J Pediatr*, **152**(4), 467–70.

8 CIOMS (2002). *International Ethical Guidelines for Biomedical Research Involving Human Subjects*. Geneva, Switzerland, CIOMS.

9 DHHS. Department of Health and Human Services. Code of Federal Regulations Title 45 Part 46. Federal Register. 56: 28012. http://www.hhs.gov/ohrp/humansubjects/guidance/45cfr46.htm (accessed August 15th 2009)

10 Wendler, D. (2006). Three steps to protecting pediatric research participants from excessive risks. *PLoS Clin Trials*, **1**(5), e25.

11 South African Medical Research Council (2006) *Guidelines on ethics in medical research*. Available: http://www.mrc.ac.za/ethics/ethics.htm. Accessed August 15th 2009.

12 Tangwa, G. B. (2009). Research with vulnerable human beings. *Acta Tropica*, **112S**, S16–S20.

13 European Parliament and the Council of the European Union (2006). Regulation (EC) No 1902/2006 of the European Parliament and the Council on medicinal products for paediatric use. Published in the Official Journal of the European Union on 27/12/2006 (L 378/20). Available at: http://www.eortc.be/Services/Doc/clinical-EU-directive-04-April-01.pdf Accessed August 15th 2009.

14 Whittle, A., Shah, S., Wilfond, B., Gensler, G., and Wendler, D. (2004). Institutional Review Board Practices Regarding Assent in Pediatric Research. *Pediatrics*, **113**, 1747–52.

15 Varma S., Jenkins T., and D. Wendler. (2008) "How do Children and Parents Make Decisions About Pediatric Clinical Research? "*J Pediatr Hematol Oncol* **30**(11), 823–8.

16 Council of Europe (2005). *Additional Protocol to the Convention on Human Rights and Biomedicine, concerning Biomedical Research*. Strasbourg, 25.I.2005: http://conventions.coe.int/Treaty/EN/Treaties/Html/195.htm

17* Gostin, L. O., C. Vanchieri, A. Pope and IOM Committee on Ethical Considerations for Revisions to DHHS Regulations for Protection of Prisoners Involved in Research (2006). *Ethical Considerations for Research Involving Prisoners*. Washington, DC: The National Academies Press.

18* Branson, R. (1977). Prison research: National Commission says 'no, unless…'. *Hastings Cent Rep*, 7(1), 15–21.

Further reading

Elger, B. S. (2008). Research involving prisoners: consensus and controversies in international and European regulations. *Bioethics*, **22**(4), 224–38.

Emanuel, E. J., Wendler, D., and Grady, C. (2000). What makes clinical research ethical? *JAMA*, **283**(20), 2701–11.

Freedman, B., Fuks, A., and Wijer C, (1993). In loco parentis : Minimal Risk as an Ethical Threshold for Research upon Children. *Hastings Ctr Rep*, **23**(2): 13–19.

Meyer, C. R. (1999). "Unwitting consent: "Acres of Skin: Human Experiments at Holmesburg Prison" tells the story of medical researchers who sacrificed the rights of their subjects for personal profit." *Minn Med*, **82**(7), 53–4.

Sammons, H. (2009). Ethical issues of clinical trials in children: a European perspective. *Arch Dis Child*, **94**, 474–7.

World Medical Association. (2008). *Declaration of Helsinki: Ethical Principles for Medical Research Involving Human Subjects*. Retrieved February 24th, 2009, from http://www.wma.net/e/policy/b3.htm (accessed October 3rd 2006).

32 The ethics of research on pain and other symptoms for which effective treatments already exist

Monica Escher and Samia Hurst

The Case

Dr. Smith is an anesthesia resident on the hospital "pain service," who has been asked to consult on a patient who has been admitted for palliative care for terminal colon cancer. The patient has had breakthrough pain on maximal oral therapy. He feels nauseous and limits his oral intake. Subcutaneous (SQ) administration of morphine is initiated, and brings partial relief. The patient requests epidural analgesia. The attending on the pain service is conducting a placebo-controlled crossover research study evaluating the efficacy of administration of SQ recombinant human hyaluronidase to improve the absorption of SQ morphine in patients with terminal illness. Each study subject will receive morphine via a different method on each of 3 days: intravenous morphine, SQ morphine plus placebo, and SQ morphine plus hyaluronidase. As part of her role on the pain service, Dr. Smith is supposed to help recruit clinical research subjects, but she is bothered by the fact that this patient is terminally ill, is in considerable pain, and is requesting a specific therapy that is not on the research protocol. Is it ethical for her to try to recruit him for this study?

Research on the management of pain and other symptoms is crucial to provide better care for acute, postoperative, and chronic symptoms, as well as better symptom management at the end of life. However, participation in clinical research places subjects at risk of harm for the benefit of others. This tension is intrinsic to all clinical research, and underlies the need for protection of human subjects. A number of national and international regulatory documents aim to protect participants in research while also taking into account the interests of future patients by allowing research to be conducted[1] All refer to similar basic principles, which have been synthesized thus: social value, scientific validity, fair subject selection, favorable risk/benefit ratio, independent review, informed consent, and respect for enrolled participants. All of the requirements are

equally necessary, and each is relevant to research on the management of pain and other symptoms, which requires the same ethical protections as any other form of research with human subjects. Some aspects, however, do present difficulties more specific to the context of symptom management studies. These include difficulties related to scientific methodology, fair subject selection, obtaining a favorable risk/benefit ratio, and informed consent.

Scientific methodology

Although individual patients may benefit indirectly from research participation, the intention of research is to generate valid data to inform the care of future patients. The research may involve delaying pain relief in participants. The investigator is responsible for minimizing risks and avoiding unnecessary harm for the patients. He/she is also accountable for the scientific validity and clinical relevance of the experimental question. Methodological issues in the design of symptom management trials, the collection of adverse effects, and the reporting of data, have ethical importance. Failure to give proper attention to these issues can make the results of a trial difficult to interpret and prevent comparisons. This limits usefulness in clinical practice, causing research to fall short of its purported goal and fail to fulfill its commitments towards patients and society. Risks to human subjects must be justified in part by the social benefit of research. Therefore any risk, however small, in a study that cannot answer its research question is excessive.

Randomized, double-blind trials have become standard in acute as well as in chronic pain trials. The inclusion of patients with moderate to severe pain at baseline may be crucial for sensitivity, i.e., the ability to detect the analgesic effect of the tested drug. Primary outcomes are usually a difference in pain

---

Clinical Ethics in Anesthesiology: A Case-Based Textbook, ed. Gail A. Van Norman, Stephen Jackson, Stanley H. Rosenbaum and Susan K. Palmer. Published by Cambridge University Press. © Cambridge University Press 2011.

intensity and a measure of pain relief. Analgesic consumption after a surgical procedure has also been used as a surrogate endpoint because it can prove more convenient to measure. Data other than pain intensity and pain relief are also useful in characterizing patients' responses. In acute pain trials onset and duration of analgesia, the time to rescue analgesia and the number of patients requiring a rescue dose at various time points all provide valuable information. Observation periods must be long enough to gather relevant data. As chronic pain impacts different aspects of the patient's life, decreasing health-related quality of life, chronic pain trials must address issues considered important by patients, such as physical and emotional functioning, sleep, relations to family, and social activities. Whenever available, a standard set of outcome measures should be used to assess these dimensions. Studies should also assess what magnitude of change brings a *meaningful* difference for the patient, as opposed to finding a statistical difference only. Defining a "meaningful difference" is therefore necessary. Such an approach enables researchers to determine which patients benefit from treatment and to perform responder analyses.

Overall patient satisfaction depends on treatment efficacy in alleviating pain, and on treatment adverse effects. Single-dose studies do not adequately characterize drug toxicity because most side effects are dose dependent and will occur only after repeated dosing. Careful monitoring of adverse effects is warranted in all pain trials to assess the balance between risks and benefits in the specific clinical context. It also helps interpret the results in trials where analgesic consumption is an outcome, as sedation, confusion, or nausea may all lead to reduced opioid use without achievement of adequate pain relief. Whatever the method, the type, frequency, and severity of adverse events should be recorded for placebo and active treatment, and the causal relationship between adverse events and the study drug should be evaluated.

For results to be readily understandable, data must be reported in a way that relates to clinical practice. Data on pain intensity and pain relief do not have a normal distribution but are highly skewed, in acute pain as well as in chronic pain trials. Giving mean values does not reflect clinical reality as some patients may benefit considerably from the intervention, while others do not experience any improvement. Analysis of individual patient data has been proposed as a more relevant way of reporting results.[2] In addition to absolute changes in pain intensity, percent change provides valuable information, and correlates with patient global satisfaction.[3]

Fair subject recruitment

Potential subjects should be selected based on the potential for generalizability of study results, and to maximize the risk/benefit ratio for enrolled subjects. They should not be recruited on the basis of misleading expectations, lesser ability to defend themselves, or because they are persons whose risk is somehow discounted.

The problem of misleading expectations

A major expectation of informed consent in clinical research is to help patients understand the difference between the goals of the research and those of medical care – the research goal is to acquire generalizable knowledge that will help improve the care of future patients, rather than providing the best care to individual patients. Chronic pain patients have often received treatments that did not satisfy them, and may welcome access to a novel treatment they believe will work better. This makes them particularly prone to "therapeutic misconception." Their hope for personal benefit can also lead them to minimize or overlook inconveniences and risks. Most chronic pain trials involve fixed-schedule drug titration, prohibit or limit the use of other pain medication, and impose constraints on nonpharmacological and alternative treatments. Moreover, chronic pain patients often experience impaired physical, emotional and social functioning, all of which have been associated with the therapeutic misconception.[4]

Therapeutic misconception is also ethically problematic because it represents misplaced trust, which can endanger the physician–patient relationship.[5] Participants may question the researcher's competence and blame him if their expectations are not fulfilled. This risk may be especially high with patients suffering from chronic pain, as it is difficult to treat, with even the best treatments available providing only partial relief. Moreover, patients may experience the side effects of medication without benefiting from its therapeutic effect. Patients' distrust towards physician investigators can extend and impact on their relationship with their own physician, thus possibly jeopardizing routine clinical care.

Is research at the end of life a special case?

The exclusion of terminally ill patients from research would not be easy to defend. Research is useful to improve therapies at the end of life and thus help the very people whom such a ban would attempt to protect. Terminally ill patients do enroll in studies, and research has shown that, when given hypothetical scenarios, a majority of palliative care patients want to participate in research[6] with motives including the hope of personal benefit, altruism towards patients going through the same ordeals[7] and the wish to maintain hope.[8] Moreover, terminal disease does not by itself invalidate the capacity for informed consent. Were it so, we would not routinely respect the choices expressed by the terminally ill in their wills.

The conduct of research with terminally ill patients is, however, often described as requiring special care due to risks of coercion or exploitation. Coercion is best described as a credible and strong threat exerted by a person that limits the options in a negative way available to another person. Having limited options through no fault of anyone's does not constitute coercion. Indeed, the possibility of enrolling in a clinical trial actually gives terminally ill patients an *additional* option.

Exploitation is the unfair distribution of the benefits and burdens of a transaction. Research participation always carries burdens. Although it can carry the prospect both of direct benefits to subjects and of benefits to their community from the social value of research, both are always uncertain in a given study. Are terminally ill patients at greater risk during research, and/or are they less likely to benefit from research participation than they should? Assessing risks and benefits of participation in research *for* terminally ill patients is a complicated question. Effects deemed sufficient by researchers – and which underlie the choice of research question and much of the methodology – may or may not reflect what terminally ill patients would consider a clinically desirable effect.[9] A patient's evaluation of both risks and benefits may shift during terminal illness, and that shift will no doubt vary between individuals. At minimum, the risks incurred by terminally ill patients should never be discounted, and the risk/benefit assessment must take into account the circumstances of terminal disease.

A favorable risk/benefit ratio

The use of a placebo control when a recognized effective treatment already exists is controversial. On the one hand, giving a placebo to subjects randomized to the control group deprives them of an effective treatment, leading to recommendations against placebo controls in such standards such as the Declaration of Helsinki.[10] On the other hand, using a recognized treatment as a control can lead to methodological difficulties. A positive noninferiority trial can mean three very different things: both treatments are equally effective, both are equally ineffective, or the trial was underpowered to detect the difference. This tension was recognized in the 2008 Helsinki declaration, which states that placebo controls can be used "where for compelling and scientifically sound methodological reasons the use of placebo is necessary to determine the efficacy or safety of an intervention and the patients who receive placebo or no treatment will not be subject to any risk of serious or irreversible harm." It then adds that "Extreme care must be taken to avoid abuse of this option."

How do we tell the difference between those situations where a placebo control is acceptable, and those where it is not? Emanuel and Miller propose that this be based on scientific rationale *and* a risk criterion.[11] Placebos should be excluded where this would deprive patients of "effective, life-saving, or at least life-prolonging treatment." While it can be justifiable to conduct a placebo-controlled trial in cases where there is *some* potential harm to patients, the methodological rationale must be compelling. Such rationale may exist if the placebo response rate is high, the condition rare, variable or with frequent spontaneous remissions, or if existing therapies are only partly effective or have serious side effects.

A scientific rationale is necessary, but not sufficient to make a placebo-controlled trial ethically justified. A placebo control should not increase the subjects' risk of death or irreversible morbidity, or disability. Nor should it substantially increase their risk of other serious harms or severe discomfort. Judging which trials are acceptable on these criteria is a delicate balance and should be specifically addressed during the ethics review. Such trials must exclude participants who are at increased risk, limit the period of placebo administration as much as possible, monitor subjects carefully, provide rescue medication, and outline specific criteria for withdrawal from the study. The use of placebo, as well as its risks and rationale, must be made clear to potential subjects during informed consent.

The question of placebo use is also relevant to research on invasive interventions like surgical treatments, sometimes raising the question of placebo surgery.[12] Sham surgery is controversial; requires placing control subjects at risk while additionally depriving them of effective treatment. Trials including sham interventions are, however, not always riskier than other accepted clinical trials, and can be important to protect future patients from the harms of ineffective interventions.

In practice, they should be assessed with at least the same criteria used for placebo-controlled drug trials. Particular care should be given to exploring alternatives, minimizing risks, and assessing the risk/benefit ratio. Informed consent should be particularly careful, as potential subjects may be more likely to confuse research with clinical care in the case of an invasive procedure. Some sham intervention trials may be justified, provided they have no valid safer alternative and respect the criteria outlined above.

Consenting to research on symptom management

Informed consent is particularly important in research, because it allow subjects to make an informed and voluntary choice to participate – or refuse to participate– in a project where they will take risks for the benefit of others.

Adequate informed consent requires that potential subjects understand the relevant aspects of their choice, are capable of decision-making and are free to accept or refuse participation. Assessment of each of these elements requires a degree of judgment. In the case of research on the management of pain and other symptoms, some of these elements can be more difficult to attain. Similarly, concerns could arise in emergency situations, or in situations where consent might be solicited during acute pain, or immediately following acute administration of anesthetic agents.

Although none of these situations necessarily represents an obstacle to informed consent, or to enrollment in research, they do require special precautions. Two aspects are particularly relevant. The first one is the risk that decision-making capacity could be affected. Since chronic pain, and chronic administration of stable doses of analgesic medication do not by themselves affect decision-making capacity, this question is most relevant in the presence of acute pain or the acute administration of analgesia. However, studies have shown that most patients perceive that they retain decision-making capacity in these circumstances.[13]

The second aspect is that, in emergency situations, there is limited time for potential subjects to think through a decision to participate in research. There are several potential solutions. First, the urgency might be reduced by the study design. If, for example, the emergency is due to severe pain rather than the need for immediate surgery, a protocol might allow treatment to proceed as usual at first, with enrollment and randomization only after the emergency has resolved. If this is not possible, care should be taken to separate those aspects of the trial that must be initiated during the emergency and those which do not. Consent should be sought at a later time for nonurgent aspects of the trial. Finally, neutral supervision of enrollment can be utilized: a clinician not involved in the trial is given veto power on the enrollment of a patient if her considered judgment is that participation is against the patient's interests. Whichever strategy is chosen, it should be described in detail in the protocol submitted for ethics review.

Case resolution

Several issues contribute to Dr. Smith's discomfort in our case scenario. (1) The patient is in pain, which she has an obligation to try to relieve. (2) The patient is terminally ill, and therefore may be vulnerable to undue pressure if he is under the therapeutic misconception that the study will necessarily provide him with better pain relief. (3) Dr. Smith understands that for portions, if not all, of the study, the patient may experience deterioration in his pain control, depending on the efficacy of SQ and IV morphine compared to his oral medications, and depending on the efficacy of the study drug, hyaluronidase. She is torn between her desire to research pain in terminally ill patients to benefit others, and her obligation to offer this patient the best and most individualized care, which could be epidural analgesia.

The solutions to some of these issues are relatively straightforward. If the patient appears competent to make medical decisions, he can certainly be informed of the risks of poorer pain control, as well as the potential benefit of better pain control for himself as well as other patients through participation in the study. Ultimately, he will have to determine if the clinical trial and its potential risks and benefits are acceptable to him. As with many terminally ill patients, the opportunity to benefit others by participating in research may have special meaning for him, and may also provide him with hope during his palliative care. While he is a "vulnerable" patient, automatically excluding him from being a clinical research subject solely on the basis of his diagnosis is arguably unethical, as long as coercion is avoided, and careful attention is paid to correcting therapeutic misconceptions he may have. Care should be taken if he agrees to be a subject to clearly outline the plans for "rescue" therapy if any, and allow for voluntary withdrawal from the study if/whenever the patient changes his mind.

However, for Dr. Smith, being both a researcher and a primary treating physician for a subject of clinical research carries several risks. The patient may be more likely to view the research study as medical care, and be unable to overcome therapeutic misconception because of Dr. Smith's dual role in his care, for example. If he is denied epidural analgesia in favor of participation in a research study, and his pain is poorly controlled, he may not only come to mistrust Dr. Smith, but transfer that mistrust to other physicians involved in his clinical care. While the study itself may be ethical, and recruitment of terminally ill patients acceptable, Dr. Smith should consider either withdrawing from the medical team caring for the patient in favor of doing the clinical research, or ask another physician to obtain consent from the patient so that she can participate solely in his clinical care and avoid the "dual" role of researcher and clinician.

Key points

- Subjects who participate in clinical research take risks for the benefit of future patients, and may not realize personal benefits themselves. It is therefore an ethical obligation of clinical researchers to pay close attention to study design to fulfil the promise of research to patients and to society, and to justify the risks to which the subjects of research are subjected.
- Researchers always have the obligation to obtain informed consent from research subjects. This can require special precautions in emergency situations, or in situations where consent might be solicited during acute pain, or immediately following acute administration of anaesthetic agents.
- Patient subjects often confuse the intention of research trials and have the misleading expectation that the research is intended to benefit them.

- Even with explicit patient consent, the researcher has the obligation to minimize risk and discomfort to the patient.
- Particular attention to subject comfort and safety is important in placebo-controlled trials.
- Research involving symptomatic relief at the end of life is ethical, but requires special considerations. Patient assessment of benefits and burdens may shift during the trial and require reconsideration.

References

1* The National Commission for the Protection of Human Subjects of Biomedical and Behavioral Research (1979); ICH Steering Committee (1996); CIOMS (2002); World Medical Association (2008); Department of Health and Human Services, (March 1983).

2 Moore, R. A., Edwards, J. E., and McQuay, H. J. (2005). Acute pain: individual patient meta-analysis shows the impact of different ways of analysing and presenting results. Pain, 116(3), 322–31.

3 Farrar, J. T., Young, J. P. Jr., LaMoreaux, L., et al. (2001). Clinical importance of changes in chronic pain intensity measured on an 11-point numerical pain rating scale. Pain, 94(2), 149–58.

4* Appelbaum, P. S., Lidz, C. W., and Grisso, T. (2004). Therapeutic misconception in clinical research: frequency and risk factors. IRB, 26(2), 1–8.

5* de Melo-Martin, I. and Ho, A. (2008). Beyond informed consent: the therapeutic misconception and trust. J Med Ethics, 34(3), 202–5.

6* Pautex, S., Herrmann, F. R., and Zulian, G. B. (2005). Is research really problematic in palliative care? A pilot study. J Pain Symptom Manage, 30(2), 109–11.

7* Todd, A. M., Laird, B. J., Boyle, D., et al. (2009). A systematic review examining the literature on attitudes of patients with advanced cancer toward research. J Pain Symptom Manage, 37(6), 1078–85.

8* Agrawal, M., Grady, C., Fairlough, D. L., et al. (2006). Patients' decision-making process regarding participation in phase I oncology research. J Clin Oncol, 24(27), 4479–84.

9* Horrobin, D. F. (2003). Are large clinical trials in rapidly lethal diseases usually unethical? Lancet, 361(9358), 695–7.

10 World Medical Association (2008). Declaration of Helsinki: Ethical Principles for Medical Research Involving Human Subjects. Retrieved February 24, 2009, from http://www.wma.net/e/policy/b3.htm (accesed October 3, 2006).

11* Emanuel, E. J. and Miller, F. G. (2001). The ethics of placebo-controlled trials – a middle ground. *N Engl J Med*, **345**(12), 915–19.

12* Horng, S. and Miller, F. G. (2002). Is placebo surgery unethical? *N Engl J Med*, **347**(2), 137–9.

13* Kay, R. and Siriwardena, A. K. (2001). The process of informed consent for urgent abdominal surgery. *J Med Ethics*, **27**(3), 157–61.

Further reading

CIOMS (2002). Guideline 4: *Individual Informed Consent. International Ethical Guidelines for Biomedical Research Involving Human Subjects*. Geneva: CIOMS.

Emanuel, E. J., Grady, C., Crouch, R. A., et al. (2008). *The Oxford Textbook of Clinical Research Ethics*. Oxford, New York: Oxford University Press.

Emanuel, E. J., Wendler, D., and Grady, C. (2000). What makes clinical research ethical? *JAMA,* **283**(20), 2701–11.

Faden, R. and Beauchamp, T. (1986). *A History and Theory of Informed Consent*. Oxford, New York: Oxford University Press.

Grisso, T. and Appelbaum, P. S. (1998). *Assessing Competence to Consent to Treatment. A Guide for Physicians and Other Health Care Professionals*. New York: Oxford, Oxford University Press.

Hawkins, J. S. and Emanuel, E. J. (2005). Clarifying confusions about coercion. *Hastings Cent Rep* **35**(5), 16–19.

International Association for the Study of Pain. *Ethical Guidelines for Pain Research in Humans*. http://www.iasp-pain.org.

33

Quality improvement initiatives: when is quality improvement actually a form of human subjects research?

Michael A. Rie and W. Andrew Kofke

The Case

Suarez et al. published an article in the Journal of Neurosurgery *examining outcomes after human albumin (HA) administration in patients with subarachnoid hemorrhage (SAH).[1] Because some believed that HA increased mortality in critically ill patients, the authors' hospital developed an administrative policy restricting its use. The authors examined patient outcomes and costs before and after the introduction of the restriction. They concluded that administration of human albumin after SAH probably improved clinical outcomes and reduced hospital costs.*

Critics argued that the decision to change the "standard of care" with regard to human albumin administration failed to take into account animal data suggesting that albumin might be neuroprotective in patients with SAH. They charged that patients had been subjected to a change in the "standard of care" because of a corporate cost containment activity that could be "more accurately described as a system level 'experiment' with the dual hypothesis of no harm and less cost." Furthermore, it was an experiment "in which no disclosure occurred, nor was informed consent obtained in an institution receiving federal funds for both patient care and clinical research. The critics questioned who would voluntarily submit to an experiment with "the main dependent variables being money saved and increased morbidity and death rate."[2,3]

Quality assurance and quality improvement

In 1980, Donabedian defined the basic elements of healthcare quality to be structure, process and outcome.[*4] Early medical quality assurance (QA) was handled in sentinel event case discussions as part of anesthesia departmental conferences and possible prospective prevention practice suggestions. The process of quality improvement (QI) was informal, collegial and educational. Accountability to assure that

professional process review would translate into prospective preventive improvements for future patients within the department's practice of anesthesia was systematically lacking.

QI/QA has evolved from an informal retrospective review of individual cases involving critical incidents, to large retrospective analyses and evaluation of physicians, departments, hospitals, and healthcare systems. Increasingly, the impetus for projects and data collection has come from extramural demands to document accountability for care, safety, quality, efficiency, and cost in all of medical care.

The root cause of nonaccountability was evident. The victim of a prior sentinel event had been possibly unintentionally injured or suffered a "near miss," and a negligence action in malpractice law was a possible consequence. Systemic analysis of quality is now recognized as a management necessity to address and distinguish system error from individual professional errors and/or patient idiosyncratic events. Thus, the incorporation of such study into "research subject protection ethics" became unavoidable.

The regulatory structure in the CFR and the powers invested in the Office for Human Subjects Research Protections (OHRP) inevitably came into operational inquiry for QI projects. The realization that system errors could produce as many as 100 000 errors of preventable nature per year came to public attention.[*5] Shortly thereafter the Joint Commission for Accreditation of Health Care Organizations (JCAHO) published its first Sentinel Event Chapter for the accreditation standards for American hospitals.

The stage was then set to revisit what QA and QI patient subject protections might be. The world had moved before clinicians had from Phase I to Phases II and III of quality improvement activities.[6] These three phases of QI are:

Clinical Ethics in Anesthesiology: A Case-Based Textbook, ed. Gail A. Van Norman, Stephen Jackson, Stanley H. Rosenbaum and Susan K. Palmer. Published by Cambridge University Press. © Cambridge University Press 2011.

(1) Reactive or descriptive QI: react to sentinel events.
(2) Outcome improvement QI: improve an already satisfactory outcome.
(3) Cost containment QI: improve efficiency leading to a satisfactory/better outcome.

A decade of conflicting OHRP interpretations of quality improvement research leaves QI project directors and institutional review boards (IRBs) predictably confused. When is patient consent prospectively necessary for a QI process? Can patients be potentially injured by delayed reporting of important data if medical publishers reject reports for lack of IRB approvals? The combined federal definitions of generalizable knowledge and publication cover virtually all conceivable prospective activities that a QI project might encompass while leaving uncertain the nature of exempt "minimal risk" projects.

The practice of population-based cost containment QI initiatives is widespread in healthcare. It is apparent that lessons from the business model (e.g., widget factory) are also commonly applied to patient care. But, unlike patients, widgets are not invested with contractual healthcare rights.

Is patient safety and quality being compromised by cost containment?

In the situation described by Suarez, the hospital imposed clinical research on a population of patients presenting with SAH, with the primary goal of reducing costs and the belief, but no proof, that no adverse change in clinical outcome would occur. Unfortunately, they have demonstrated the very nature of research itself: a hypothesis cannot *a priori* state the outcome of the research in a specific group of patients until the data are analyzed after the experiment is over.

The publication and responses to the Suarez scenario command a unique position in academic medical publication morality. If negative outcomes occur by corporate actions, then how are critical care practitioners able to speak and professionally publish such data? How do they assure that lessons learned from negative outcomes in one institution are promulgated to prevent the same mistakes in other hospitals? One could argue that any information derived from a negative outcome QI study should be mandated for generalization as a matter of organizational ethics. A similar public safety nondisclosure issue in publication occurred in aviation safety, resulting in an airliner crash into a mountain.[7]

Critical care professionals work in complex organizational environments in which documentation of negative outcome data for safety and quality purposes pose risk for public discovery of the cases, negligence malpractice litigation, and conflict with hospital corporate management. In many academic hospitals, there is a formal organizational structure in which the medical faculty is employed by corporate entities directly linked with hospital management and budget directors, creating intractable conflicts of interest.

Thus, there exists a culture of silence in advancing QI initiatives driven by cost containment. These professionals are in an untenable master–servant relationship when they want to report negative (as opposed to positive) data necessary for the advancement of medicine, science, and the public welfare.

Is patient safety and professional integrity threatened by state interests?

In the *Suarez* matter more than 25 years of animal experiments supported the use of human serum albumin to diminish intracranial ischemia and stroke propagation in patients with ruptured cerebral aneurysms. A fundamental principle of the Nuremberg Code is that human experimentation should be based on previous animal experiments, and that experiments that pose risk of serious injury to human subjects cannot be ethically conducted. The publication by Suarez led to the awarding of an NIH research grant regarding the use of human albumin in patients with ischemic stroke, and a national multi-center trial was initiated.

The *Suarez* matter further reveals "the moral abuse of evidence-based medicine" (EBM) in the pursuit of cost containment. The vast majority of treatments utilized in critical care medicine lack level I and II evidence to support them. To suggest (via a pharmacy and therapeutics committee) that such a lack of evidence may mandate banning of a pharmaceutical in contradiction of what is thought to be an existent standard of care without evidence-based support is to use EBM in a fashion antithetical to the welfare of patients and their abilities to participate or decline cost-driven corporate experimentation. Conversely, because there was insufficient evidence to warrant the use of serum albumin, policy makers might argue for albumin's elimination and say that the patients were not given an appropriate consent option to decline serum albumin because it was an unproven therapy. Generalization of this approach throughout the healthcare system might drive a cost-containment-driven wedge into the fiduciary trust relationships that are the legal and moral bases for the delivery of individual healthcare.

Should we simply eliminate therapies that do not have sufficient evidence-based support?

It is quite a different matter to delay FDA approval for new therapeutics that are of unproven benefit than to proscribe historically based treatments until better ones are found. Were this a reality, digoxin might never have entered the pharmacopeia and both the FDA and physicians everywhere have been negligent in continuing to use it.

The *Suarez* matter was referred to the OHRP for review. Their response was:

> "… it appears that the restriction on the administration of the human albumin by the University Hospitals in Cleveland was not research as defined by federal regulations at 45CFR 46.102 … from the information submitted to OHRP it appears that the hospital's restrictions on the administration on human albumin was not a systematic investigation and was designed to reduce hospital costs and perhaps reduce morbidity."

We interpreted this OHRP response in the *Suarez* matter to indicate that the federal government presently has neither legal interest nor congressional mandate to ensure that a return to pre–Nuremberg Code practices does not develop in the practice of QI in the United States.

As rationing becomes reality, the IRB will increasingly be perceived to be under corporate economic pressure, although the converse may be as likely. This would place upon the QI-IRB of the future an apparent moral and legal conflict of interest concerning human subject protection. It seems that conflict for professionals, IRBs, and corporate officials will be unavoidable if negative outcomes derived from cost containment quality improvement activities of the institution were never subject to human subject protections by independent review.

The OHRP has reduced the definition of research for QI in such a fashion as to deputize itself as final arbiter of what systematic clinical observations may be lawfully permitted publication. A former editor of the *Annals of Internal Medicine*, Dr. Frank Davidoff, has stated publically, "you can be punished if you try to publish the results of your QI work but you will avoid punishment if that same work goes unpublished."

The coming of healthcare reform and heightened concerns for patient privacy with the explosion of clinical information technology will now awaken concerns for governmental control of professional free speech in publication by healthcare investigators and QI data analysts. As Bosk *et al.*[*8] point out, the art of medicine will be more complex and costly in achieving true improvement than Gawande's sensational exposé on checklists.[9]

What should be the responsibility of IRBs with regard to QI initiatives?

Many cost-containment activities occasioned either by professionals or hospital corporations constitute human experimentation by accidental but predictable intent.[*10] Such activities demand vigorous scientific peer review and some form of independent extramural funded ethical oversight beyond hospital control under the existing rule of law. Unfortunately, the most comprehensive review on this subject proposes only an extension of the existent IRB structure called a QI-IRB to perform the determination of exempt or non-exempt study for consent procedures.[11] Keeping such activities within hospital management that has a cost containment integrity conflict related to the care of individuals and its public mission is not likely to prove legally or morally acceptable in the long run. In Sabin's "Accountability for Reasonableness" illustration, there is diminishing fidelity to individuals as decision-making occurs increasingly in boardrooms rather than exam rooms, and diminishing stewardship of resources as the focus on individuals increases (Fig. 33.1).

The Electronic Medical Record (EMR), QI initiatives and privacy issues

As the US prepares for healthcare reform, the 2009 Emergency Federal Relief Budget and The Health Information Technology for Economic and Clinical Health Act allocated 19 billion dollars for electronic medical records (EMRs) for patients in every physician's office and acute care hospital by 2014.[12] Already, 1.4 billion dollars have been spent to develop regional federal extension centers to assist providers in creating the EMR and its local integrated development.

Defining a "recompensible EMR" and requirements for integrated connectivity upon manufacturers of hardware and software for local and national databases is a first step to future QI evaluation projects using the EMR. QI analysts in the "reform era" and health system leaders await these definitions to produce the "data-driven cultural change" of healthcare delivery.

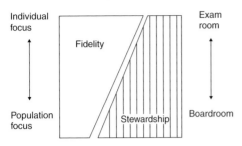

Figure 33.1. Reproduced by permission from J. Sabin. Cost-containment ethics requires fiduciary trust of both physicians and institutions to disclose their summative integrity for patient care under rationing policies.

QI projects in this new world require new ethical/legal regulatory architecture. If there is to be privacy and confidentiality of shared information between patients and providers, then the Office of the National Coordinator for Health Care Information Technology (ONC) should publish the specifics of lawfully maintaining that privacy. QI activities requiring both collection and transparent data dissemination will be in conflict with existent regulations of the OHRP placed on present-day IRBs.

Plans to define efficiency and quality value performance will be morally challenged if quality measures defining payment of institutions and physicians are recognized as social policy experimentation that violates the existent Code of Federal Regulations (CFR). Such policy questions require review and revision of the Belmont Report structure for QI organizational ethics and law interpretations, since such issues were not existent when the Belmont Report was issued in 1979. Defining "meaningful usage" of the EMR in national health policy awaits the necessary regulatory revision. These conceptual issues are the major unknowns for people conducting QI activities in anesthesiology and acute care hospital medicine. Resolving these unknowns are prerequisite to integrating primary care and acute care databases under healthcare reform.

At the operational level, QI project design needs concrete definitions of "meaningful usage."[12] Meaningful QI projects need meaningful end-point definitions of quality in order to define enhanced payments to providers to accomplish those endpoints and to determine what performance data will be deemed of lower payment priority. Detailed definitional output from ONC is an urgent emerging national QI priority.

At the most basic clinical level, QI projects must ask "Will EMRs truly cut costs and find efficiencies without decrements in the quality and accessibility of care?" Contemporary EMRs provide major cost savings and revenue enhancements for billing and coding systems integrated into provider payments.[13] Physicians clearly see computers as helpful when they facilitate rapid access to laboratory data and imaging diagnostic results. What has proved burdensome to patients and professionals is the time needed to properly enter computerized physician order entry (CPOE) and the nonmonetarized costs of added professional time.

Users of hospital computer information systems need ongoing real-time transparent flowcharts for ICU, emergency room, operating suites, and procedure area patients on hospital-based computers. The records must fulfill the seamless availability of ongoing minute-to-minute flow sheets to facilitate information transfer across shifts of individuals and nursing personnel to physicians. If these flow records cannot meet these standards of clinical necessity, they should be accounted for as quality and safety decrements in performance evaluation.

Future QI ethics projects will be more easily understood and rewarded when efficiency is properly measured and held financially accountable to maximize professional quality/time inputs and outputs.

A primary care physician in a remote office will need the same enhanced EMR time maximizing efficiency. Leveraging system productivity requires funded connectivity telemedicine applications in offices and patient residential sites that will permit physician extenders to leverage and maximize higher complexity decision-making activity by primary care physicians liberated from present-day documentation inefficiencies. Primary care physicians will need swift telemedicine consultation with specialists when necessary to efficiently solve chronic disease management issues in the home setting to prevent additional hospitalizations. Meaningful usage criteria here should carry the ability of the EMR to produce demonstrable cost savings and efficiency, on the one hand, while providing negative efficiency documentation of redundant functions not captured in deficient EMR hardware and software on the other.

Other nations have been implementing EMR integration with direct caregivers for several years. Successful smaller nations have required local integration. Vast data composites to assess the national productivity or net aggregate costs are a political imperative but will not offer a delivery cultural transformation. Smaller QI projects undertaken by QI analysts going forward will offer the necessary guidance to effect real change in individual services, hospitals and communities as a whole. Thus, the data-driven EMR, defined as "meaningful usage" will be fundamental in illuminating the legislative revision of CFRs and OHRP's legal accountability in advancing efficiency, safety, quality, and privacy in clinical medicine.

Key points

- QI/QA has evolved from an informal retrospective review of critical incidents to large retrospective analyses and evaluation of physicians, departments, hospitals and healthcare systems.
- These three phases of QI are:
  - Reactive or descriptive QI: react to sentinel events.
  - Outcome improvement QI: improve an already satisfactory outcome.
  - Cost containment QI: Improve efficiency leading to a satisfactory/better outcome.
- Some forms of QI activity actually represent human subjects research, with potential for patient harm. As such, similar ethical imperatives should apply in protecting patients from unconsented research when QI initiatives involve significant changes in patient care.
- As rationing and cost-containment efforts increase, IRBs may come under increasing pressure, and therefore experience conflicts of interest, with regard to evaluation of cost-containment QI activities.
- The Electronic Medical Record (EMR) carries powerful potential as a tool in QI and cost-containment efforts. Use of patient records carries risk for future privacy conflicts necessitating revision of the CFR and OHRP's regulatory authority in federal policy creation.

References

1 Suarez, J.I., Shannon, L., Zaidat, O.O., *et al*. (2004). Effect of human albumin administration on clinical outcome and hospital cost in patients with subarachnoid hemorrhage. *J Neurosurg*, **100**, 585–90.

2 Heros, R. (2004). Fluid management. *J Neurosurg*, **100**, 581–2.

3 Rie, M.A., Fahy, B.G., and Kofke, W.A. (2005). Human serum albumin. *J Neurosurg*, **101**, 564–6; author reply 566.

4* Donabedian, A. (1980). *Definition of Quality and Approaches to Its Assessment*. Ann Arbor, Michigan: Health Administration Press.

5* To Err Is Human. (1999). A Report of the Institute of Medicine. Washington, DC: National Academy Press.

6 Bellin, E. and Dubler, N.N. (2001). The quality improvement–research divide and the need for external oversight. *Am J Public Health*, **91**(9), 1512–17.

7 Aviation Safety Network. http://aviation-safety.net/database/record.php?id=19741201-0.

8* Bosk, C.L., Goeschel, C.A., and Pronovost, P.J. (2009). The art of medicine: reality for checklists. *Lancet*, **374**, 444–5.

9 Gawande, A. (2007). A life saving checklist. Opinion, *New York Times* December 30. Available at www.nytimes.com/2007/12/30/opinion/30gawande.html?/.

10* Kofke, W.A. and Rie, M.A. (2003). Research ethics and law of healthcare system quality improvement: The conflict of cost containment and quality. *Crit Care Med*, **31**(Suppl), S143–52.

11* Baily, M.A., Bottrell, M., Lynn, J., and Jennings, B. (2006). The ethics of using QI methods to improve quality and safety. *Hastings Cent Rep*, **36**, S1–40.

12 http://healthit.hhs.gov/.

13 Haig, S. Electronic records: will they really cut costs?. http://www.time.com/time/health/article/0,8599,1883002,00.html/.

Further reading

Childress, J.F., Meslin, E.M., and Shapiro, H.T. (2005). *Belmont Revisited*. Washington, DC: Georgetown University Press (p.vii).

Grady, C. (2007). Quality improvement and ethical oversight. *Ann Int Med*, **146**(9), 680–1.

Miller, F. and Emanuel, E. (2008). Quality improvement research and informed consent. *NEJM*, **358**(8), 765–7.

Rie, M.A. and Kofke, W.A. (2007). Non-therapeutic quality improvement: The conflict of organizational ethics and societal rule of law. *Crit Care Med*, **35 (Suppl)**, S66–84.

Rodwin, M.A. (1993). *Medicine, Money and Morals: Physicians' Conflicts of Interest*. New York: Oxford University Press.

Tapp, L., Edwards, A., Elwyn, G., *et al*. (2010). Quality improvement in general practice: enabling general practitioners to judge ethical dilemmas. *J Med Ethics*, **36**(3), 184–8.

US Department of Health Education and Welfare. (1979). Protection of human subjects: Belmont Report. Ethical principles and guidelines for the protection of human subjects of research. *Fed Reg*, **44**, 23192–7.

34

Conflicts of interest in research funding

Michael Nurok and Carl C. Hug, Jr.

The Case

An academic physician has a long history of receiving industry support for clinical research on a medication that she had helped to develop. The university sold the patent rights to a local biotechnology company. The company is small but rapidly growing, and the physician knows most of the founding members. She and her husband are friendly with the Chief Executive Officer, and their children attend the same school along with children of other company members.

To date, clinical reports have supported the new drug as superior to the much less costly and generically available alternative. But data analysis from her recent clinical trial yields no statistical difference between the two products. She discusses her findings with members of the sponsoring biotechnology company, and they suggest that she allow one of their statisticians to check the results.

The company's statistician segregates the study population according to age and finds that there is greater variability in the group less than 40 years of age. He then repeats the standard statistical test after omitting the under 40 group and shows a clear statistical difference in favor of the new drug. Reanalysis of the data for the entire group with a novel statistical test also shows a definite benefit for the new product compared to the generic drug. A statistician at the university tells the physician that the novel statistical test was done correctly, but points out that this is an unusual – but not incorrect – statistical test to apply to this body of data. Because it is very important to prospective investors, the company officers urge that the positive data based only on the novel statistical method be published as soon as possible.

The investigator is an associate professor at the university and, with one additional peer-reviewed publication, feels confident that her promotion to professor will go through. She knows that her chances of publishing a paper on the study are greatly increased if the study findings are positive. In addition, she is in discussion with the biotechnology company about funding a large project to develop another drug. Without this funding she would be required to do more clinical work to support her salary and probably would have to dismiss members of her laboratory because no other future funding is envisaged. The economy is slow and two members of her laboratory are the sole support of their families.

The United States Institute of Medicine defined conflict of interest as:

Circumstances that create a risk that professional judgments or actions regarding a primary interest will be unduly influenced by a secondary interest. [1]

The report defines *primary interest* as promoting and protecting the integrity of research, the quality of medical education, and the welfare of patients. *Secondary interests* are listed as financial, the pursuit of professional advancement and recognition, and the desire to do favors for friends, family, students, or colleagues.

A number of different sources of potential conflicts of interest can be identified in the introductory case. These can be divided between *financial* and *non-financial* conflicts.

There is a risk that the physician's professional judgments or actions with respect to her duty to promote and protect the integrity of research could be unduly influenced by the following *financial* motivations:

- Reliance on the company for partial support of her salary.
- Reliance on the company for financial support of her laboratory.

Sources of *non-financial* conflict exist with respect to this physician and include:

- Desire for publication of positive findings to facilitate academic promotion.
- Personal and spousal relationships with members of the biotechnology firm and its CEO.
- Children's social relationships with company members' children.
- Sense of responsibility towards members of her laboratory in regard to continued employment.

Clinical Ethics in Anesthesiology: A Case-Based Textbook, ed. Gail A. Van Norman, Stephen Jackson, Stanley H. Rosenbaum and Susan K. Palmer. Published by Cambridge University Press. © Cambridge University Press 2011.

Discussions of financial conflicts of interest tend to be based on certain assumptions. Stossel[2] describes these as beliefs that:

(1) Academic–industrial relationships promote research misconduct.

(2) Commercial intrusion leads to subtle or overt bias in the interpretation of research data, limitations of academic freedom, degradation of quality of research, and violation of important research values.

(3) If commercial intrusions even appear to compromise scientific integrity, public trust in and support for research will be eroded.

Stossel also points out that there is little empiric evidence to support these assumptions. Many point to the positive effects on medical innovation that academic relationships with industry have produced in contrast to the often-noted theoretical effects of conflicts of interest. Nevertheless, potential conflicts are apparent in the above scenario and are common in the practice of academic medicine. The most concerning effect of a financially motivated conflict of interest is that it may introduce bias into science and medicine.

The clinician investigator in this case has a number of potent incentives to publish positive findings of the trial using the novel statistical test. She would please the pharmaceutical company and enhance her ability to receive further research funding from the company. She would likely acquire the additional publication needed to be promoted. The social problems that may arise between her family members and their network of friends would be avoided. In addition, if her laboratory is funded, all of her employees would retain their jobs.

Disincentives to using the novel statistical test and publishing the positive findings include the risk to her reputation as an investigator and the increased costs of health care resulting from reliance on her study as support for prescribing the drug in question. More broadly, maintaining the public's trust in research is critical to ensuring participation in studies that may lead to new medical breakthroughs and also to ensuring faith in science and medicine. Using only the novel statistical test risks jeopardizing this trust.

A number of facts support the concerns that financial conflicts influence the integrity of medical research. Corporations in general, and industry and drug companies in particular, are focused on their responsibility to stockholders and some have acted aggressively to increase profits through various mechanisms such as controlling the use of data concerning their products.[3] A 2003 meta-analysis found that industry-associated clinical trials were significantly more likely to report product-favorable results than those in which industry relationships did not exist.[4]

Contracts between industry and academic institutions have included restrictions on the publication and other use of data without advance permission of the sponsor. Examples of the various contractual provisions related to publications of industry-sponsored trials were published in 2005.[5] A minority of institutions allowed sponsors to decide whether a study should or should not be published. Many institutions allowed contractual provisions to permit the sponsor to insert its own statistical analysis, and sometimes even to draft the manuscript.

Conflicts of interest are not just limited to researchers. In a recent study, 94% of physicians reported some sort of relationship with industry. Interestingly, anesthesiologists were less likely to have received samples, reimbursements, or payments than were family practitioners, internists, pediatricians, cardiologists or general surgeons who write more prescriptions for long-term use of drugs.[6] Psychiatrists have been a major focus of the investigations by US Senator Charles E. Grassley (R-Iowa), a sponsor of The Physician Payment Sunshine Act, 2009 (S.301). Despite evidence to support public concern regarding conflicts of interest, with the exception of isolated cases, little evidence points towards actual harm having been caused by conflicts.

Physicians have multiple loyalties, interests, and obligations that go beyond their professional role. These relationships lead to the potential for competing interests that are *non-financial* in their nature. Non-financial conflicts – although inherent to research and the practice of medicine – are more difficult to manage. Critics who perceive the focus on financial conflicts to be overzealous, have argued that industry is subject to scrutiny by the FDA and other regulatory bodies whereas academics are not.

Because the potential for nonfinancial conflicts is so ubiquitous, it is a challenging subject to study and there are far fewer data to assess their impact. Ideally, nonfinancial conflicts should be disclosed and acknowledged. However, criteria for doing so have not been established, and further research is needed to determine the magnitude of the problem and its consequent effects.[7]

Recommendations

Several options are open to the academic clinician in this case.

Option 1

The clinician may chose to publish using only the novel statistical test and to make the raw data from her study available online. This puts any uncertainty about the findings into the public domain and renders it available for transparent discussion and debate in addition to allowing other statistical analysis based on the raw data. The industry sponsor may not like this approach; however, it would most likely be better received by the company officers than Option 2. In addition, this approach would mitigate the social and professional risks discussed previously. An ethically defensible argument for this approach is that the novel statistical test is not inaccurate, simply unusual.

Option 2

The clinician may choose to use only the conventional statistical test and attempt to publish the negative findings of her results along with the raw data from her study. This approach may be difficult to achieve if the contract with the sponsor specifies limits on publication without the sponsor's approval. In addition, this option may antagonize the industry sponsor and expose the researcher to many of the social and professional risks noted above. Another important risk of this approach is that, if the conventional test is providing a false-negative result, use of this test may lead to the product being abandoned when it could provide a clinically important benefit. Placing the raw data in the public domain may mitigate this risk.

Option 3

The clinician may chose not to publish any results from her study. This is an ethically acceptable stance provided that the clinician is motivated by genuine uncertainty regarding her results in the face of opposing statistical interpretations. This stance is harder to justify if it is motivated by avoiding the social and professional conflicts brought about by her predicament. In addition, this approach means that data from her study are not available in the public domain.

Option 4

The clinician may choose to apply for additional funding either (1) to expand the number of patients in the under 40 group; or (2) to conduct another, better powered clinical trial in an attempt to answer the question definitively.

Option 5

The clinician may choose to publish using only data from the over 40 groups which represent the vast majority of people for whom the new drug would be prescribed. This approach is neither scientifically nor ethically appropriate because it is misleading and motivated by conflicting interests. It exposes the clinician to the lowest risk of adverse financial, social and professional consequences of all options at the cost of jeopardizing her professional reputation with respect to the duty to promote and protect the integrity of research.

Mitigating conflicts of interest

The potential for conflicts of interest can never be eliminated, but conflicts of interest can be managed and, in some cases, reduced. Strategies for doing so are most useful when they are matters of institutional and editorial policies that are focused on preventing the adverse effects of conflict of interest and are not unduly burdensome.

The first and most common step in managing conflicts involves disclosure. Following recent scandals in the United States, several institutions are voluntarily publishing information regarding conflicts of interest online.[8] Agreement is needed on criteria and thresholds for disclosure. Another mechanism for managing conflicts is monitoring of research by independent bodies, and public disclosure of raw scientific data. This step would help prevent (by functioning as a deterrent) or detect the most concerning effect of conflicts of interest – the introduction of bias. Research on other mechanisms for preventing bias is needed.

Managing financial and other types of conflicts of interest extend beyond the individual investigator to the academic institutions themselves, because the institutions have become dependent on research productivity, scientific, and medical advancements for their financial well-being and enhancement of their reputations.[9] The American Bayh-Dole Act of 1980 (pub L. No. 96–517) and the Federal Transfer Act of 1986 (Pub L. No. 99–502) provided strong incentives to investigators and institutions to patent findings of publicly funded research, and led to an explosion of academic–industry interactions highlighting that academia and industry have different as well as common interests (Table 34.1).

Table 34.1. Diverse and common interests of academic anesthesiology and industry

	Academic Anesthesiology →	Common Interests	←Industry

Incentives	**Professional recognition**
	• Promotion
	  • Increased income
	  • Increased resources
	    • Research space
	    • Assistants
	• **Increased extracurricular activities**
	  • Lectures
	  • Consulting
	  • Prestige
		• New knowledge
		• Research and Development
		• Improved Quality of Life
		• Improved Patient Care and Safety
			• **Attract Customers**
			• **Attract Investors**
			• **Increased Valuation**
			• **Pay Dividends and Bonuses**

Methods	• **Financial support**
	  • Mentors
	  • Space, Staff
	  • Equipment, Supplies
	  • Travel, publications
	• **Publication**
	  • "Selling" ideas
		• Attract bright people
		• Find experts
		• Recognize need and find solution
		• Develop products
		• Collaboration
		• Promote ideas and products
		  • Journals
		  • Meetings (CME and social)
		  • Mailings
		  • Personal contacts
			• **Operations**
			  • Build facilities
			  • Hire Staff
			• **Obtain Approvals FDA**
			• **Advertise**
			  • Selling ideas and products
			  • Public media
			  • Annual reports

Resources	• **Grants**
	  • University
	  • Foundations
	  • Industry
	  • Government
			• **Investors**
			• **Sales**

Checks and Balances	• **IRBs**
	  • Research
	  • Human, clinical
	  • Animal
	• **Compliance, regulations**
	• **Peer review**
	  • Grant applications
	  • Publications
	• **Misconduct Reports**
		• **Ethics, morals**
		  • Individual
		  • Institutional
		• **Legal actions**
		• **Public censure**
			• **Government regulations**
			• **Negative publicity**
			• **Lawsuits**

Policies and guidance on conflicts of interest are changing rapidly. The United States the National Institutes of Health[10] and the Department of Health and Human Services Office of Human Research Protection offer updated guidelines.[11] In the United Kingdom, the General Medical Council offers such guidance.[12]

Key points

- One of the most harmful adverse consequences of conflicts of interest in research is the potential introduction of bias into the science of medicine and the denigration of the integrity of scientific research.

- The potential for conflicts of interest in research can never be eliminated, but can be managed, and in many cases reduced.
- Strategies for reducing conflicts of interest in research are most effective if they involve clear institutional and editorial policies.
- Disclosure is the most common first step in managing conflicts of interest.
- Public disclosure of raw scientific data and independent monitoring of research are additional mechanisms for managing conflicts of interest.

References

1* Institute of Medicine. (2009). *Conflict of Interest in Medical Research, Education, and Practice*. Washington, DC: National Academies Press.

2* Stossel, T.P. (2005). Regulating academic-industrial research relationships – solving problems or stifling progress? *N Engl J Med*, **353**, 1060–5.

3* Angell, M. (2004). *The Truth about the Drug Companies: How They Deceive Us and What to Do about It*. 1st edn. New York: Random House.

4* Bekelman, J.E., Li, Y., and Gross, C.P. (2003). Scope and impact of financial conflicts of interest in biomedical research: a systematic review. *JAMA*, **289**, 454–65.

5* Mello, M.M., Clarridge, B.R., and Studdert, D.M. (2005). Academic medical centers' standards for clinical-trial agreements with industry. *N Engl J Med*, **352**, 2202–10.

6* Campbell, E.G., Gruen, R.L., Mountford, J., *et al.* (2007). A national survey of physician–industry relationships. *N Engl J Med*, **356**, 1742–50.

7* The *PLoS Medicine* Editors. (2008). *Making Sense of Non-Financial Competing Interests*. PLoS Med 5(9): e199. doi:10.1371/journal.pmed.0050199

8* Steinbrook, R. (2009). Online disclosure of physician–industry relationships. *N Engl J Med*, **360**, 325–7.

9* Johns, M.M.E., Barnes, M., and Florencio, P.S. (2003). Restoring balance to industry–academia relationships in an era of institutional financial conflicts of interest. Promoting research while maintaining trust. *JAMA*, **289** (6), 741–6.

10 NIH Guidelines. (Accessed 2 April 2009, at http://grants.nih.gov/grants/policy/coi/.)

11 DHHS Guidelines. (Accessed 2 April 2009, at http://www.dhhs.gov/ohrp/special/conflict.html.)

12 GMC Guidelines. (Accessed 2 April 2009, at http://www.gmc-uk.org/guidance/current/library/conflicts_of_interest.asp#1.)

Further reading

Levinsky, N.G. (2002). Nonfinancial conflicts of interest in research. *N Engl J Med*, **347**, 759–61.

35

Publication ethics: obligations of authors, peer-reviewers, and editors

Gail A. Van Norman and Stephen Jackson

The Case

An anesthesia pain management researcher submits abstracts for two studies. It is discovered that he did not obtain prior approval for human subjects research. In addition, a colleague finds he is listed as a co-author on one of the studies, although he did not participate in the research. Investigation reveals that the anesthesiologist had fabricated data in some or all of 21 published studies dating back over 13 years. This uncovered what arguably is one of the most wide-ranging research fraud cases in history. His reports had been favorable to several drugs under investigation as "replacements" for postoperative narcotic therapy, and also had refuted animal studies suggesting that one of these medications interfered with bone healing after orthopedic surgery.

Not only are all of this researcher's findings now in question, but also those of numerous studies by other investigators that relied upon these findings for subsequent research design and comparisons. A medical journal editor remarked that "these retractions clearly raise the possibility that we might be heading in the wrong directions or toward blind ends in attempts to improve pain therapy."[1] A prominent academic anesthesiologist stated that the fraudulent research had affected "millions of patients worldwide," and possibly led to the sale of "billions of dollars worth of potentially dangerous drugs."[2]

Ethical principles of beneficence and nonmaleficence require that physicians strive to improve medical knowledge to improve patients' lives (beneficence) and avoid harmful or ineffective treatments (nonmaleficence). Medical research seeks to find truths that support these principles, and medical literature should be a map illuminating that search. The integrity of research involves more than simply the just and honest conduct of research, but also honest and fair reporting and analysis of results, peer review, and publication of research findings. Investigators and authors have primacy over the ethical conduct and reporting of research, but the publication process also involves ethical obligations on the part of reviewers, editors, and publishers. Fraudulent research and publication practices divert the search for truth, and corrupt the medical literature.

Publication also serves other critical processes in promoting the integrity and efficacy of the medical profession, and thereby in promoting patient well-being. Scientific enterprise is built on a foundation of trust. "If science is to flourish and attain its appropriate role in aiding human progress, it is incumbent upon…the scientific community to help provide a research environment that, through its adherence to high ethical standards…will attract and retain individuals of outstanding intellect and character."[3] Synthesis, debate, and discussion are all integral to the intellectual process required for analyzing and validating the relevancy of scientific findings in the context of medical care. Medical publications educate physicians through reviews and synopses of complex research findings, distilled for application in clinical practice.

Publication is a critical part of academic medicine, and sets scholarly work apart from the practice of medicine. Authorship is integral to obtaining credit for one's research, creative thoughts, and educational efforts, and it is essential for achieving a successful academic career. Publications influence promotions and can affect recruitment opportunities and future research funding. As the gatekeepers to publication, reviewers and editors wield power over whether academic credit is justly apportioned, and thereby can affect academic careers. They also determine which research is "relevant" enough to see the light of publication, and may thereby indirectly determine which patient groups benefit from research efforts.

Investigation of scientific fraud

Scientific misconduct is internationally recognized as a serious problem, but few countries have regulatory

---

Clinical Ethics in Anesthesiology: A Case-Based Textbook, ed. Gail A. Van Norman, Stephen Jackson, Stanley H. Rosenbaum and Susan K. Palmer. Published by Cambridge University Press. © Cambridge University Press 2011.

systems in place to evaluate scientific fraud. Widely publicized cases of scientific misconduct led the US Congress to establish the Office of Scientific Integrity (later named the Office of Research Integrity, or ORI) in 1989. Denmark, Norway, Finland, and Sweden all established formal review councils in the early 1990s to investigate scientific fraud. In the UK, medical fraud is reported to the General Medical Council (GMC). A voluntary organization, the Committee on Publication Ethics (COPE), which includes publishers and editors of over 300 journals in Europe and Asia, reviews instances of misconduct. However, it functions as an advisory body and cannot apply sanctions. Other countries calling for institutional or other reviews and sanctions include Canada, Japan, India, Croatia, Germany, and China, although none has regulatory agencies.[4]

In practice, the reporting, investigation, and (potential) sanctioning of fraudulent research and publication practices falls largely to professional peers, individual institutions, and the actions of journal reviewers and editors.

Ethical obligations of authorship and author misconduct

The International Committee of Medical Journal Editors (ICMJE) defines an author as one who has made substantial contributions in all of the following areas: concept, design and acquisition of data or analysis and interpretation of data, drafting or critical revision of the publication, and final approval of the version that is published.[5]

Medical authors have ethical obligations of veracity, or to be truthful and nonmanipulative, in the reporting of research results. In addition, authors have obligations to be just in allocating credit for what often is a collaborative effort among colleagues. Author misconduct has the potential to cause detrimental treatment of patients, as well as to mislead other researchers in the construction and implementation of their subsequent research designs. It also may harm academic colleagues by failing to properly credit their work, or by inappropriately crediting them with work they did not do.

Types of author misconduct in research publication include, but are not limited to: (1) fabrication (the invention of false results); (2) falsification (the manipulation or omission of critical data so as to inaccurately represent the research record or results); (3) plagiarism (appropriation of another's ideas, processes, results or words without appropriate attribution); (4) ghost authorship (the acceptance of credit for publications written by another or the assignment of credit to a non-author); and (5) redundant publication (the submission of the same study in more than one publication, or the deliberate splitting of results from one study into several publications).

Fabrication and falsification of data

The harm caused by falsification and fabrication of data is self-evident. False information may cause practitioners to expose patients to ineffective, or worse, harmful treatments. Other researchers may be diverted from productive paths of inquiry in the pursuit of fictional results. One study of researchers suggests that nearly 2% admit to at least one career episode of fabricating, falsifying or modifying data. However, when asked about the behavior of colleagues, about 14% admitted to knowing of falsifications. Medical and pharmacological researchers more frequently report misconduct than other researchers.[6] Another study confirmed these discouraging results, finding that 4.7% of authors surveyed stated they had participated in research that involved fabrication or misrepresentation. In only about half of cases had the misconduct ever been discovered. Over 17% of the authors indicated that they knew of instances of falsification, fabrication or misleading reporting involving other academics. In a large proportion of these cases, the conduct also remains undiscovered, suggesting that the authors themselves had not reported the misconduct.[7]

Plagiarism: theft of intellectual property, or the sincerest form of flattery?

A basic definition of plagiarism is the appropriation of someone else's words and/or ideas as one's own. It is nearly always wrong,[a] because it damages the true author (by denying credit and disrespecting their efforts), it harms readers (by deceiving them, and by making it harder for them to trace the true route by which an idea was developed) and it accumulates benefits to the undeserving (the plagiarist). Plagiarism raises questions of trust in scholarly work: if an author copies some material, how do we know they didn't copy something else?

A review conducted at Harvard found that complaints over medical authorship, including the plundering of noncredited work of junior academicians, had more than quadrupled over a period of one decade. A larger total proportion of complaints came from females, although they represented a minority of the academic population. There was also a trend toward more complaints from non-US citizens,[8] suggesting that plagiarism may more often "victimize" academically vulnerable populations. A notorious example of scientific plagiarism is the surreptitious acquisition by Watson and Crick of unpublished data, "photograph 51," from Rosalind Franklin's research on DNA structure as well as of a confidential research progress report about her work. Both elements were essential to their development of the double helix model.[9,10] Crick later acknowledged that their work was based on Franklin's data in 1961, sadly 3 years after her death.[11]

Plagiarism violates ethical principles of nonmaleficence and justice. While it is easy to condemn plagiarism, it nonetheless is technically challenging to identify precisely what constitutes plagiarism. It also is questionable whether all forms of plagiarism are equally culpable.

Words versus ideas

The verbatim copying of an entire thesis of another is easy to identify as plagiarism, because it steals both the words and ideas that comprise the creative work of the original author. But words and ideas do not in all instances have similar weight in determining originality. For example, a great love poem is not great because of an original concept (love), but is exceptional for its *expression* of the concept. Paraphrasing such a poem would not constitute plagiarism because it is the original *wording* that makes it unique. Bouville points out that science and scholarship, on the other hand, are about new *knowledge and ideas*. "An experimental result that is described using different words is not a different result."[12] Therefore, in medicine and science, the wording might be less important than the ideas that the words convey in determining if a scientific thesis has been plagiarized.

Is all plagiarism equally wrong?

Is self-plagiarism (when an author makes duplicate statements in two different publications) ethically as concerning as plagiarizing the work of another? Self-plagiarizing original research results is the same as redundant or duplicate publication and it is harmful in ways that are discussed below. But what about scholarly reviews, synthesis, and opinion publications? Ideas can only be expressed in so many ways. While some have labeled the practice "intentional fraud,"[13] Chalmers points out that an author may deliberately

use similar styles and wording in different venues to express particularly important concepts, simply because repetition also represents emphasis, and thereby underscores an idea's importance.[14] The self-plagiarist is not stealing original ideas or words from anyone else. Publishers have reason to expect that their copyrights will be honored, but concerns about the integrity of the scholarly work itself appear to be less serious in such cases.

Redundant publication

Redundant publication includes the practice of publishing the same results in different journals, publishing a review of those results nearly simultaneously in a different journal, or splitting a study into two or more parts to publish in separate journals. While the last practice may be acceptable when a study involves large populations studied over many years, overlapping or split manuscripts are usually not justified.

Redundant publication may be undertaken to distort academic accomplishments in a "publish or perish" system. Almost 1 in 20 scientists admit to publishing the same data in two or more sources in order to enhance their curriculum vitae.[15] Some authors claim that they merely were trying to reach different audiences. However, duplicate publication has detrimental effects that may be visited on patients, and on colleagues trying to sort through a mass of information for meaningful results. Redundancy adds inconsequential material to the medical literature, may wrongly emphasize the importance of findings, and burdens an already overladen publication review system.

Ghost authorship and honorary authorship

"Ghost writing" and "honorary" authorship both involve the improper attribution of authorship or credit to someone who did not actually participate in the research or the review and synthesis of ideas on which a publication is based. "Ghost writing" is the practice of failing to name an individual who substantially contributed to a publication. The term often refers to the practice of attaching a researcher's name to a paper that was written by a professional writer who is not named. In "honorary authorship," the name of (often) a senior academic is included among the true authors although that academician did not have a principle role in the publication. Both of these practices are common. In one study, approximately 29% of articles had honorary authors, ghost authors, or both.[16] In the case of industry-related trials, one study demonstrated a prevalence of ghost authorship approaching 91%.[17]

Improperly assigning or concealing authorship violates ethical guidelines for authorship, and is harmful to the medical publication process in a number of ways. It may falsely elevate the perceived significance and reliability of a study if well-respected researchers are inappropriately credited with the findings. Ghost writing can hide conflicts of interest that may affect the balance and veracity of the material presented – as, for example, when the writer is a pharmaceutical company employee discussing an important new drug that the company is developing. Knowing the identities of the true author(s) of a study is important with respect to both accountability, and also to the ability to retrospectively examine results in light of new data, such as newly recognized adverse outcomes. Basic trial data can be difficult to review after the fact, particularly if the authors of the record did not write the original report and no longer have access to original trial data.[18] An author who knowingly agrees to allow his or her name to be attached to work in which he/she did not participate is engaging in an act of fraud.

Ethical obligations of peer reviewers

Peer review is encountered throughout medicine. It is used to judge clinical performance and quality outcome measures, as well as to determine the allocation of research grants and the quality of research design. It is also a key process in medical publications. Peer review satisfies the practical need to determine if research and reviews are well-designed, ethically executed, and present significant new information that will lead to better patient care. Peer review also serves professional interests in maintaining autonomy within the specialty to evaluate professional performance. Peer reviewers have the power not only to impact career advancement among authors, but also to directly affect which studies and opinions find their way into the medical literature and thereafter influence the practice of medicine.

Expertise

Although it seems self-evident that peer reviewers require appropriate expertise in the field being reviewed, incompetent review is one of the most common complaints among researchers. More than 60% of researchers polled in one study indicated that they had experienced incompetent reviews, defined as the reviewer being unfamiliar with the subject matter, not

carefully reading the article, or making mistakes of fact or reasoning in the review.[19]

Confidentiality and trust

Reviewers are in a position of trust, receiving advance notice of potentially important discoveries prior to their publication. Breach of confidentiality exposes the author to the risks of plagiarism, and also to the risks that commercially sensitive information could be inappropriately released, either to the public or to investor interests. Examples of plagiarism and theft by peer reviewers, while not common, are not very difficult to find.[20] One-tenth of researchers who were surveyed indicated they believed that a reviewer had deliberately delayed approval of one of their manuscripts so that the reviewer could publish an article on the same topic.[19]

Respect and protection of dignity of colleagues

No author relishes a poor review or rejection, but surprisingly, *abusive* reviews, that is ones in which the author, and not the idea, comes under attack, are not uncommon.[19] One article reports abusive reviewer comments that included an unsupported accusation that a new primary investigator had submitted a senior researcher's ideas as their own, a statement that revisions to a paper should "start by burning the entire manuscript," and actual name calling.[21] Clearly, peer reviewers have obligations not only to confine their critiques to the manuscript, but also to respect the dignity of their colleagues, lest the peer review process become mired in personal attacks and retributive behavior.

Ethical obligations of journal editors

Editors have considerable power: their decisions about what gets published – whether research results, reviews or editorial opinion – significantly impact perceptions and practice in medicine and medical research. They control what criticisms may be launched against authors, and how authors may respond when criticized. As the ultimate gatekeepers on publication, they hold considerable sway over academic careers. Despite such influence, the ethical responsibilities of editors only recently have been considered in depth.

In parallel to authors and peer reviewers, editors have ethical obligations to assure as far as possible that published material is accurate and not fraudulent, that research adheres to ethical guidelines with regard to protection of human and animal subjects, that confidentiality of manuscript submissions is maintained,

Table 35.1. Responsibilities of journal editors*

General responsibilities
- Strive to meet the needs of readers and authors
- Constantly improve the journal
- Ensure the quality of published material
- Champion freedom of expression
- Maintain the integrity of the academic record
- Preclude business needs from compromising intellectual standards
- Willingly publish corrections, clarifications, retractions and apologies when needed

Relations to readers
- Inform readers about who had funded research and the role of the funders in the research

Relations with authors
- Ensure the quality of published materials, recognizing that journal and sections within journals have different aims and standards
- Decisions to accept or reject a paper should be based only on the paper's importance, originality, and clarity, and the study's relevance to the journal
- A description of the review process should be published and any deviation from the published process justified
- There should be a declared mechanism for author appeal
- There should be published guidelines of expectations to authors that are regularly updated
- Acceptance of submissions should not be reversed except in cases where serious problems are identified
- New editors should not overturn acceptances by previous editors unless serious problems are identified

Relations with reviewers
- There should be published guidelines to reviewers of what is expected of them; these guidelines should be regularly updated
- Editors should assure that reviewers' identities are protected unless they have an open review system that is declared to authors and reviewers

The peer-review process
- Systems should be in place to assure that submitted materials remain confidential while under review

Complaints
- Editors should follow the COPE flowchart
- Editors should respond promptly to complaints. Mechanisms for further management of complaints should be published, and unresolved matters referred to COPE

Encouraging debate
- Cogent criticisms of published works should be published unless there are convincing reasons why they cannot be.
- Authors of criticized material should be given opportunity to respond

* summarized from the Committee on Publication Ethics
http:www.publicationethics.org/files/u2/New_Code.pdf.

and that any potential personal conflicts of interest are avoided or at least made transparent.

COPE has outlined a code of conduct for journal editors, listing essential responsibilities (see Table 35.1). While much of this effort concentrated on the administrative duties and transparency of medical editorship, the code included important responsibilities to assure that allegations of misconduct are properly investigated.

A critically important, and difficult responsibility of medical editors is one of "cleansing" the medical literature when instances of publishing misconduct

are proven. This is especially important if the reliability of data is in question, since erroneous or fraudulent results has ramifications for both patient care and future research. Although the COPE published code of conduct for editors charges them with retraction of fraudulent or unethical research (see Table 35.2), barriers to such retractions may include protracted investigation processes, author disagreement, threats of litigation, and misunderstandings by editors themselves of appropriate actions to take. COPE emphasizes that the purpose of retraction should always be correction of the literature, and not punishment of the author,

Table 35.2. Guidelines for retracting articles*

Editors should consider retraction when
- There is clear evidence that the findings are unreliable, due to misconduct or honest error
- Findings have been previously published elsewhere without proper reference, permission or justification
- The publication is plagiarized
- The study reports unethical research

Editors should consider an expression of concern when
- There is inconclusive evidence of research or publication misconduct
- There is evidence the findings are unreliable, but the authors' institution will not investigate
- They believe an investigation into misconduct has not been – or would not be – fair and impartial, or conclusive
- An investigation is underway, but judgement will not be available for a considerable time

Editors should consider issuing a correction when
- A small portion of an otherwise reliable publication proves to be misleading
- The author/contributor list is incorrect

Retractions are NOT usually appropriate if
- A change of authorship is needed, but there is no reason to doubt the findings

Notices of Retraction should
- Be linked to the retracted article electronically
- Clearly identify the retracted article
- State clearly that it is a retraction (i.e. not a correction or comment)
- Be published promptly to minimize harms
- Be freely available to all readers (i.e. not only available to subscribers)
- State who is retracting the article
- State the reasons for the retraction
- Avoid statements that are potentially defamatory or libellous

* summarized from the COPE guidelines on retracting articles
http: publicationethics.org.

because problems in publishing can occur due to honest mistakes as well as willful misconduct. Investigation and punishment are best referred back to the author's institution for further action.

Case resolution

The introductory case is an example of fabrication of data. Moreover, the anesthesiologist improperly involved an unknowing colleague in the fraud by attaching his name to the research. The concerns about the anesthesiologist's research were raised at his home institution, which then notified journals in which his publications appeared. *All* of the researcher's articles were retracted. However, "scrubbing" the literature of all citations of this research as well as managing derivative publications from related research is an ongoing task that may never be complete. The effects on patients are unknown. Because the research results encouraged the use of medications that may have had detrimental effects on bone healing, both physical and financial harms to patients on a large scale remain possible.

Key points

- Publication serves physicians' ethical duties to improve medical knowledge, provide continuing benefits to patients, and avoid harmful or ineffective treatment.
- Publication is an integral part of academic medicine – crediting research, creative thoughts, and educational efforts.
- Few regulatory bodies exist globally to investigate scientific fraud.
- Authors have ethical obligations to be truthful regarding credit for the work and outcomes of research.
- Fabrication and falsification of data, plagiarism, misleading assignment of authorship and redundant publications all are detrimental to the mission of medical publication.
- Peer reviewers have obligations to be competent, fair, and balanced, and free of

conflicts of interest in reviewing medical manuscripts. Breaches of confidentiality and abusive review tactics are not consistent with ethical review.

- Journal editors have parallel responsibilities to assure accuracy in the medical literature. They have additional responsibilities to try to assure that appropriate investigation occurs if fraud is suspected, and to retract suspect material when it is discovered.

Notes

[a] Authors' comment: plagiarism that is encouraged and condoned by the original author may not always be wrong.

References

1   Winstein, K.J. and Armstrong, D. Top pain scientist fabricated data in studies, hospital says. *The Wall Street Journal*. March 11, 2009. http://online.wsj.com/article/SB123672510903888207.html.

2   Borrell, B. A medical Madoff: anesthesiologist faked data in 21 studies. *Scientific American*, March 10, 2009. http://www.scientificamerican.com/article.cfm?id=a-medical-madoff-anesthesiologist-faked-data.

3   Alberts, B. (2010). Promoting scientific standards. (Editorial). *Science*, **327**, 12–3.

4   Council of Science Editors. White paper on promoing integrity in scientific journal publications. Approved by the CSE Board of Directors, March 29, 2009. http://www.councilscienceeditors.org/editorial_policies/whitepaper/3-2_international.cfm.

5   Uniform requirements for manuscripts submitted to biomedical journals; ethical considerations in the conduct and reporting of research: authorship and contributorship. International Committee of Medical Journal Editors. ICMJE.org. http://www.ICMJE.org./ethical_1author.html.

6   Fanelli, D. (2009). How many scientists fabricate and falsify research? A systematic review and metaanalysis of survey data. *PLoS One*, **4**(5), e5738.

7   Gardner, W., Lidz, C.W., and Hartwig, K.C. (2005). Authors' reports about research integrity problems in clinical trials. *Contemp Clin Trials*, **26**(2), 244–51.

8   Wilcox, L. (1998). Authorship. The coin of the realm, the source of complaints. *JAMA*, **280**(3), 216–17.

9   Fuller, W. (2003). Who said 'helix'? *Nature*, **424**, 876–8.

10 Watson, J.D. (1968). *The Double Helix: A Personal Account of the Discovery of the Structure of DNA*. New York: Athenaeum.

11 Zallen, D.T. (2003). Despite Franklin's work, Wilkins earned his Nobel. *Nature*, **425**(6951), 15.

12* Bouville, M. (2008). Plagiarism: words and ideas. *Sci Eng Ethics*, **14**, 311–22.

13 Editorial: Self-plagiarism: unintentional, harmless, or fraud? (2009). *Lancet*, **374**(9691), 664.

14 Chalmer, I. (2009). Intentional self-plagiarism. *Lancet*, **374**(9699), 1422.

15* Khanyile, T.D., Duma, S., Fakude, L.P., *et al.* (2006). Research integrity and misconduct: a clarification of the concepts. *Curationis*, **29**(1), 40–5.

16 Flanagin, A., Carey, L.A., Fontanarosa, P.B., *et al.* (1998). Prevalence of articles with honorary authors and ghost authors in peer-reviewed medical journals. *JAMA*, **280**(3), 222–4.

17 Gotzsche, P.C., Hrobjartsson, A., Johansen, H.K. *et al.* (2007). Ghost authorship in industry-initiated randomized trials. *PLoS Med*, **4**, e19.

18 Johansen, H.K. and Gotzsche, P.C. (1999). Problems in the design and reporting of trials of antifungal agents encountered during meta-analysis. *JAMA*, **282**, 1752–9.

19 Resnik, D.B., Gutierrez-Ford, C., and Peddada, S. (2008). Perceptions of ethical problems with scientific journal peer review: an exploratory study. *Sci Eng Ethics*, **14**, 305–10.

20 Dalton, R. (2001). Peers under pressure. *Nature*, **413**, 102–4.

21 Hadjistavropoulos, T. and Bieling, P.J. (2000). When reviewers attack: ethics, free speech, and the peer review process. *Can Psychol*, **41**(3), 152–9.

Further reading

Committee on Publication Ethics (COPE) http://publicationethics.org/ International Committee of Medical Journal Editors http://www.icmje.org.

Ross, J.S., Hill, K.P., Egilman, D.S., and Drumholz, H.M. (2008). Guest authorship and ghost writing in publications related to rofecoxib. *JAMA*, **299**(15), 1800–12.

Sox, H. and Rennie, D. (2006). Research misconduct: retraction and cleansing the medical literature: lessons learned from the Poehlman case. *Ann Int Med*, **144**(8), 609–13.

Wager, E., Barbour, V., Yentis, S., and Kleinert, S., on behalf of COPE Council. *Retractions: guidance from the Committee on Publication Ethics*. http://publicationethics.org/guidelines (accessed Dec 1, 2009).

World Association of Medical Editors. Dalla Lana School of Public Health, University of Toronto, Ontario, Canada http://www.wame.org/.

Section 5

Practice issues

36

The impaired anesthesiologist – addiction

Thomas Specht, Clarence Ward, and Stephen Jackson

The Case

A 43-year-old male anesthesiologist has been drug-free for 6 years following initial treatment for his sufentanil addiction and an extensive rehabilitation program administered by his state medical board. He has re-entered private practice with the support of his department and colleagues. His tightly monitored recovery program was considered to be a model of success. After 5 years, his monitoring intensity was loosened, although he continued to take naltrexone in a witnessed environment, regularly attended Narcotics Anonymous meetings, submitted witnessed random abstinence-urines for testing when required, and met every 3 months with an addiction specialist who reported his findings to the medical staff impaired physician chair. During the past 2 months, suspicion of relapse was raised by several close colleagues, but no evidence for narcotic diversion could be substantiated. Shortly after his last urine test submission, he was found unconscious in a bathroom with an empty 20 ml syringe and ampoule of propofol. This relapse was immediately followed by appropriate treatment for 18 months, once again serving as a "model" patient in recovery. He again expresses his desire to return to practice, but this time there is sharp disagreement within his department and group over re-entry.

Chemical dependence in the form of addiction is a chronic relapsing disease characterized by the overwhelming compulsion (both genetic and behavioral in origin) to use drugs in spite of adverse consequences. Drug addiction, unless identified and treated skillfully, will lead to disability and often to death. The practice of anesthesiology provides the setting for a susceptible "host" by offering an environment in which powerfully addictive drugs are immediately available for abuse.

Addiction in the specialty of anesthesiology

Prevalence

Addictive disease in the form of chemical dependency is present in all classes, cultures, and professions, including healthcare professionals. Its lifetime prevalence in the physician population is estimated to be 10%–12%, essentially the same as that of the general population.[1] Among anesthesiologists, the prevalence *appears* to be even higher. However, support for this perception is based on diagnosis from treatment programs for chemical dependence where the specialty of anesthesiology is over-represented in relation to most other medical specialties, at least with regard to drugs other than alcohol. This may be because the specialty of anesthesiology is particularly attuned to the issue, monitors its members more closely, and therefore detects chemical dependency more often than specialties that have lower vigilance.

Furthermore, recent trends in prescription drug abuse in the US suggest that perceptions regarding drug abuse that are based on literature from past decades is no longer relevant.

Outcomes

The historic approach to the addicted anesthesiologist has been to assume that those who complete treatment for addiction should be returned to practice. But a 1990 study of chemically dependent anesthesiology *residents* indicated that prolonged abstinence following treatment is unusual. Startlingly, 7% of those cases *presented with death*. Two-thirds of the residents who were allowed to reenter their programs after treatment relapsed, and perhaps most frightening, in 16% of those who relapsed, *death* was the presenting sign.[2] However, this study was criticized because of its poor design and inadequate inpatient treatment times. Nonetheless, its conclusion are likely to be valid, as a 2005 publication found that less than half of anesthesiology residents who attempted reentry successfully completed their residency, while 9% of those attempted reentrants *died*.[3] Such statistics raise the question of whether reentry by residents after treatment for substance abuse should

Clinical Ethics in Anesthesiology: A Case-Based Textbook, ed. Gail A. Van Norman, Stephen Jackson, Stanley H. Rosenbaum and Susan K. Palmer. Published by Cambridge University Press. © Cambridge University Press 2011.

even be attempted, or whether there is an ethical obligation of anesthesia training programs to prohibit residents from returning. This debate remains unresolved, but hopefully will lead to the development of effective standardized guidelines for appropriate evaluation, treatment, monitoring and aftercare (monitoring if returning to work) of the addicted anesthesiologist.

Is addiction a disability?

Addiction is approached from the perspective of a disease model in the United States, but it is not treated entirely as a disability. The Americans with Disabilities Act of 1990 prohibits discrimination based on disability, defined as "physical or mental impairment that substantially limits a major life activity." While physicians who are in current treatment for substance abuse are afforded some legal protections by the act, current substance abuse is excluded as a protected condition.

Ethical issues

The ASA *Guidelines for the Ethical Practice of Anesthesiology*[4] recognizes that anesthesiologists have professional responsibilities to patients, to colleagues, to facilities at which they practice, to self (meaning the duty to maintain physical, mental and emotional abilities necessary to good patient care), and to community and society. In the case of the addicted anesthesiologist, these obligations are further complicated by the fact that the anesthesiologist is not only a healthcare provider, but is also a patient, with ethical duties owed to them by others.

Anesthesiologists' ethical responsibilities to patients and themselves

All physicians have as their primary ethical responsibility the obligation to place their patients' interests foremost while providing competent medical care with compassion and respect for human dignity. This obligation, in turn, invokes anesthesiologists' ethical responsibilities to themselves. According to the American Society of Anesthesiologists' *Guidelines for the Ethical Practice of Anesthesiology*, they are required to

> "*maintain their physical and mental health and special sensory capabilities [and] if in doubt about their health … seek medical evaluation and care … [and further] during this period of evaluation or treatment … should modify or cease their practice.*"[4]

The unethical and illegal behavior inherent to the impaired anesthesiologist's addictive disease leads to a gradual inability to provide safe and competent care to the patient. Due to the progressive nature of drug addiction, the anesthesiologist-patient becomes subservient to the incessant demands of the disease. The addicted anesthesiologist may have tangential awareness of this fact, but the same rationalization that accepts or excuses his/her diversion of drugs dims awareness of the declining quality of patient care. Feeding addiction reorders a physician's priorities, pushing honesty and patient responsibility into the background.

As the disease progresses, there eventually is a degradation of the physician's personal health, and the physician commonly develops organic neuropsychiatric impairment that further clouds his/her ability to provide competent and compassionate care. This failure to place a patient's interests foremost represents a stark violation of the primary ethical obligation of any physician. It frequently is only after diagnosis and successful treatment that there is any direct awareness or acknowledgment of this inverted priority by the addicted physician.

During the course of the disease, the development of chemical (alcohol or drugs) tolerance demands ever-increasing doses and frequency of use. The pattern of use escalates, often rapidly, from off-duty occasional use to consumption while directly involved with patient care in the healthcare facility or operating room. Chemical impairment of anesthesiologists while they are involved in direct patient care clearly places patients at increased risk from cognitive errors in decision-making, diminished capacity for vigilance, and chemically induced physical discoordination. The incessant compulsion to obtain drugs is accompanied by both the continuous stress of disguising the addiction and the anxiety of impending withdrawal. In addition, the opiate-addicted anesthesiologist may divert drugs from patient use, potentially leading to inadequate postoperative pain control for patients. The potential for patient harm caused by the impaired anesthesiologist is the major impetus for prompt and effective action by the medical community.

Anesthesiologists' ethical responsibilities to their colleagues

In the course of their disease, the addicted anesthesiologist often violates many obligations to their colleagues. These include duties of honesty and fidelity to the profession. The addicted physician is induced by self-interest to conceal their addiction (thus preventing treatment), lest they be removed from the work place – and in most cases, away from their drug supply. In addition, the anesthesiologist abusing operating room (OR) drugs (e.g., fentanyl, sufentanil, ketamine or propofol) often turns to the theft of those drugs from the OR to maintain their supply. Alternatively, they may obtain drugs using actual or forged prescriptions. Not only are such activities frankly illegal, but they are a betrayal of the trust placed in physicians by society and by their colleagues, and thus a breach of duty.

ASA guidelines also describe the ethical responsibilities of anesthesiologists to their colleagues.

> *"Anesthesiologists should advise colleagues whose ability to practice medicine becomes temporarily or permanently impaired to appropriately modify or discontinue their practice. They should assist, to the extent of their own abilities, with the re-education or rehabilitation of a colleague who is returning to practice."* [4]

These obligations by extrapolation include the detection of addiction, intervention, treatment, and eventually rehabilitation of a colleague who is returning to practice. However, the response of an addicted physician's colleagues to addictive behavior, as in society, reflects a wide range of understanding of the relevant issues. Even with the reported high incidence of addiction in the specialty of anesthesiology, individuals in a department often are most influenced by their own personal experience with this problem, by the broader view society takes, or even other factors such as religious beliefs, rather than by full understanding of the addictive disease process.

Because chemical dependency is a disease, in the case of an impaired anesthesiologist there are actually two patients: the patient receiving anesthesia care, and the anesthesiologist him or herself. Conflicts may arises among colleagues of the addicted provider, between concern for the safe provision of care for patients by the impaired anesthesiologist, and the support of the impaired anesthesiologist's well-being in the event of a relapse. For physician colleagues trained to view illness with compassion, this conflict can present difficult choices.

Further complicating this matter is the potential for bias in decision-making due to lack of acceptance of the disease model for addiction, and a perception of the issue as rather a moral problem or deficiency of willpower. Moral judgments of addictive behavior may greatly influence the decision of whether or not to support the addicted colleague professionally. Concern may principally be for the care of the patient and, perhaps, for the safety of the anesthesiologist, with little

consideration over the fate of the colleague professionally. Placing concerns for patients first is important, but the professional fate of the addicted provider is also a legitimate ethical concern of their colleagues. If the recovering anesthesiologist is not well respected or is thought to be professionally substandard, greedy, manipulative, or possessing a genuine personality disorder, then it is almost impossible to expect that these factors will not influence or even dominate group decision-making with respect to re-entry.

Anesthesiologists' ethical obligations to healthcare facilities

Anesthesiologists personally handle and have easy access to many controlled and potentially addictive substances. The ASA ethical guidelines declare that:

> *"Anesthesiologists personally handle many controlled and potentially dangerous substances and, therefore, have a special responsibility to keep these substances secure from illicit use. Anesthesiologists should work within their healthcare facility to develop and maintain an adequate monitoring system for controlled substances."* [4]

Increased awareness of addiction and diversion of controlled substances in anesthesiology has been fostered by educational efforts, particularly during residency. All anesthesiologists, whether in training or not, have an ethical responsibility to learn to recognize the signs and symptoms of addiction in order to avert a possible tragic outcome, either to that individual or one of his/her patients. Unfortunately, educational efforts to raise awareness of addiction among anesthesiologists apparently have not resulted in a decreased incidence of the disease. Increased reporting and diagnosis may reflect an actual increase in addiction, or simply reflect increased awareness, adding to the confusion.

Ethical considerations regarding re-entry into the anesthesia workplace

Addiction is not only a life-threatening, but also a career-threatening disease. Many are concerned about whether the addicted anesthesiologist should return to practice or training once treatment has been completed. Opioid abusers with co-morbid psychiatric conditions (dual diagnosis) and/or a family history of drug addiction/abuse present greater risk for at least one relapse. Recidivism is a characteristic of addictive disease and focuses discussion of re-entry on the safety for both the recovering anesthesiologist and his/her patients.

Post-residency addicted physicians have years, even decades, invested in professional training and practice. This intensifies the real dilemma of deciding whether or not to support and advocate for that colleague's return to practice.

On the other hand, the impaired provider's substantial investment also represents enormous leverage to "encourage" compliance in recovery. There is much more literature regarding the addiction experience in academic training programs than that of the majority of anesthesiologists who are in private practice. Furthermore, information from academic programs is almost exclusively concerned with trainees, who have been in the profession for only a short period of time and have the least substantial career investment. The differences in addiction and recovery between trainees and those in long-time practice may be substantial, but are currently poorly understood and under-studied.

Does a practicing anesthesiologist have an ethical obligation to inform patients about past addictive behavior?

Although this ethical issue has received little if any comment, it certainly is a physician-impairment topic worthy of discussion. Two court rulings in the United States were divided in their legal opinions regarding such disclosure as an integral part of informed consent. Those who support informed consent disclosure by physicians who have been treated for chemical dependence build their argument on the apparent "materiality" of the risk of relapse to informed treatment decisions by patients. According to this line of belief, when the personal health problems of an anesthesiologist *may* endanger the welfare of the patient, this constitutes an identifiable material risk about which a patient would want to know when deciding upon a decision about treatment. In fact, however, the probability is extremely remote that a properly rehabilitated practicing anesthesiologist who is being appropriately monitored would relapse *and* injure a patient. Taken to the extreme, a mandate for such disclosure by a recovering anesthesiologist could be extended to a multitude of other medical diagnoses and personal situations that conceivably could have a negative impact on quality of anesthesia care. Relevant to this discussion is the fact that a significant pool of professionals with obvious impact on public safety – commercial airline pilots – includes a subset of several thousand aviators rehabilitated back to work with little or no direct mention of this fact to the flying public.

Key points

- Addiction to drugs is a chronic, relapsing disease best characterized by the overwhelming compulsion to use drugs despite adverse personal and professional consequences.
- A major occupational hazard of anesthesiologists is the development of addictive disease, which, in the light of the specialty's powerful drugs, often involves a rapidly progressive, life- and career-threatening pattern of behavior.
- Addiction prevents the anesthesiologist from his/her primary ethical responsibility of placing the interests of his/her patients foremost, providing competent and compassionate care.
- Anesthesiologists have an obligation to themselves as well as to their patients and their health care facility to maintain their physical and mental health and special sensory capabilities.
- Anesthesiologists have an ethical responsibility to be knowledgeable about addiction, to detect it in its earliest stages, and to support the treatment, rehabilitation, and eventually, if appropriate, reentry into the workplace of a recovering colleague.

References

1* Berge, K.H., Seppala, M.D., and Schipper, A.M. (2009). Chemical dependency and the physician. *Mayo Clin Proc*, **84**(7), 625–31.

2 Menk, E.J., Baumgarten, R.K., and Kingsley, C.P. (1990). Success of reentry into anesthesiology training programs by residents with a history of substance abuse. *JAMA*. **263**, 3060–2.

3 Collins, G.B., McAllister, M.S., Jensen, M., and Gooden, T.A. (2005). Chemical dependency treatment outcomes of residents in anesthesiology: results of a survey. *Anesth Analg*, **101**, 1457–62.

4* Guidelines for the Ethical Practice of Anesthesiology (2008). American Society of Anesthesiologists, www.asahq.org.

Further reading

Ackerman, T. (1996). Chemically dependent physicians and informed consent disclosure. *J Addictive Dis*, **15**, 25–42.

Baldisseri M. (2007). Impaired healthcare professional. *Crit Care Med*, **35(No 2 suppl)**, S106–16.

Berge, K., Seppala, M., and Lanier, W. (2008). The anesthesiology community's approach to opioid- and anesthetic-abusing personnel: time to change course. *Anesthesiology*, **109**, 762–4.

Booth, J., Grossman, D., Moore, J., *et al.* (2002). Substance abuse among physicians: A survey of academic anesthesiology programs. *Anesth Analg*, **95**, 1024–30.

Bryson, E. and Silverstein, J. (2008). Addiction and substance abuse in anesthesiology. *Anesthesiology*, **109**, 905–17.

Chemical dependence in anesthesiologists: what you need to know and when you need to know it. (1998). Park Ridge, IL: American Society of Anesthesiologists.

Domino, K., Hornbein, T., Pollisar, N., *et al.* (2005). Risk factors for relapse in health care professionals with substance use disorders. *JAMA*, **293**, 1453–60.

Gallegos, K., Lubin, B., Boweres, C., *et al.* (1992). Relapse and recovery: five to ten year follow-up study of chemically dependent physicians: the Georgia experience. *Md Med J*, **41**, 315–19.

Model Curriculum on Drug Abuse and Addiction for Residents in Anesthesiology. (2003). Park Ridge, IL: American Society of Anesthesiologists.

Oreskovich, M. and Caldeiro, M. (2009). Anesthesiologists recovering from chemical dependency: Can they safely return to the operating room? *Mayo Clin Proc*, **84**, 576–80.

Specht, T. (2009). Reentry after addiction treatment: Research or retrain? *Anesthesiology*, **110**, 1423–4.

37

The impaired anesthesiologist – sleep deprivation

Steven K. Howard

The Case

At 3 am, a first-year anesthesia resident was providing an anesthetic to a young adult male undergoing exploratory laparotomy for presumed appendicitis. The resident had started his shift 20 hours earlier at 7 am at this very busy county hospital. There were cases to follow and it was obvious that this resident would be busy until being relieved of duty the following day. As the case was finishing, the resident was drawing up medications to reverse neuromuscular blockade. He drew up 3 mg of neostigmine. He intended to draw up 0.6 mg of glycopyrrolate but instead drew up 30 mg of phenylephrine. The two drugs were in adjacent bins in the drug cart and were packaged in similar appearing vials. Prior to administering the likely lethal concoction, the resident described feeling that "something was not right." Upon checking the empty vials on the anesthesia cart, the near miss was discovered and the syringe disposed of. The intended reversal agents were then drawn up and administered to the patient without incident. The resident completed two more cases during his call until being relieved the following morning. This incident was not reported to the residents' supervisor. In three years of anesthesia training, this resident was offered the opportunity to nap on call only once by faculty.

The ASA Guidelines for the Ethical Practice of Anesthesiology outline the ethical responsibilities of anesthesiologists. Section IV.2 states:

The practice of quality anesthesia care requires that anesthesiologists maintain their physical and mental health and special sensory capabilities. If in doubt about their health, then anesthesiologists should seek medical evaluation and care. During this period of evaluation and treatment, anesthesiologists should modify or cease their practice.[1]

Sleep deprivation has a negative impact on performance, including the "special sensory capabilities" mentioned in the ethical guidelines. Anesthesia care providers are required to care for patients around the clock, presenting special problems for human physiology. Specific strategies have been used in other domains to mitigate the impairing affect of fatigue.

Human error

In 1999, the Institute of Medicine (IOM) published a treatise *To Err is Human* which uncovered a previously unappreciated level of patient mortality and morbidity associated with human error of health care providers.[2] Although the IOM report did not specifically address the issue of care provided by sleep-deprived practitioners, it is likely that a fraction of the preventable errors that occur are secondary to this performance shaping variable. Error investigation in healthcare and in other industries has shown that fatigued workers make errors, although exact rates are difficult to quantify. Physicians are not able to withstand the impairing effect of sleep deprivation. Even though sleep deprivation and fatigue could not be proven to have contributed to the near miss in the case scenario, sophisticated accident investigation performed in other industries would conclude that it played a role.[3]

Basic sleep physiology

A basic primer in sleep physiology is important to understand the issues of sleep deprivation and its effect on performance. Sleep is a reversible behavioral state of perceptual disengagement from and unresponsiveness to the environment, and it is vital to human survival. It is comprised of two states – non-rapid eye movement (NREM) and rapid eye movement (REM) sleep that cycle throughout the night and can be differentiated electrophysiologically. Both NREM and REM sleep are required for optimal alertness, though the body will preferentially replete lost sleep with slow wave sleep (NREM stages 3 and 4). REM sleep is the stage when dreaming takes place. REM sleep periods get longer

---

Clinical Ethics in Anesthesiology: A Case-Based Textbook, ed. Gail A. Van Norman, Stephen Jackson, Stanley H. Rosenbaum and Susan K. Palmer. Published by Cambridge University Press. © Cambridge University Press 2011.

as the sleep period extends – the longest REM periods coming before awakening in the morning.

Physiologic sleepiness

Sleep is a basic human need similar to eating and drinking. When deprived of food or drink, we develop hunger or thirst. Similarly, if we obtain less sleep than we require, sleepiness becomes marked and our brain becomes "pressured" to acquire sleep –extreme sleepiness during hazardous activities can become manifest. In these situations the brain may shift uncontrollably between wake and sleep with little or no awareness from the individual. These short sleep episodes (called microsleeps or attentional failures) create safety risks especially when envisioning them occurring in the operating room during patient care or upon driving home after a long call period. This level of sleepiness occurs in all humans if pressed to extremes.

Subjective sleepiness

Subjective sleepiness (how sleepy we feel) often underestimates the level of physiologic sleepiness. It is conceivable that this subjective – physiologic disconnect makes critical decision making more challenging. This disconnect might help explain why the incidence of single vehicular automobile accidents is higher from 2–6 am, during times of increased physiologic vulnerability. Though we may think we are "OK" to perform, we are often less than optimally alert. The two primary determinants of sleepiness are modulated by sleep homeostasis and circadian rhythms.

The homeostat

Sleep homeostasis refers to the sleep–wake balance of an individual. This balance is a function of sleep need, offset by the quantity and quality of sleep obtained. An individual's sleep propensity (i.e., sleep pressure) changes when this equilibrium is tipped in either direction. For example, if an individual's sleep need is 8 hours per night but sleep achieved is 7 hours per night a sleep debt develops and sleep propensity increases. Average adults require greater than 8 hours of sleep per 24-hour period to maintain optimal alertness and function at peak levels. Population studies reveal that sleep need is normally distributed so that for every person who needs 6 hours of sleep for optimal alertness another will require 10 hours. Importantly, humans are notoriously poor at determining their true level of sleep need.

An individual's sleep need is genetically determined and cannot be trained. As adults age, sleep need remains constant but obtaining adequate quantity and quality of sleep becomes more difficult. Sleep disorders increase with age and other benign issues associated with aging (e.g., urinary frequency in males and menopausal symptoms in females) make sleep consolidation increasingly difficult.

The circadian pacemaker

A circadian pacemaker located in the suprachiasmatic nucleus of the brain governs alertness. Humans are programmed for two nadirs of alertness between 2–6 am and 2–6 pm and these times represent periods of increased vulnerability to performance impairment due to pacemaker-induced sleepiness. The circadian clock is very resistant to alterations and does not adjust rapidly. For healthcare providers, the clock's resiliency to change is best evidenced by those who work the night shift. It is often difficult to maintain alertness during the night when the body's clock is "turned off" and similarly it is difficult to gain adequate sleep during the day when clock is "turned on" (e.g., attempting to sleep during the day after an on-call period). Working in opposition to circadian physiology is necessary in the round-the-clock work of health care providers but it comes at the risk of decreased alertness.

Fatigue affects performance

Fatigue adversely affects performance.[4] Examples include slowing of cognition, increased performance variability, and decreased motivation. The learning of new information slows, memory is impaired, and nonessential activities are neglected. Picture the fatigued anesthesiologist at 3 am after being awake for a number of hours trying to safely care for patients with these very real constraints of human physiology. These are precisely the special sensory capabilities alluded to in the ASA's Guidelines for Ethical Practice, and are critical for safe provision of care.

Performance is proven to be altered in sleep-deprived physicians. The Harvard Work Hours, Health and Safety Group showed that reducing shift duration by interns from 30 to less than 17 hours decreased serious medical errors by 35.9%.[5] Simulation research of anesthesiologists supports the findings that a clinician's performance is negatively impacted by sleep deprivation and that increasing sleep (either by prioritizing or napping) can improve performance.[6]

A robust finding in similar studies is that mood is dramatically affected by sleep loss and fatigue. Negative moods (e.g., anger, depression, fatigue, tension) increase and positive moods decrease as sleep loss accrues.[7] The impact of impaired mood on interpersonal interactions between health care providers and between providers and patients has been inadequately studied but is likely to have an overall negative effect.

Comparison of sleep deprivation to ethanol usage

Results of research correlating the affect of sleep loss and alcohol consumption are alarming. Dawson showed that after 17 hours of wakefulness that performance on a tracking task declined to a level of impairment equivalent to a blood alcohol concentration (BAC) of 0.05%.[8] After 24 hours of wakefulness, the decline in performance was equivalent to a BAC of 0.1% – over the legal level for driving everywhere in the US. This amount of wakefulness is commonly seen in medical professionals who take "in house" call and creates a source for systemic latent errors thus increasing system vulnerability.[9]

A study comparing the effects of sleep loss and alcohol consumption on performance of a simulated driving task further supports the correlation.[10] With increasing blood alcohol concentration, simulated driving performance became progressively impaired. Speed variability, and off-road events increased, while speed deviation decreased, the result of subjects driving faster. Wakefulness of 18.5 and 21 hours produced changes of the same magnitude as 0.05 and 0.08% BAC, respectively. Finally, wakefulness prolonged by as little as 3 h can produce decrements in the ability to maintain speed and road position as serious as those found at the legal limits of alcohol consumption.

Arendt and colleagues found that the neurobehavioral performance of residents after a "heavy" (every fourth or fifth night) call was comparable to that of residents after alcohol ingestion to BAC of 0.04 to 0.05% during "light call" conditions.[11]

Caring for patients while under the influence of alcohol is not ethical and would be viewed as abhorrent behavior. Professionals caring for patients "under the influence" of alcohol would likely lose their license to practice and be shunned by society. Threats to patient safety would be clear. Yet similar levels of impairment are now known to be caused by sleep loss. Are we routinely harming patients because of impaired decision making due to sleep deprivation?

No direct link between fatigue due to sleep loss and patient morbidity and mortality has yet been made, and this is one reason for the maintenance of the status quo. If 4 hours of sleep predict poor patient outcome (or driving off the road after call) healthcare providers would have to prioritize sleep as an important component of professionalism. Instead, in the current culture of health care, staying up all night on call, is still thought of by many as a rite of passage and a badge of honor. If anesthesiologists better recognized the level of impairment engendered by sleep loss, perhaps these behaviors would change.

Ethical responsibilities of anesthesiologist

Responsibilities to patients

Anesthesiologists have an ethical responsibility to be optimally prepared to safely care for patients and this includes avoidance of impairments from any cause. Optimal performance in part depends on level of alertness and this is largely under the control of the individual. There is no BAC equivalent marker for sleepiness and no "sleep police" to deter poor sleep habits, so it is the individual's responsibility to come to work optimally prepared – not impaired. Excellent sleep habits form the most important strategy for each physician. A variety of strategies have been proven to increase alertness.

Recuperative sleep

Average adults require at least 8 hours per 24-hour day. Sleep blocks less than this can be supplemented by nap periods both at work and after work shifts. Every attempt should be made to mitigate sleep debt prior to call periods by prioritizing sleep. The sleep environment should be conducive to sleep by allowing control over ambient light, noise, and temperature. Pre-sleep routines that give cues for relaxation and sleep should be employed and distractions such as electronic devices, pets, children, etc. should be minimized.

Strategic napping

Napping has been shown to improve alertness and performance.[12] As little as 10–15 minutes of sleep will improve performance and longer sleep periods have a more substantial effect. Naps address physiologic sleep need by decreasing sleep debt. Unfortunately, naps are not utilized in our society for mostly cultural reasons – the most common reason given is that napping is a sign of weakness or laziness. Strategic napping has been piloted in a few healthcare facilities but have not reached widespread use at the present time.[13]

Strategic use of caffeine

Caffeine is the most widely used drug to improve alertness. Chronic use of caffeine limits its strategic use as tolerance develops to routine exposure. Strategic use of caffeine includes: (1) limiting chronic ingestion hence tolerance; (2) ingesting when you have be awake (e.g., during circadian low points); (3) knowing its onset (15–30 minutes) and duration of effect (3–4 hours); and (4) avoiding its use if close to a sleep opportunity. Combining the effect of a nap and caffeine can be used to improve alertness.[14]

Mindful intake of food and drugs

Use of caffeine, alcohol, and nicotine close to sleep opportunities will impair initiation, consolidation, and maintenance of sleep. Attempting to sleep either hungry or on a full stomach will negatively impact sleep.

Exercise

Regular exercise improves sleep, but exercise within a few hours to the sleep period can impair sleep. It is best to complete exercise routines 2–3 hours before sleep to avoid this.

Diagnose and treat sleep disorders

There are more than 80 different sleep disorders, the most common of which is obstructive sleep apnea (OSA). Almost all of the disorders have impaired alertness as a common presenting finding. Anesthesiologists with excessive daytime somnolence should consider being evaluated by a sleep medicine professional.

Optimize scheduling

The most contentious issue to attempt to change is that of individual work schedules. Monetary and time at work issues are central to most decisions regarding scheduling and often compete with what might be "correct" for both physiological and patient safety reasons. Important factors that need to be taken into account are:

- Length of shift
- Length of rest opportunities while off duty
- Number of consecutive duty periods
- Start and end time of shifts
- Periodic days off of clinical work

Modafinil – an alertness enhancing drug

Modafinil is a non-amphetamine stimulant with low physiologic addictive potential.[15] Its current FDA approval is for excessive daytime sleepiness due to narcolepsy, OSA, and shift work sleep disorder. Use of modafinil in these populations is associated with improvements in daytime alertness and small improvements in performance. The development of these types of drugs is creating controversy in the medical profession regarding the ethical use of such stimulants while performing patient care activities. Cephalon, the maker of modafinil issued a statement that the drug is "not intended for use in helping residents work longer hours."

Physicians' ethical responsibilities to each other

In an ideal world patients would not suffer consequences of care from impaired providers. Honest dialogue between colleagues regarding coverage if sleep deprivation is present could improve system safety. This type of discussion occurs infrequently, most likely because of ego and a lack of understanding of the impairment caused by sleep loss and the consequent decrease in safety.

Rest breaks

Rest breaks are common in many anesthesia practices. These breaks interrupt the monotony of care, allow for personal time (food and bath room breaks) and allow for brief physical activity. Rest breaks have been shown to transiently improve alertness but they do not alter sleep pressure.[16] Longer rest breaks can be used for strategic napping. Strategically placed rest and nap breaks could improve alertness, performance and likely morale and should be built into anesthesia practice when the situation allows.

Work schedules should be created with homeostatic and circadian processes in mind. Anesthesia groups should allow for flexibility to accommodate schedule requests that the providers desire but also have this balanced by the science of sleep medicine.

Hospital responsibilities to groups and physicians

Hospitals have an important role in how providers practice. Production pressure (case throughput) and a culture of safety are important factors especially in anesthesia practice. In hospitals where production pressure is high and a culture of safety is lacking, fatigue related problems are more likely be prevalent. Pressure to perform elective surgery in the middle of the night is but one example of how a hospital can increase the collective sleep pressure of all of its providers – not just the anesthesiologists. Some hospitals have acted proactively to address fatigue-related risk. The Veteran's Administration has piloted strategic napping in the high acuity areas of its intensive care units and operating rooms.[13]

Key points

- Professional (and ethical) behavior begins with the practitioner who should come to work prepared and not impaired. Sleep deprivation is an important example of a common and preventable disorder negatively impacting the performance of anesthesiologists.
- Sleep is a basic human need. Sleep deprivation causes increasing physiologic pressure to acquire sleep, and resultant uncontrollable "microsleeps" create the risk of performance lapses and safety risks. In the case of anesthesiology practice, these risks are visited upon patients.
- Fatigue has been shown to affect performance to a similar degree that is associated with legal intoxication with alcohol.
- Anesthesiologists have ethical obligations to patients to obtain appropriate levels of sleep, and to work to optimize work schedules within groups to minimize sleep-disordered performance degradation.
- Anesthesiologists have ethical obligations to each other to promote work breaks, and discourage sleep deprivation among colleagues.
- Anesthesiologists also have obligations to work with hospitals to promote a culture of patient safety and proactively address fatigue-related risks.

References

1   ASA Guidelines for Ethical Practice of Anesthesiology. HOD October 2008. www.asahq.org.

2* Kohn, L.T., Corrigan, J.M., and Donaldson, M.S. (1999). *To Err is Human: Building a Safer Health System.* Washington, D.C.: National Academy Press.

3   Rosekind, M.R., Gregory, K.B., Miller, D.L., *et al.* Aircraft Accident Report: Uncontrolled Collision with Terrain, American International Airways Flight 808, Douglas DC-8, N814CK, US Naval Air Station, Guantanamo Bay, Cuba, August 18, 1993. (Report #NTSB/AAR-94/04). Washington, D.C., National Transportation Safety Board, 1994.

4   Philibert, I. (2005). Sleep loss and performance in residents and nonphysicians: a meta-analytic examination. *Sleep*, **28**, 1392–1402.

5   Landrigan, C.P., Rothschild, J.M., Cronin, J.W., *et al.* (2004). Effect of reducing interns' work hours on serious medical errors in intensive care units. *N Engl J Med*, **351**, 1838–48.

6* Howard, S.K., Gaba, D.M., Smith, B.E., *et al.* (2003). Simulation study of rested versus sleep-deprived anesthesiologists. *Anesthesiology*, **98**, 1345–55.

7   Howard, S.K., Gaba, D.M., Rosekind, M.R., and Zarcone, V.P. (2002). The risks and implications of excessive daytime sleepiness in resident physicians. *Acad Med*, **77**(10), 1019–25.

8* Dawson, D. and Reid, K. (1997). Fatigue, alcohol and performance impairment [Scientific Correspondence]. *Nature*, **388**: 235.

9   Reason, J. (1990). *Human Error*. Camridge, Great Britain, Cambridge University Press.

10   Arnedt, J.T., Wilde, G., Munt, P., and MacLean, A. (2001). How do prolonged wakefulness and alcohol compare in the decrements they produce on a simulated driving task? *Accid Anal Prev*, **33**, 337–44.

11* Arnedt, J.T., Owens, J., Crouch, M., *et al.* (2005). Neurobehavioral performance of residents after heavy night call vs after alcohol ingestion. *JAMA*, **294**, 1025–33.

12   Sallinen, M., Harma, M., Akerstedt, T., *et al.* (1998). Promoting alertness with a short nap during a night shift. *J Sleep Res*, **7**, 240–7.

13   Joint Commission Resources: Strategies for Addressing Health Care Worker Fatigue. (2008). Oakbrook Terrace, IL, The Joint Commission on Accreditation of Healthcare Organizations.

14   Bonnet, M.H. and Arand, D.L. (1994). Impact of naps and caffeine on extended nocturnal performance. *Physiol Behav*, **56**, 103–9.

15   Czeisler, C.A., Walsh, J.K., Roth, T. *et al.* (2005). Modafinil for excessive sleepiness associated with shift-work sleep disorder. *N Engl J Med*, **353**, 476–86.

16   Neri, D.F., Oyung, R.L., Colletti, L.M., *et al.* (2002). Controlled breaks as a fatigue countermeasure on the flight deck. *Aviat Space Environ Med*, **73**, 654–64.

Further reading

Borbely, A.A. and Achermann, P. (2005) Sleep homeostasis and models of sleep regulation, in *Principles and Practice of Sleep Medicine*, 4th Edition. Edited by Kryger MH, Roth T, Dement WC. Philadelphia, PA, Elsevier Saunders. pp. 405–17.

Carskadon, M.A. and Dement, W.C. (2005). Normal Human Sleep: An Overview, in *Principles and Practice of Sleep Medicine*, 4th Edition. Edited by Kryger MH, Roth T, Dement WC. Philadelphia, PA, Elsevier Saunders, pp. 13–23.

Lockley, S.W., Cronin, J.W., Evans, E.E., et al. (2004). Harvard Work Hours H, and Safety Group: Effect of reducing interns' weekly work hours on sleep and attentional failures. *N Engl J Med*, **351**, 1829–37.

National Sleep Foundation: 2008 Sleep in America Poll, 2008 website: http://www.sleepfoundation.org/article/press-release/sleep-america-poll-summary-findings. Accessed June 1, 2009

Rosekind, M.R., Graeber, R.C., Dinges, D.F., et al. (1994). Crew Factors in Flight Operations IX: Effects of Planned Cockpit Rest on Crew Performance and Alertness in Long-Haul Operations. NASA Technical Memorandum #108839. Moffett Field, CA, NASA Ames Research Center

Van Dongen, H.P. and Dinges, D.F. (2005). Circadian rhythms in sleepiness, alertness, and performance, in *Principles and Practice of Sleep Medicine*, 4th Edition. Edited by Kryger MH, Roth T, Dement WC. Philadelphia, PA, Elsevier Saunders, pp. 435–43.

38 Ethical considerations regarding the disabled anesthesiologist

Jonathan D. Katz

The Case

Dr. X is a 63-year-old right-handed, previously healthy, male anesthesiologist who suffered a stroke, resulting in a mild speech deficit and right-sided weakness. He underwent intensive rehabilitation with 90% recovery of his speech and other motor functions. However, as his physical status improved, a personality change became apparent, marked by uncharacteristic emotional swings and subtle errors in cognition and judgment. He was placed on a course of anti-depressants, which narrowed the mood swings and further improved his cognitive function sufficiently so that his physician declared him fully recovered. Family members and close friends, however, remained aware of cognitive deficits that manifested as forgetfulness and faulty decision making.

Dr. X claimed that he was "100%" back to his pre-stroke status. His close friends and family believed otherwise. Three months after his stroke he notified his partners of his intention to return to the full time practice of anesthesiology.

All individuals, if they live long enough, will suffer a disability for some period during their life. Physicians are no exception. At least one-third of all physicians will experience a disabling illness or injury during their professional careers.[1] At any given time, 2%–10% of practicing physicians are suffering from some degree of disability.[2]

Identifying an individual as "disabled" is a complex diagnosis with profound personal, professional, and societal ramifications. Similar degrees of impairment can result in significant disability to one individual or a mere inconvenience to another or even to the same individual in different circumstances. For example, many wheel-chair users do not consider themselves disabled. And many deaf individuals consider themselves *advantaged* by possessing unique communication skills. It can require a ruling by the Supreme Court to determine ultimately whether or not an individual is "disabled."

Definitions

Impairment is "any loss, loss of use, or derangement of any body part, organ system, or organ function." The degree of impairment is an objective determination that is based upon both physical and psychological loss.[3]

Disability is "an alteration of an individual's capacity to meet personal, social, or occupational demands, because of impairment." Disabling conditions result from physical, mental, emotional, sensory, or developmental etiologies. Disabilities can have an acute onset, as occurs with injury or acute illness, or a more progressive onset, as occurs with many chronic diseases.[3]

Work disability is a subgroup in which an individual's ability to perform his/ her expected work role is compromised as a result of impairment. Work disability is the result of a complex interaction between individual characteristics and behavior and the work environment.

An *impaired physician* is one who is unable to practice medicine with reasonable skill and safety because of mental illness, physical illness or condition, or the habitual or excessive use or abuse of alcohol or other substances that would adversely affect cognitive, motor, or perceptive skills.[4]

An *incompetent* physician is one who lacks the minimally acceptable levels of knowledge and skills needed to practice medicine. One can be incompetent without being impaired or impaired without being incompetent.

Legal considerations

There are several, often conflicting, principles that frame the legal environment in which an impaired physician finds him/herself.

A physician who accepts the privileges afforded by a state license to practice medicine also accepts many

Clinical Ethics in Anesthesiology: A Case-Based Textbook, ed. Gail A. Van Norman, Stephen Jackson, Stanley H. Rosenbaum and Susan K. Palmer. Published by Cambridge University Press. © Cambridge University Press 2011.

legal responsibilities. Paramount among these is the responsibility to remain physically, mentally and emotionally competent in his/her profession. The medical practice acts in most states include a requirement that physicians self-report if they become aware that their professional skills may be compromised. Most states also include a provision that provides certain protections to physician–patients who voluntarily enter into an appropriate program of rehabilitation. If a physician-patient successfully completes the prescribed rehabilitation program all information surrounding the episode of impairment remains confidential and protected from public disclosure.

The treating physician of an impaired physician-patient also has potentially conflicting legal obligations. To the extent that the disabled physician is a patient, he or she is entitled to the same rights and protections of privacy that are provided to non-physician patients. The confidentiality of the physician-patient's medical history is recognized by federal and most state laws. The sanctity of medical records is also recognized by the American Medical Association (AMA) and most state medical societies.

On the other hand, considerations of patient confidentiality are superseded in situations where a patient poses a threat to him/herself, or to others. In many states there is an affirmative "duty to report" that would require a treating physician to report to the state licensing board any physician who is considered impaired for any reason. In many cases failure to report is potentially grounds for disciplinary action.

Disability law can impact the future practice decisions of an anesthesiologist who has suffered a disabling illness. Disability is one of the protected classes under United States federal nondiscrimination law. The most important of these statutes that directly bear on disabled anesthesiologists are the Rehabilitation Act of 1973,[5] the Americans with Disabilities Act of 1990 (ADA),[6] and the Family and Medical Leave Act.[7] These laws prohibit covered employers from discriminating against applicants and employees solely because of disability. All aspects of employment are encompassed, including hiring and firing, training, advancement, compensation, and benefits. The laws go further by requiring that employers proactively offer equal opportunity to disabled employees by providing reasonable accommodations that do not cause them "undue hardship."

Title II of the ADA pertains specifically to medical licensure. It prohibits state and local governments and their agencies from excluding a disabled individual from any government program, such as medical licensure or renewal. Title III of the ADA further extends the law to protect applicants to both public and private institutions, for example, medical schools.

There are notable exceptions to protections afforded by the ADA. Most important for this discussion is that an individual who poses a direct threat to the health and safety of others is not considered a "qualified person" with a disability.

In addition to the legal obligation to self-report if medical competence is compromised, the medical practice acts in many states also require that a physician report his or her colleague who they suspect of incompetent practice. The requirements and details of reporting vary from state to state and most states provide a framework to permit confidential reporting with immunity from civil lawsuits.

Ethical considerations

The medical profession is a moral community that is charged by society with the ethical duty to treat disease in such a manner as "to help, or at least to do no harm" (*primum non nocere*). Each of the individual components of the medical community must fulfill specific ethical duties in order to meet that public trust.

Ethical obligations of the physician

The ethical responsibility of each physician to maintain the highest standards of professional conduct is deeply ingrained in all ethical constructs for physicians. Thomas Percival articulated this obligation and the remedy that must be applied to those who do not meet it: "Let both the Physician and Surgeon never forget that their professions are public trusts, properly rendered lucrative whilst they fulfill them, but which they are bound by honor and probity to relinquish as soon as they find themselves unequal to their adequate and faithful execution."[8]

The ethical codes of virtually all medical societies contain language that requires that members maintain mental and physical fitness in order to enable them to meet their ethical obligation of providing competent medical care. For example, the Code of Medical Ethics of the AMA specifies that physicians have an obligation to maintain their own health and wellness, by preventing and/or treating diseases including mental illness, disabilities, and occupational stress. The Code further explains that the effectiveness and safety of the medical care that is rendered is likely to be compromised if the health of the physician is in question.

Finally, "[P]hysicians whose health or wellness is compromised should take measures to mitigate the problem, seek appropriate help as necessary, and engage in an honest self-assessment of their ability to continue practicing." [9]

The Ethics Manual of the American College of Physicians (ACP) makes a similar assertion that any impaired physician must refrain from assuming patient responsibilities. If there is any doubt of a physician's capabilities he or she is required to seek assistance in caring for his or her patients. [10]

The Guidelines for the Ethical Practice of Anesthesiology of the American Society of Anesthesiologists (ASA) (Section IV.2) also specifically addresses this obligation to maintain physical and mental health and "special sensory capabilities" as a prerequisite to providing quality anesthesia care. [11] The guideline continues by encouraging anesthesiologists to seek medical care if there is any doubt about their health. Moreover, during the period of medical evaluation and treatment, anesthesiologists are urged to modify or cease practice.

Ethical obligations to colleagues

Physicians have an ethical obligation beyond the legal requirement to intervene if they believe a colleague's performance is impaired. This duty to report in part stems from each physician's obligation to protect patients from harm – in this case at the hands of an impaired colleague. This requirement is also grounded in professionalism and the physician's responsibility to self-regulate. This has been clearly articulated in the AMA's written positions on physician impairment wherein all physicians are reminded of their ethical responsibility to "take cognizance of a colleague's inability to practice medicine adequately" if that colleague is compromised by physical or mental illness." [12] The AMA's Code of Ethics further reminds physicians of their ethical duty to report impaired, incompetent, and/or unethical colleagues and to ensure that these physicians cease practice and seek appropriate treatment.

Similarly, the code of ethics of the ACP states that it is the obligation of each physician to protect patients from any impaired colleague. [10] There is a clear ethical imperative to report a physician who shows evidence of impairment to an appropriate authority.

The Guidelines for the Ethical Practice of Anesthesiology of the ASA (Section II.4) also requires of anesthesiologists that they advise impaired colleagues to modify or discontinue their practice/ Section III.2 declares that anesthesiologists have the ethical obligation to "observe and report to appropriate authorities any negligent practices or conditions which may present a hazard to patients or healthcare facility personnel." [11]

Hand in hand with their duty to report, physicians also have a moral obligation to aid their colleagues in seeking help with disabling conditions. For example, the ASA guidelines include the additional ethical responsibility of assisting with the re-education or rehabilitation of a colleague who is returning to practice. This is an important moral duty that demonstrates respect and compassion for disabled colleagues and facilitates their ability to continue contributing to their profession and society. This duty was clearly articulated by Dr. Ulla Nielsen, of the Canadian Association of Physicians with Disabilities in a presentation to the Federation of Medical Licensing Authorities of Canada in June 2001:

> It is easy to say "It's (the problem of disability among physicians) not a big problem." "It's not my problem." The problem is easy to ignore – out of sight, out of mind. But these are your colleagues. They deserve the respect you give to your other colleagues. They deserve to hear the questions, "What CAN you do? What can we do to help? How can we keep you involved? The worse disrespect of all is the ignoring, the dismissal, of the person. It could be you in those shoes tomorrow." [13]

In practice, intervention with an impaired colleague can be a daunting task. Although it is widely recognized that competence and self- regulation are cornerstones of professionalism, little has been written on how to implement these lofty goals on a day-to-day basis. When a physician is treating a colleague, the ethical mandate to report can come into direct conflict with the treating physician's obligation to protect the physician–patient's confidentiality. On the one hand, the AMA Code of Medical Ethics asserts that some form of intervention or reporting to a licensing or disciplinary board is required if the physician is impaired, incompetent or behaving unethically. On the other hand, the treating physician is bound by contract to secrecy and may not disclose any aspects of the physician-patient's medical care, except as required by law or when essential to protect patients from harm. Even when required by law, the treating physician is bound to only reveal the minimum amount of information that is required.

The ACP code also addresses this conflict between the dueling obligations to protect confidentiality and to report. The code makes the recommendation that a third party, independent of the treating physician, should monitor the impaired physician's fitness for duty.[10]

Ethical duties of professional organizations

Professional and specialty societies have a duty to ensure that their members are capable of providing safe medical care. The AMA Code of Ethics specifies that this obligation is discharged by promoting health and wellness among physicians and intervening promptly when a colleague's health or wellness is compromised. The Code also calls for the establishment of physician health programs. The importance of this obligation to ASA is evidenced by the fact that the Ethical Guidelines are the *only* ASA documents that are binding upon all of its members.

Case resolution

Dr. X has suffered a significant illness with residual disability that threatens to compromise his ability to provide safe anesthetic care. The burden of proof is on Dr. X to demonstrate that his skills are once again adequate to the challenging tasks of providing a safe anesthetic. His professional obligations to his patients require that he discontinue or at least curtail his practice until such time as it is clear to himself and to his advisors that he is once again capable of providing competent care.

If Dr. X is incapable or unwilling to accept an objective assessment of his limitations, his colleagues and the organizations of medicine share a duty to ensure that he does not return to practice until his level of competence is assured. This obligation might have to be exercised through legal channels.

Key points

- Up to one-third of physicians will suffer from a disabling injury or illness during their professional careers.
- Medical licensure carries ethical and legal responsibilities to maintain physical, mental and emotional abilities necessary to the safe practice of medicine.
- Physicians have ethical obligations to self-report problems that may compromise their ability to practice, and to take measures to mitigate the problem, seek appropriate help and honestly assess their ability to continue practice.

- Physicians have obligations of respect and compassion for disabled colleagues; to intervene if a colleague's performance is impaired, and to engage disabled colleagues to the degree that they can in continued contribution to the profession.
- Professional organizations have duties to ensure that their members are capable of providing safe medical care.

References

1   Leape, L.L. and J.A. Fromson. (2006). Problem doctors: is there a system-level solution? *Ann Intern Med*, **144**(2), 107–15.

2   DeLisa, J.A. and Thomas, P. (2005). Physicians with disabilities and the physician workforce: a need to reassess our policies. *Am J Phys Med Rehabil*, **84**(1), 5–11.

3* American Medical Association. (2001). *Guides to the Evaluation of Permanent Impairment*. 5th edn. Chicago: American Medical Association.

4* Federation of the State Medical Boards of the United States, Inc. (1995) *Report of the Ad Hoc Committee on Physician Impairment*. [cited 2009 5/27]; Available from: http://www.fsmb.org/pdf/1995_grpol_ Physician_Impairment.pdf.

5   29 U.S.C. § 701 *et seq*.

6   42 U.S.C. § 12101 *et seq*

7   29 U.S.C. § 2601 *et seq*

8* Percival, T. (1803). *Medical Ethics; Or, a Code of Institutes and Precepts, Adapted to the Professional Conduct of Physicians and Surgeons*. London: Johnson and Bickerstaff

9* American Medical Association. (2008) *Code of Medical Ethics: Current Opinions with Annotations, 2008–2009*. [cited 2009 5/28]; Available from: http://www.ama-assn.org/ama/pub/physician-resources/medical-ethics/code-medical-ethics.shtml.

10* Snyder, L. and Leffler, C. (2005). Ethics manual: fifth edition. *Ann Int Med*, **142**(7), 560–82.

11* American Society of Anesthesiologists. (2009). *Guidelines for the ethical practice of Anesthesiology* [cited 2009 5/27]; Available from: http://www.asahq.org/ publicationsAndServices/standards/10.pdf.

12* The sick physician. Impairment by psychiatric disorders, including alcoholism and drug dependence. (1973). *JAMA*, **223**(6), 684–712.

13 Nielsen, U.D. How big is the problem of disability among physicians? June, 2001 [cuted 2010 1/06]; Available from: http://www.capd.ca/How_BIG_is....htm.

Further reading

Rich, C.F. (1999). Physician licensing and the Americans with Disabilities Act. An update on the Minnesota Board of Medical Practice. *Minn Med*, **82**(1), 30–1, 43.

Rosenbaum, J.R., Bradley, E.H, Holmboe, E.S., *et al.* (2004). Sources of ethical conflict in medical housestaff training: a qualitative study. *Am J Med*, **116**(6), 402–7.

Steinberg, A.G., Lezzoni, L.I., Conill, A., and Stineman, M. (2002). Reasonable accommodations for medical faculty with disabilities. *JAMA*, **288**(24), 3147–54.

DISCOVERY LIBRARY
LEVEL 5 SWCC
DERRIFORD HOSPITAL
DERRIFORD ROAD
PLYMOUTH
PL6 8DH

39 The abusive and disruptive physician

Stephen Jackson

A hospital's busiest surgeon is universally disliked because of his persistent negative demeanor, punctuated by harsh and abusive outbursts that spare no category of healthcare provider, and often upset the efficient functioning of patient care areas. Over the years, this behavior has been tolerated without any effective attempt at correction or control by the medical staff. His list of surgeries has been delayed because the preceding surgeon (who is slow and marginally competent) took 2 hours longer than anticipated. The surgeon berates the OR secretary, technician and circulating nurse. Then as the anesthesiologist is transferring his patient to the recovery department, the surgeon demands that his case get started in short order.

The surgeon has stated in his workup that his patient is having a right inguinal herniorrhaphy – but the patient has related to the admitting nurse that she has left-sided symptoms and was told by the surgeon in his office that she has a left-sided hernia. In the preoperative unit the surgeon marks the right side as the operative site and convinces a somewhat recalcitrant – but otherwise timid – patient to sign an informed consent for a right-sided herniorrhaphy. The preoperative nurse, known herself for harsh verbal attacks against physicians and co-workers, calls the anesthesiologist to warn him of this potential for wrong-site surgery, and rails against the head nurse for assigning her to this surgeon's patients. In the background the anesthesiologist can hear the surgeon berating her for making the phone call to him.

The behavior described in this scenario is experienced by many physicians during their professional careers. It is termed *abusive and disruptive*, and adversely impacts the ethical practice of medicine. *Abusive* behavior signals the treatment of others harshly, cruelly and unremorsefully. *Disruptive* behavior indicates interference with the integrity and continuity of functions necessary for the provision of quality care. One may encounter nonabusive but disruptive behavior, represented by the slow surgeon in our case. Or, one may encounter abusive but nondisruptive behavior, represented by the preoperative nurse in the case scenario. The focus of this chapter, however, is mean, abusive, and disruptive (MAD) behavior of medical professionals in the workplace.

The importance of respect and civility in assuring good patient care is a foundation of the American Medical Association's *Code of Medical Ethics*.[1] MAD behavior subverts the ethical obligation of healthcare professionals from consistently placing the interests of the patient foremost, by interfering with the normative processes of collegiality, cooperation, communication, and teamwork. This sabotages the viability of an effective and efficient institutional culture of safety and quality care. Indeed, there is ample evidence of the linkage of MAD behavior to adverse events, medical errors and compromise of patient safety.[2]

MAD behavior – definition and consequences

MAD behavior encompasses an extreme degree of uncivil and unprofessional demeanor. It violates ethical standards of practice and impedes patient safety and quality improvement. It is a pattern of personality flaws and traits that interferes with a physician's effective clinical performance and can be directed at any member of the healthcare team, as well as patients and/or their family and friends. Manifestations include, but are not limited to:

(1) Verbal abuse – threats; intimidation; insults; degrading, demeaning, or foul language; or unwarranted yelling, tone or innuendo.

(2) Physical abuse – inappropriate physical contact that is threatening, humiliating or intimidating, or actual physical violence (from finger poking to battery).

(3) Invasion of the space or boundaries of others, physically and/or psychologically.

Clinical Ethics in Anesthesiology: A Case-Based Textbook, ed. Gail A. Van Norman, Stephen Jackson, Stanley H. Rosenbaum and Susan K. Palmer. Published by Cambridge University Press. © Cambridge University Press 2011.

(4) Visual abuse – threatening or humiliating movements; or inappropriate writings, drawings or photographs, including electronic transmissions.

(5) Harassment or discrimination against any individual on the basis of race, religion, color, ethnicity, national origin, ancestry or culture, socioeconomic status, physical, mental or other medical disability, marital status, gender or sexual orientation.

The MAD physician controls others through intimidation, bullying, belittling, berating, and condescendence. They manifest impulsive and unexpected anger, behave with arrogance, inconsideration and inflexibility, blame others rather than accepting responsibility, and are intolerant of those they deem to be "incompetent."

MAD behavior's harmful impact on workplace staff increases the risk for substandard care and adverse patient consequences. It amplifies stress; diminishes productivity; lowers self-esteem and morale; increases absenteeism, turnover, "sick" leave and worker compensation claims; and impedes the hiring of new staff. MAD behavior encourages failures to follow policies and procedures – for example by causing fear, disinclination or disinterest in questioning a MAD physician's orders no matter how illegible, inappropriate or incorrect they may appear to be. MAD behavior decreases or aborts normative communication regarding patient care and polarizes staff into those who are deemed as "favored" versus "not favored." The adverse impact on healthcare institutions includes time-consuming, unpleasant, and frustrating medical staff investigations; malpractice claims; and legal suits because of creation of a hostile work environment.

The aberrant personality of the MAD physician

MAD behavior is an Axis II psychiatric classification (which is *not* a psychiatric diagnosis or illness) characterized by an underlying personality with maladaptive behaviors that deviate markedly from normative expectations. This behavior poses a *direct* danger to patients as well as an *indirect* one by disrupting institutional and professional cultures of safety. This personality disorder is one of enduring traits, that is, it is part of the person's innate character, and not merely a response to environmental factors. Cultural factors, concomitant substance abuse, or a dual psychiatric

diagnosis may play a contributing role. But, because they suffer from lack of insight, the MAD physician is impervious to psychotherapy. The only potential treatment is to hold the MAD physician to strict limits of acceptable behavior. Unfortunately, the medical community's history has been one of impotence, permissiveness, frustration and a collective unwillingness to act decisively to address these antics.

Quelling MAD behavior – a standard for assuring quality of care

The Joint Commission has declared that MAD behavior constitutes a "Sentinel Event Alert" because of the potential to "foster medical errors, contribute to poor patient satisfaction and to preventable adverse outcomes."[3] Indeed, in the new "Leadership Standard" requirements, they state that

> "The hospital [must have] a code of conduct that defines acceptable and disruptive and inappropriate behavior … [and that] … leaders [should] create and implement a process for managing disruptive and inappropriate behaviors."[4]

Two of the six core competencies for which The Joint Commission and the Accreditation Council for Graduate Medical Education (ACGME) want every physician to be regularly appraised relate to MAD behavior: "*interpersonal and communication skills … that enable [physicians] to establish and maintain professional relationships with patients families, and other members of the healthcare team;*" and *professionalism*, especially for "behaviors that reflect a commitment to continuous professional development, ethical practice, and understanding and sensitivity to diversity, and a responsible attitude towards their patients, their profession, and society."[4]

Ethics, morals, and professionalism

Moral precepts and dilemmas involve actions that may harm or benefit others. Ethics is the study of society's moral challenges, precepts and codes – a scholarly effort to analyze rules, customs and beliefs, and how to achieve the moral good. Ethics focuses on the study of *intentional* human actions that we choose to carry out with sufficient knowledge with respect to their being right or wrong.

In Western literature concerning morality, some philosophers describe the qualities of character that lead to praise or blame. Others reflect on the duties and obligations that bind humans to perform certain actions and to refrain from performing others. Still others consider how the existence of communities is related to the purpose of individuals. These three themes – character, duty and social responsibility – are recurrent topics of ethical reflection, serving as the threads that also bind medicine and morality.

The writings ascribed to the School of Hippocrates describe characteristics of the "good physician." Physicians should be gentle, pleasant, comforting, discreet, and firm, and these qualities represent true values. A more grave morality involves the injunctions that define the duty of the good physician: to benefit the sick and do them no harm, to keep confidences, to refrain from exploiting patients, and to show concern and caring, even at the cost to one's own wealth and health. These duties are more profoundly linked to deep moral beliefs than to the admonitions of decorum, and the paradigm of these moral imperatives are embodied in the Hippocratic Oath. Finally, as ethical professionals, physicians must define their place in society, by demonstrating their worthiness of social trust, social authority, and reward.

Becoming a physician involves the acceptance of specific moral responsibilities. Physicians are members of a learned profession defined by its educational breadth, importance in satisfying fundamental human needs, and society's permission to use their special knowledge, powers, and privileges. In return, societies have expected that physicians will hold as their primary concern the welfare of their patients. The covenant of trust established by physicians with patients serves as the basis for the physician's privileged contract with society. The special claim of the medical profession lies *less* in physicians' knowledge and expertise, and *more* in their altruistic dedication to something other than self-interest or self-indulgence. The insistence on clinical competence, caring and trustworthiness define the core of medicine's professional responsibilities, but it is a physician's unique commitment – his or her promise and dedication to the welfare of those who seek their help – that makes medicine a moral enterprise.

As a structurally stabilizing, morally protective force in our society, *professionalism* protects vulnerable persons and social values. The ideal of professionalism has succinctly been described as a "set of values, *behaviors*, and relationships that underpin the trust the public has in doctors."[5] The ACGME includes in its compellation of the essence of professionalism the "adherence to ethical principles."[6] Indeed, the expectations of ethical behavior are stated in professional codes such as

the American Society of Anesthesiologists' *Guidelines for the Ethical Practice of Anesthesiology*,[7] which also incorporate the American Medical Association's *Principles of Medical Ethics*. The ASA *Guidelines* speak to an anesthesiologist's ethical responsibilities to their patients, themselves, their colleagues, their healthcare institutions, and society.

Curbing MAD behavior: an ethical responsibility

Section I.1 of the ASA's ethical guidelines addresses an anesthesiologist's primary ethical responsibility to patients: "The patient–physician relationship involves special obligations for the physician that include *placing the patient's interests foremost*, faithfully caring for the patient and being truthful." Because MAD behavior creates a practice atmosphere in which quality of patient care is threatened, it is not consistent with this primary ethical responsibility.

With respect to ethical responsibilities to colleagues, Section II.1 declares "Anesthesiologists should promote a cooperative and respectful relationship with their colleagues that facilitates quality medical care for patients. This responsibility respects the efforts and duties of other care providers including physicians, medical students, nurses, technicians and assistants." MAD behavior clearly fails to conform to this ethical duty.

Anesthesiologists also have ethical responsibilities to themselves, as addressed in Section IV.2: "The practice of quality anesthesia requires that anesthesiologists maintain their physical and mental health … [,and] … if in doubt about their health, then anesthesiologists should seek medical evaluation and care,… [and furthermore,]… during this period of evaluation or treatment, anesthesiologists should modify or cease their practice." A practical problem with MAD behavior is that MAD physicians are largely incapable of acknowledging it, and equally unable to gain meaningful understanding or insight through treatment.

Finally, Section III.2 iterates that anesthesiologists have ethical responsibilities to the health care facilities in which they practice and should "share with all medical staff members the responsibility to observe and report … any potentially negligent practices or conditions which may present a hazard to patients or health care facility personnel."[7] Detection and documentation of a physician's MAD behavior is the first of the requisite steps to curb this harmful institutional infestation.

Civility and social capital

Relationships with colleagues and staff involve overlapping responsibilities and obligations centering on the care of patients. Our diverse healthcare community is composed of a wide spectrum of personalities, knowledge bases, intelligences, competencies, motivations, backgrounds, cultures, races, ethnicities, religions, and value systems. Given this reality, disagreement, tension, and even conflict are not only anticipated, but welcome when managed civilly, because they can contribute to improving quality of care. Yet, no matter how well honed our coping skills may be, it is extremely challenging to circumvent the distasteful aftermath of unprofessional and uncivil behavior.

Civil, the root word for civilization, connotes an advanced stage of social development.[8] "Civil" is generally thought of as being "polite" or "courteous," each synonym referring to behaving with manners necessary in social situations and interactions. Civil behavior increases *social capital*, which is the well of interpersonal trust, sense of obligation, strength of norms, and unrestrained information pathways that accrue from robust relationships among members of a community.[9] Social capital produces communities of cooperation, fosters communication, enhances achievement of common goals, and facilitates successful realization of complex and dynamic relationships. MAD behavior, on the other hand, weakens social capital and breaks down cooperation, communication, and achievement of common goals – the very essence of a well-functioning medical team.

Managing MAD behavior

Accrediting authorities mandate that every medical staff have bylaws that delineate a credible and effective policy to deal with the MAD physician.[3,4] Identification and documentation of MAD behavior is the point of initiation of this process. This presupposes a workplace educated about the endangerment to patient care wrought by such behavior *and* the ethical responsibility to respond to quell it. Personnel should be urged to bring allegations, concerns or complaints to the attention of medical staff leadership. The entry point for incident reports must be simple, easily accessible, and free of impediments. The complainant must be fully protected, and fear of retaliation and/or retribution dispelled.

Investigation of the incident report is the ethical responsibility of the medical staff. The review and verification of this report must be free of bias or prejudice, yet thorough. It should include interviewing the initiator of the report as well as any other relevant third parties. The medical staff leadership must adhere to its bylaws, policies and procedures. The physician under investigation must be treated with respect and in compliance with due process rights under relevant law. The law protects medical staff review of actions that affect quality of care from discovery.

When appropriate, intervention should incorporate an attempt to resolve the allegations with simple solutions – first pursuing collegial steps without necessarily progressing to disciplinary measures or facilitative rehabilitation. One example is an interview and counseling by the department chair. If that approach is impractical or impossible (there already exists an adverse relationship with the chair, or they are economic competitors), then the medical staff president with at least one other medical staff leader should conduct an interventional meeting. All conversations must be documented.

For a first offense, depending on the tone and responses during the interventional meeting, the MAD physician might simply be warned that the process for the medical staff's abusive/disruptive policy will be invoked upon another reported incident. However, if warranted by the severity of the initial incident and/or the response of the MAD physician in the first "interventional" meeting, then the full body of the disruptive/abusive policy can and should be enforced immediately. If particularly egregious, then the MAD physician should be placed on summary suspension.

The "repeat offender" would, upon judgment of leadership, have to enter a process of further investigation, counseling and advice. Ultimately, the medical staff bylaws addressing repeated MAD deportment must lead to a referral for evaluation and recommendation for treatment by a psychiatrist with experience in providing a comprehensive "fitness-for-duty" evaluation or its equivalent. The full force of imminent suspension of medical staff privileges – and its attendant report to state and national authorities – may suffice to induce the MAD physician to comply with this mandate. The MAD physician's options, consequences for failure to comply, and potential sanctions, must be made crystal clear.

A contract for treatment and monitoring in accordance with the recommendations of the evaluator must establish absolute boundaries for acceptable behavior, and clear and meaningful consequences for their violation. The institution's Well Being Committee or its equivalent can be consulted for advice and assistance. Anger management therapy often is one of the elements included in these recommendations. *The goal of therapy and monitoring is behavioral compliance, not psychological insight.* Expert legal counsel's advice at each procedural step is prudent.

Constructive problem solving and avoidance of future incidents can be achieved without a change of attitude, by compelling compliant behavior. However, some MAD physicians may not achieve substantial changes in attitude or behavior, and even may retaliate, escalate MAD behavior or even pursue litigation. Despite this, there should be no laxity in applying the expectations and limits of acceptable demeanor. Recidivism is not unusual and must be handled according to its severity and frequency. Monitoring adherence to behavior contracts is crucial to success: it should include montoring attendance at "therapeutic" sessions (individual or group), reviewing reports from therapists (or psychologist "coaches"), and requiring the physician to meet regularly with medical staff leadership to review compliance with the contract.

Abuse of disruptive/abusive policies

In the US, physicians may participate in business arrangements that hospitals might view as unfair or unwanted competition, such as physician-owned surgery or procedural centers. Professional competition and animosity has, on occasion, created incentives for hospital administrators to use the disruptive/abusive label inappropriately in a ruse to remove such competitors from the medical staff. Physicians should not be labeled as MAD if they violate onerous, overly broad, or sham "codes of conduct" that are created to squelch medical advocacy, target competitors, or otherwise have no nexus to improving patient care.

Key points

- MAD behavior violates ethical standards of practice and impedes patient safety and quality of care.
- MAD behavior is a manifestation of a personality disorder that is characterized by maladaptive behavior and lack of personal insight. It is not amenable to psychotherapy.
- The American Society of Anesthesiologist's Guidelines for the Ethical Practice of Anesthesiology outlines obligations to patients, colleagues, self and health care

institutions that are incompatible with MAD behavior. In fact, it is the ethical obligation of anesthesiologists to work to eradicate MAD behavior from the workplace.
- Investigation of MAD behavior should be thorough, unbiased, and respectful of the accused physician.
- The goal of intervention and monitoring of the MAD physician is behavioral compliance and not psychological insight.
- In order for MAD physicians to continue to practice, they must be strictly be held to exert a sufficient degree of control over their behavior that precludes their adversely impacting the culture of safety.

References

1* American Medical Association. Council on Ethical and Judicial Affairs. (2003). Code of Medical Ethics.

2* Rosenstein, A. and O'Daniel, M. (2006). Impact and implications of disruptive behavior in the perioperative arena. *J Am Coll Surg*, **203**, 96–105.

3 The Joint Commission on Accreditation of Healthcare Organizations. Sentinel Event Alert. Issue 40, July 9, 2008.

4 The Joint Commission on Accreditation of Healthcare Organizations. Hospital Accreditation Standards. 2009. LD.03.01.01; MS.06.01.03; PC.01.03.05.

5* Wass, V. (2005). Doctors in society. Medical professionalism in a changing world. *Clin Med*, **5(Suppl 1)**, S5–40.

6* Accreditation Council on Graduate Medical Education. (2006). Outcome Project: Enhancing residency education through outcomes assessment. Available at www.acgme.org.

7* American Society of Anesthesiologists. (2009). Guidelines for the Ethical Practice of Anesthesiology. Available at www.asahq.org.

8* Jackson, S. (2005). Civility and professionalism in anesthesia. In *Principes de Reanimation Chirurgicale*, 2nd edn. J-L Pourriat, C Martin, eds. Paris: Arnette, pp. 1420–24.

9* Waisel, D. (2005). Developing social capital in the operating room: the use of population-based techniques. *Anesthesiology*, **103**, 1305–10.

Further reading

Jackson, S. (1999). The role of stress in anaesthetists' health and well-being. *Acta Anaesthesiol Scand*, **43**, 583–602.

40

Sexual harassment, discrimination, and faculty–student intimate relationships in anesthesia practice

Gail A. Van Norman

The author wishes to thank Rosemary Maddi MD for her contributions to the author's understanding of discrimination and harassment in the anesthesia workplace. Regretfully, due to illness Dr. Maddi was unable to participate personally in the writing of this chapter, which is nevertheless a direct result of her previous writings, teaching, and discussions with the author.

The Case

Dr. Frances K. Conley held a tenured professorship in Neurosurgery at Stanford University. She was the first woman to complete a surgical internship at Stanford in 1966, and the first woman appointed to a tenured professorship at any US medical school in 1986. In 1991 she abruptly resigned when a male colleague with a widely publicized pattern of misogyny, harassment and disrespect of female physicians and staff members was appointed Acting Chair of her department. In a letter to the Los Angeles Times, *Dr. Conley described a workplace that was relentlessly hostile and demeaning. She related stories from her own illustrious career: a male colleague who repeatedly suggested in front of colleagues that she "go to bed" with him, professional presentations she had attended in which images of Playboy centerfolds "spiced up" the lectures, and male physicians who groped female colleagues and staff members at will in the operating room. She described finding that "any deviation on my part from the majority view often was prominently announced as being a manifestation of either PMS syndrome or being 'on the rag.' She ultimately rescinded her resignation, but not before her office had been rifled, her name had been summarily removed from the university stationery (even before her resignation had taken effect), and her research lab had been dismantled. Only 12 years ago Dr. Conley wrote, "I have acquired a curious inner peace … realizing, in my lifetime, I will not see women obtain the equality that should be theirs."*[1]

Frances Conley's story is a sadly familiar one to the more than 80% of female academic physicians who report sexual harassment or discrimination on the job.[2] Sexual harassment and discrimination represent only the tip of an iceberg of similar issues in the medical workplace that include discrimination based on race and sexual orientations, and bullying.

Sexual harassment

In the US, sexual harassment is considered sexual discrimination and violates the Civil Rights Act of 1964 – Title VII. Sexual harassment is anti-social and unacceptable behavior defined as unsolicited sexual advances or requests for sexual favors, or any verbal or physical conduct of a sexual nature. Sexual harassment is independent of the gender of the offender or the recipient. It can occur between members of the same or opposite sex, and between workers of any rank. The victim is defined as *anyone* who is offended by the behavior, not just the person toward whom the behavior is directed. It can take the form of inappropriate jokes or stories, touching, or subtle or overt pressure for sexual activity. Sexual harassment is deemed to exist if the victim's job performance is adversely affected by the behavior, or if an offensive, hostile, or intimidating work environment results from it.

In the US, federal law recognizes two forms of sexual harassment. The first is "quid pro quo" harassment, in which the offender demands verbal or physical sexual behavior from an employee in return for job benefits or advancement. The second is the creation of "a hostile work environment" in which no quid pro quo exists.[3] The law also recognizes retaliation against an employee for resisting or complaining about offensive conduct as unlawful.

In 2005, Great Britain amended the Sex Discrimination Act of 1975 to include sexual harassment, defined as verbal, nonverbal, or physical conduct

Clinical Ethics in Anesthesiology: A Case-Based Textbook, ed. Gail A. Van Norman, Stephen Jackson, Stanley H. Rosenbaum and Susan K. Palmer. Published by Cambridge University Press. © Cambridge University Press 2011.

based on sex that has the effect of violating [her] dignity or creating a hostile, degrading, humiliating, or offensive environment. British courts further recognize that women suing for sexual harassment need not show that a man would have been treated differently in order to prevail. The European Union defines sexual harassment as unwanted conduct of a sexual nature affecting the dignity of women and men at work.[4]

Sexual discrimination is more commonly directed against women, but male students are not immune from mistreatment. In pediatrics, obstetrics, and gynecology, for example, men report frequent discrimination with regard to mentoring, educational opportunities, and even general support for entering these specialties.[5]

How is this behavior harmful?

Many ethical principles and values are breached, whether intentionally or not, when sexually charged and discriminatory behavior is tolerated in the workplace. Discrimination flies in the face of social principles that hold that all persons have intrinsic value, and that equals should be treated equally. It also violates principles of justice, beneficence, nonmaleficence, and respect for individual autonomy.

Discrimination creates exclusionary classes of persons – unfairly bestowing benefits on some while harming others – and thus violates the ethical principle of justice. Unfair benefits to a "privileged" group include a greater sense of power and control, lower stress, greater access to educational and promotional opportunities, and by extension, professional and financial advancement, job security, and greater social acceptability. By excluding some individuals, members of the privileged class also proportionally increase the remaining benefits to themselves.

Exclusion from the privileged class assures lower quality education, personal and professional insecurity, higher stress secondary to bullying and harassment, lower rates of promotion and lower rates of pay. In the case of Frances Conley, the "privileged" class was male physicians, and the "excluded" class was women on the healthcare team. But unfair discrimination can just as well be described for any racial, ethnic, financial, or social divisions in which professionally and intellectually comparable persons are treated unequally due to qualities that are unrelated to their ability to perform the job required of them.

Discrimination restricts the individual autonomy of members of the "excluded" class. They do not have the same freedom that the members of the "privileged" class have to choose their associates or their profession – discrimination reduces even their ability to acquire mentors who could advocate for them. The oppressive environment increases stress and limits the individual's emotional ability to cope with bullying. In extreme cases, some individuals may feel compelled to engage in unwanted sexual acts to secure a benefit or promotion they desperately want or need.

Tolerance of discrimination is harmful to patients as well as to the medical profession as a whole, while conferring few if any benefits. When talented future physicians are excluded from training or practice due to discrimination, advancements for the profession that these individuals might have contributed are never achieved. Physicians as a whole are less able to understand and advocate for their patients when the profession is restricted to a sexually and ethnically narrow group of individuals that is not reflective of the population of patients they serve. Restriction of access to the profession gives everyone in the "privileged" group the short-term gain of a larger share of "benefits," but at the expense of long-term degradation of physician resources for patient care – the very reason for which the medical profession exists.

It has been shown that trainees who experience or witness sexual harassment or discrimination in the workplace become accepting of it, and more likely to commit abuses themselves in the future.[6] Thus the harasser of today not only harms today's trainee, but the trainees of tomorrow as well. Physicians often justify the presence of hostile work elements as "routine" and even a "rite of passage," implying that mistreatment and abuse of staff and trainees is not merely acceptable, but somehow *necessary* because it toughens the trainee to a demanding occupation. This further entrenches discriminatory behavior, even while being antithetical to the training of empathetic, compassionate physicians. Furthermore, demeaning any victim who objects to such treatment as "too sensitive" or "not able to play with the boys" violates the values of respect and preservation of dignity of individuals – values that are integral to the ethical practice of medicine.

These harms are not merely theoretical, and certainly are not trivial. In one study,[7] more than 80% of women medical students had heard jokes in the workplace demeaning to women, 71% had experienced subtle sexual comments, 62% had heard overtly sexual comments, 22% had received unwanted sexual advances, and 36% had seen printed sexual material such as magazines or "pin-up" images of women in sexual situations in the workplace. Such behaviors were more common on surgical rotations (74%) and rare on anesthesia rotations (2%). However, the specialty of anesthesia was not exempt: one student described an attending anesthesiologist who asked her about "the sexy things" she was wearing under her scrubs and then told her to "lighten up" when she was offended. Another study found that anesthesiology residency was fourth among specialties (following only surgery, internal medicine, and emergency medicine) in frequency of sexual harassment of residents.[8]

Sexual harassment undermines the victim's sense of self-confidence and dignity. Female trainees report feelings of confusion ("Did he really mean that?" "Did he touch me by accident?"), self-blaming ("I'm too sensitive"), and fear of reprisals ("They'll say I'm a 'bitch,'" "They won't work with me").[7] The belief that reporting harassment is a sign of weakness, and that a "strong" woman would put up with the behavior and "just go on," undermines attempts to identify and punish offenders. Society tends to view "victims" in a negative light (as powerless outsiders or angry zealots), and it is often easier for individuals to ignore harassment or blame themselves for the problem than report it. Failing to act to prevent harassment grants legitimacy to the beliefs that such behavior is benign or innocuous. Frances Conley admitted that she may have herself contributed to the problem when she "put up" with such behavior and "shut up" rather than taking action against it.

Research has shown that the perception of being sexually harassed results in increased cynicism, lessened professional commitment, poor self-esteem, depression, and increased risk of posttraumatic stress disorder. Psychological manifestations are seen in 90% of women who experience sexual harassment, although few seek professional help. In one study involving European physicians, suicidal ideation among female physicians was three times more commonplace among those who had experienced degrading or harassing experiences at work.[9]

Are consensual sexual relationships in the workplace the same as sexual harassment?

A third-year female anesthesia resident falls behind her peers in clinical performance. Although her technical skills are average, she does not appear to be studying, is far below her peers in her objective knowledge, and regularly comes to the operating room poorly prepared. Her faculty advisor warns her that unless her performance improves, she will be put on academic probation, and ultimately graduation

from residency is in question. The resident tells her advisor that she is dating a male faculty member, who has assured her she is doing fine and will graduate. Her partner attends faculty evaluation meetings where her performance is reviewed, and participates in performance evaluations of her. Although faculty evaluation meetings are confidential, he has revealed some of their confidential discussions to her.

Ethical boundaries in the medical student–teacher relationship are complex. The participants are adults, and Western culture values freedom of choice for mature individuals. Freedom of association is a basic tenet of democracy and centers of higher learning. Romantic and/or sexual pairing is intensely private, and scrutiny by governments and regulators of such relationships generally is discouraged in both the US and Europe. Regulatory interference in private relationships is therefore usually restricted to those situations in which behavior is perceived to clash with critical social values, or when vulnerable persons may be exploited. Examples include domestic abuse, marital rape, and incest.

Although intimate relationships between teachers and adult students are not illegal, they are problematic, sharing some issues in common with sexual harassment. Such relationships may intentionally or unintentionally exploit unequal power dynamics. They run the risk of creating actual or perceived favoritism, and may cast doubt on the integrity of the faculty member or institution. Overt sexual harassment of *either* party can also occur. Such relationships are therefore risky for both the student and the teacher, and are at minimum imprudent in most cases.

Faculty–student consensual sexual relationships appear to be common. In one report, up to 17% of psychology students admitted to engaging in "consensual" sexual activity with teachers.[10] Most students later reported an impaired sense of well-being, and many took action to avoid certain teachers, even changing specialties or dropping out of training as a consequence of such relationships. Many students who engage in a sexual relationship with a teacher report that they feel coerced to some degree, and such feelings increase over time.[11] Importantly, many do not feel free to break off the relationship while the teacher is in a position to supervise or evaluate them.

Deceiving someone – such as promising positive evaluations, or professing emotional commitment where there is none – in order to engage them in a sexual relationship is a form of exploitation. Sexual exploitation is wrong, because it is an example of one person using coercive or manipulative influence over another, thus violating their autonomy. Are consensual faculty student relationships truly "consensual" or are they actually exploitative?

Many professionals argue that faculty–student relationships are never truly consensual if the teacher is in a position to affect the student's evaluations or future career prospects. Even if the teacher does not *intend* to coerce or deceive, the student may *believe* that their evaluations will suffer if they do not participate, or be elevated if they do. The student may be desperate for a particular benefit from a teacher, and therefore believe they are not truly free to refuse a sexual advance. Even if such relationships begin consensually, many students later report fear, regret and disproportionate guilt. Furthermore, studies show that when a student participates in such a relationship they are more likely to commit future sexual misconduct with their own patients and future students.[6]

Quid pro quo relationships between a teacher and an adult student, even if voluntary, are clearly unethical because they are unjust to other students who actually perform the necessary academic work to receive the academic recognition. Favorable evaluations that are awarded in return for sex corrupt the academic process by disconnecting academic evaluation from academic performance. Furthermore, teachers may be unconsciously unable to assign even "fair" grades to students with whom they are intimately involved, or from whom they have recently severed a sexual relationship.

When a teacher agrees to pursue a "voluntary" sexual relationship with a student, the "rightness" or "wrongness" of that decision depends in part on how accurately they have assessed that the student is behaving in a truly "voluntary" manner. Self-deception may prevent an instructor from being able to truly recognize problems of coercion and academic fairness. Even the *perception* of unfairness among colleagues and students can cause institutional harm by casting doubt on the objectivity of the academic process. These issues can be difficult to judge from the "inside" of an intimate relationship, and ethical considerations therefore weigh against faculty engaging in such relationships with students as a general rule.

In the 1990s, almost half of US 4-year academic institutions had adopted or were considering adopting policies restricting intimate relationships between faculty and students. In 2003, the University of California instituted a policy that prohibits teachers from dating either students in their classes, or *students that they might reasonably expect in the future to be in their classes.*[12] Many universities now proscribe intimate relationships between faculty members and students so long as the supervisory relationship is intact or has the potential to occur in the future. If an intimate relationship develops between a student and instructor, the teacher has at minimum an ethical obligation to withdraw from any supervisory and evaluation processes involving their partner.

Case resolution

In the case example, the relationship between the student and faculty member presents several serious problems. The student has developed an unrealistic faith in her partner's reassurances, or she may believe that their sexual relationship "guarantees" her graduation. The student is not learning what she needs to learn to perform her duties well, and may therefore harm future patients. She may even fail to graduate by not attending to her studies, and her peers may discredit her if they believe that she received academic favors in return for sex, regardless of her actual ability to do her job.

The faculty member has broken fidelity with his faculty colleagues to keep confidences, and may be deceiving the resident about his intentions or ability to guarantee her graduation. He is harmed by the negative impact these actions have on how others perceive his professional and personal integrity. The institution is harmed if other trainees believe that such relationships are tolerated and can corrupt the integrity of the academic process. The faculty member should withdraw immediately from any role in his partner's evaluations, and should observe the confidentiality of faculty meetings. The resident must be informed that her graduation is in jeopardy, and be held to the academic goals that must be met in order to graduate.

Key points

- Sexual discrimination and harassment in the workplace are examples of a broader group of antisocial and unethical behaviors that include discrimination on the basis of race and sexual orientation, and general bullying.
- Sexual harassment is antithetical to the values of medicine which promote respect for autonomy, beneficence, nonmaleficence, justice, respect for others, and promotion of human dignity.

- Physicians have ethical obligations to avoid discriminatory behavior as well as to take measures to banish it from the workplace when it occurs.
- Not all consensual sexual relationships in the workplace are automatically unethical, but all have the potential for harm through exploitation of vulnerable persons and degradation of the educational process. The proven, harmful effects on students, faculty and institutions suggest that such relationships are imprudent and generally should be discouraged.
- When a consensual sexual or romantic relationship develops between a teacher and student, the teacher is ethically obliged to withdraw from any process involving evaluation or promotion/demotion of the student.

References

1* Conley, F. (1998). *Walking Out on the Boys.* New York: Farrar, Straus and Giroux.

2   Carr, P.L., Ash, A.S., Friedman, R.H., *et al.* (2000). Faculty perceptions of gender discriminatin and sexual harassment in academic medicine. *Ann Intern Med*, **132**(11), 889–96.

3   Title VII, Civil Rights Act of 1964.

4   Directive 2002/73/EC of the European Parliament and of the Council of 23 Sept 2002.

5* Stratton, T.D., McLaughlin, M.A., Witte, F.M., *et al.* (2005). Does students' exposure to gender discrimination and sexual harassment in medical school affect specialty choice and residency program selection? *Acad Med*, **80**(4), 400–8.

6* Robinson, G.E. and Stewart, D.E. (1996). A curriculum on physician-patient sexual misconduct and teacher-learner mistreatment Part 1: Content. *CMAJ*, **154**, 643–9.

7* Hinze, S.W. (2004). Am I being too sensitive? Women's experience of sexual harassment during medical training. *Health (London)*, **8**(1), 101–27.

8* Nagata-Kobayashi, S., Maeno, T., Yshizu, M., and Shimbo, T. (2009). Universal problems during residency: abuse and harassment. *Med Edu*, **43**(7), 628–36.

9* Fridner, A., Belkic, K., Marini, M., *et al.* (2009). Survey on recent suicidal ideation among female university hospital physicians in Sweden and Italy (the HOUPE study): cross-sectional associations with work stressors. *Gend Med*, **6**(1), 314–28.

10* Biaggio, M., Paget, T.L., and Chenoweth, M.S. (1997). A model for ethical management of faculty-student dual relationships. *Prof Psychol Res Prac*, **28**(2), 184–9.

11 Glaser, R.D., and Thorpe, J.S. (1986). Unethical intimacy: a survey of sexual contact and advances between psychology educators and female graduate students. *Am Psychol*, **41**(1), 43–51.

12 Paulson A. (2004). Student/teacher romances: off limits. *Christian Science Monitor*, February 17.

Further reading

Bumiller, K. (1988). *The Civil Rights Society: The Social Construction of Victims.* Baltimore MD: The Johns Hopkins University Press.

Changing the Face of Medicine: Dr. Frances K. Conley. shttp://www.nlm.nih.gov/changingthefaceofmedicine/physicians/biography_68.html

Conley F. *Why I'm leaving Stanford: I wanted my dignity back – sexism: a brain surgeon gives up her teaching job in protest over a system that reinforces men's ideas that they are superior beings. The Los Angeles Times,* June 9, 1991.

Maddi, R. (2000). Sexual Harassment. In *The ASA Syllabus on Ethics.* Park Ridge, IL: American Society of Anesthesiologists.

Robinson, G.E. and Stewart, D.E. (1996). A curriculum on physician–patient sexual misconduct and teacher–learner mistreatment Part 2: Teaching method. *CMAJ*, **154**, 1021–5.

Witte, F.M., Stratton, T.D., and Nora, L.M. (2006). Stories from the field: students' descriptions of gender discrimination and sexual harassment during medical school. *Acad Med*, **81**(7), 648–54.

Zippel, K.S. (2006). *The Politics of Sexual Harassment: A Comparative Study of the United States, the European Union, and Germany.* Cambridge, UK: Cambridge University Press.

41

Conflicts of interest – industry gifts to physicians

Murali Sivarajan

The Case

Dr. Daniel Carlat, a practicing psychiatrist, published an article entitled, 'Dr. Drug Rep' in the New York Times Sunday Magazine *in November, 2007.*[1] *In it, he wrote of his experience acting more or less as a drug company detail man going to physicians' offices and giving lunch-time talks to primary care physicians and psychiatrists extolling the virtues of Effexor®, an antidepressant, while the audience feasted on gourmet luncheons supplied by the maker of Effexor®. Wyeth Pharmaceuticals had recruited him to do this by inviting him and his wife to attend a conference in New York City, plying them with expensive dinners and theater tickets and, in addition, paying him an honorarium of $750.00. He was given a set of slides on Effexor® prepared by Wyeth to use for his talks and he was promised a fee for each talk that he delivered. He admits to being somewhat uneasy about this arrangement but nevertheless decided to participate.*

In his talks, Dr. Carlat pitched Effexor® as a better antidepressant than other drugs on the market. This was based on a meta-analysis presented at the conference by an esteemed academic psychiatrist who was a paid consultant to Wyeth. The co-authors were Wyeth employees. As the year went by, new data emerged showing that Effexor® was only marginally better than other drugs in improving depression. It also had a significant side effect – a 50% greater incidence of hypertension than with other antidepressants – and serious withdrawal effects as well. Dr. Carlat realized that these undesirable properties of Effexor® had been downplayed at the conference but he still continued to pitch the drug to his audiences because he was "concerned that the reps would not invite him to give talks if he divulged any negative information." He came to the realization that he was just a "drug rep with an MD" when he was challenged by one of the psychiatrists in the audience on the incidence of hypertension with Effexor®. After a year of giving an average of one talk a week, earning him a supplemental income of $30 000.00, he quit being a drug rep. At the end of the article, he raised several questions:

Did I contribute to faulty medical decision-making? Did my advice lead doctors to make inappropriate drug choices, and did their patients suffer needlessly?

And he provides his own answers

Maybe. I'm sure I persuaded many physicians to prescribe Effexor®, potentially contributing to blood-pressure problems and withdrawal symptoms.

Dr. Carlat's ethical lapses are obvious; misrepresenting and evading the truth, prevarication if not outright lying. One could argue that there was no conflict of interest because Dr. Carlat did not misrepresent himself as any one other than a speaker for Wyeth paid to promote its product. However, a conflict resides in a general sense because the payments he accepted from the drug company to sustain or increase its market share were against the interests of patients he is sworn to protect as a physician. In his confessional, Dr. Carlat acknowledges his own ethical lapse in "dancing around the truth…," but he ignored the larger problem of drug companies trying to influence physicians by plying them with gifts.

As part of promotion aimed at physicians, drug companies have always given out gifts. In 1985, this author observed that these gifts were "no longer cheap ball-point pens but something moderately priced, such as a document case, with the name of the company emblazoned on it."[2] Subsequently, the gifts became even more extravagant. Expensive dinners at local restaurants, all-expenses-paid trips to resorts to attend quasi-scientific meetings where the company's products were heavily promoted, and cash offerings to sit through promotional presentations became commonplace. In response to concern expressed in the peer-reviewed literature about drug companies' influences on physician practice and behavior, the American College of Physicians[3] and The American Medical Association[4] published position papers that sought to limit, but not eliminate, drug companies' gifts to physicians. They found trivial gifts such as pens and calendars, modest dinners, drinks and hospitality related to

---

Clinical Ethics in Anesthesiology: A Case-Based Textbook, ed. Gail A. Van Norman, Stephen Jackson, Stanley H. Rosenbaum and Susan K. Palmer. Published by Cambridge University Press. © Cambridge University Press 2011.

an educational event, even trips to educational meetings chosen for their convenience and not for recreation still acceptable. It was suggested that whether a gift is acceptable or not may be guided by the answer to the question, "would you be willing to have these gifts generally known?"[3]

In spite of position papers and guidelines, the practice of feting physicians with expensive gifts continued unabated. The print media began to take note. Numerous articles, editorials and Op-Ed commentaries in major newspapers and magazines led the Pharmaceutical Research and Manufacturers of America (PhRMA) to publish a voluntary code of conduct for interactions with health professionals in July 2008.[5] It prohibits small gifts (e.g., logo-embossed pens and coffee mugs), and recreational and entertainment gifts, (e.g., tickets to shows and sporting events that have no educational value). But it does not prohibit drug reps from providing office-based and hospital-based meals and educational material less than $100.00 in value. Does the acceptance of these gifts, such as the office-based meals that Dr. Carlat presided over, constitute conflicts of interest? Do these gifts influence physicians' practices and potentially harm patients?

The obligation of gifts

Most physicians who accept gifts from drug companies deny that they are influenced to prescribe that company's drug over other, or generic, drugs of equal merit. But to expect them to admit being influenced by gifts is unrealistic. Their natural and instinctive response is denial because admission reflects poorly on their character or professionalism. In behavioral psychology this response is attributed to "self-serving bias" that tends to favor one's own self interests:[6] an individual's judgments of appropriate behavior are biased in favor of their own actions. Yet, in fact, both philosophical reasoning and empirical evidence *do* implicate drug company gifts in influencing the prescribing behavior of physicians.

A reasonable body of enquiry in moral philosophy has defined the obligation that gifts impose.[7] In some Native American tribes, gifts entail no reciprocal obligation on the part of the recipient. However, gifts in our society have a more personal meaning. The giver offers a personal relationship and the receiver in accepting the gift, accepts the relationship that carries an obligation to reciprocate. Camenisch also describes the tension between the giver and the receiver if the gift is not reciprocated; the recipient in accepting the gift

without reciprocating assumes an inferior or dependent relationship.[7] The desire to reciprocate is a powerful emotional response to maintain an equal relationship with the giver. Partaking of food in the company of others is a social event that most enjoy; therefore gifts of food, in particular are more entangling because of the camaraderie and the good feelings that accompany it. It has been said that food is "the most commonly used technique to derail the judgment aspect of decision making."[8] Obviously, the doctor who accepts a drug company gift is not expected to respond by giving a gift to the drug rep. Physicians' desire to reciprocate results in their favoring the company's product when prescribing from a bewildering formulary of similar, equally effective drugs.

Empirical evidence supports the contention that physicians favor the products of the company that provided gifts to them. One study examined the prescribing patterns of 20 physicians before and after their attendance at a drug company sponsored seminar. They found that prescription for the index drug increased after the drug company sponsored event compared with that before the event and also compared with national trend at the same time. All but one of the physicians denied that the seminar would affect their behavior.[9] A critical analysis of the studies on the influence of drug company interactions with physicians on their practice patterns demonstrated that: (1) physicians' meetings with drug company representatives are associated with increased requests for adding the drugs promoted by the drug reps to the hospital formulary; (2) continuing medical education (CME) programs sponsored by a drug company preferentially promoted the sponsor's drug compared to non-sponsored CME programs; (3) physicians who attended drug company sponsored CME programs and accepted travel funds from sponsors were more likely to write prescriptions for the drug(s) made by the sponsor and less likely to prescribe generic drugs; and (4) resident physicians attending drug company sponsored luncheon lectures were more likely to have inaccurate information about the sponsor's and the competitor's products.[10]

Social science and marketing research support the view that the insidious obligation that gifts impose is not related to the size and cost of gifts. Studies show that even trinkets with brand names etched on them, such as key chains, ball-point pens, refrigerator magnets and coffee mugs, increase sales of the brand products.[6] A simple indication of their effectiveness is the fact that the drug companies would not be doing it if the resulting increase in sales did not warrant the cost of these promotions. From a behavioral perspective, small gifts with brand logos create brand-awareness and implicit associations in memory. This results in their name being recalled when purchasing a product or writing a prescription. Another study demonstrated that two small pharmaceutical promotional items, namely a clipboard and a notepad with brand logos, skewed the treatment preferences of medical students who were exposed to them when compared to students who were not.[11]

The cost of the obligation created by accepting gifts

The *financial* costs of these obligations are impressive. Annual marketing expenditures by pharmaceutical companies are approximately $ 20 billion, 90% of which is directed at physicians.[12] In 2004, Blumenthal reported that drug companies spent $8 000 to $15 000 per physician every year to promote their products.[13] The money to pay for such promotions comes from the sale of products, paid for by patients in one way or the other. During this decade, when inflation was approximately 1%–3%, drug company profits increased by double-digit percentages every year, and over 30% of their budgets were spent on marketing. Inevitably, this adds to the cost of healthcare overall.

The *moral* cost of the obligation of gifts is the erosion of the physician's professional image. The drug companies declare these expenses as legitimate marketing, but there is a crucial moral difference between the marketing of pharmaceuticals to physicians and the marketing of consumer products such soaps, cosmetics and cars directly to consumers. In pharmaceutical marketing to physicians, gifts are given to physicians to influence their practices while the patients, who are the consumers, pick up the tab. In stark mercenary terms, physicians decide the medicine or treatment for which the patients pay and then receive tax free gifts for those decisions. There is the injustice of redistribution of wealth from the patients, some of whom are least able to afford it, to doctors, who are considerably better off.

Anesthesiologists are less likely to write prescriptions than other physicians but are still the target of drug companies and medical equipment manufacturers. A survey of physicians in the US revealed that, on the average, anesthesiologists met with drug and equipment sales representatives about two times a month. They were as likely to have received gifts – such as free meals and entertainment tickets – as surgeons, internists, pediatricians, family practitioners, and cardiologists. In general, anesthesiologists were less likely to have received travel reimbursement and payment for consulting than cardiologists, internists, and family practitioners.[14]

Cartoon by Paul Noth, published in the July 7, 2008 edition of *The New Yorker*. Reproduced with permission.

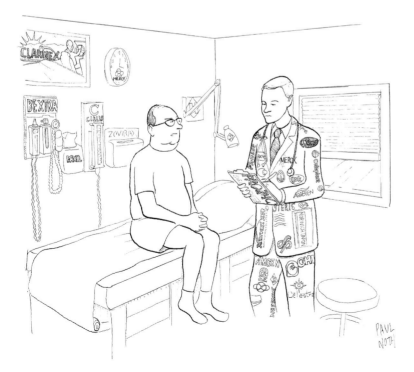

Physician obligations to the profession

Voluntary guidelines and policy statements published over the last 15 years have had some effect in curbing some of the practices, such as all-expenses paid vacation in luxury resorts, that could be seen as blatant bribes. But, by pharmaceutical industry's own guidelines, gifts will continue to be given especially in professional meetings in which the company's products are promoted. Because voluntary guidelines have had only limited success, a group of academic physicians and representatives from the Association of American Medical Colleges have called on academic medical centers to take a leadership role in abolishing potential sources of unwanted influence by drug companies.[12] The hope is that academic medical centers, which have responsibility for educating and training physicians, will have an influence in shaping the attitude of future physicians toward these conflicts of interests. There is some validity to this assumption. A recent study reported that students at a medical school that had policies prohibiting gifts from drug companies were less likely to be influenced by drug company promotional items than students from medical schools that had no restriction on gifts from drug companies.[11]

Some years ago, the Marketing Executive of a large drug company was invited by the author's institution to debate their promotional activities. He declined the invitation but confided that there were two reasons for their gift program: (1) that the rival companies were doing it in a fierce competitive market, and (2) that without some gifts to catch their attention, doctors would not give them their time of day. Surveys of resident physicians confirm the view that without meals as inducement they were less likely to attend drug company sponsored CME meetings.[13] Physicians are therefore at least somewhat complicit with the drug companies in perpetuating these activities. But physicians' obligations to the medical profession demand that they put patients' interest ahead of material gain outside of regular remuneration. If physicians rejected the overtures of commercial medical companies with as much indignation as they display when accused of being influenced by them, then these practices and conflicts of interest would probably cease. In the words of Goldfinger, "In this world of medical commerce, it still takes two to tango".[15]

Key points

- Drug companies exert influence on physicians' practice behaviors by bestowing a wide variety of gifts on them, from trinkets to gourmet dinners and travel reimbursements to attend company sponsored meetings.
- Even inexpensive gifts influence physician behavior by creating "brand awareness" and implicit associations with the products of the companies that provide the gifts.
- Accepting gifts creates obligations for physicians that are in direct conflict with their obligations to patients.
- Company gifts are funded from the sale of companies' products to patients. Hence patients suffer additionally by having to pay for these gifts.
- Voluntary guidelines by professional medical organizations have had very little effect in curbing drug companies' influences on physician practices.
- Academic medical centers might have a role in shaping the attitudes of future physicians to drug industry influence on physician behavior.
- Individual resolve is essential if physicians are to preserve their professional image and dignity.

References

1* Carlat D. (2007). Dr. Drug Rep. *New York Times*, November 25. http://www.nytimes.com/2007/11/25/magazine/25memo-t.html?_r=1&emc=etal Accessed October 27, 2009.

2* Sivarajan, M. (1985). Tarnishing the medical profession's image. *N Engl J Med*, **312**, 1132.

3* Physicians and the pharmaceutical industry: A position paper of the American College of Physicians. (1990). *Ann Intern Med*, **112**, 624–6.

4* Gifts to physicians from industry (editorial). (1991). *JAMA*, **265**, 501.

5* Pharmaceutical Research and Manufacturers of America. (2008). Code on interactions with healthcare professionals. http://www.phrma.org/files/PhRMA%20Marketing%20Code%202008.pdf Accessed October 27, 2009.

6* Dana, J. and Lowenstein, G.A. (2003). Social science perspectives on gifts to physicians from industry. *JAMA*, **290**, 252–5.

7* Camenisch, P.F. (1981). Gift and gratitude in ethics. *J Religious Ethics*, **9**, 1–33.

8* Katz, D., Caplan, A.L. and Merz, J.F. (2003). All gifts large and small: towards an understanding of the ethics of pharmaceutical industry gift-giving. *Am J Bioeth*, **3**, 39–46.

9* Orlowski, J.P. and Wateska, L. (1992). The effects of pharmaceutical firm enticements on physician prescribing patterns: there is no such thing as a free lunch. *Chest*, **102**, 270–3.

10* Wazana, A. (2000). Physicians and the pharmaceutical industry: is the gift ever a gift? *JAMA*, **283**, 373–80.

11* Grande, D., Frosch, D.L., Perkins, A.W., and Kahn, B.E. (2009). Effect of exposure to small pharmaceutical promotional items on treatment preferences. *Arch Intern Med*, **169**, 887–93.

12* Brennan, T.A., Rothman, D.J., Blank, L., *et al.* (2006). Health industry practices that create conflicts of interest: a policy proposal for academic medical centers. *JAMA*, **295**, 429–33.

13* Blumenthal, D. (2004). Doctors and drug companies. *N Engl J Med*, **351**, 1885–9.

14* Campbell, E.G., Gruen, R.L., Mountford, J., et al. (2007). A national survey of physician-industry relationships. *N Engl J Med*, **356**, 1742–50.

15* Goldfinger, S.E. A matter of influence. (1987). *N Engl J Med*, **316**, 1408–9.

Further reading

Brody, H. (2010). Drug detailers, professionalism, and prudence. *Am J Bioeth*, **10**(1), 9–10.

Disclosure of medical errors in anesthesiology practice

Karen Souter

The Case

A 45-year-old woman presents for laparoscopic cholecystectomy. She is healthy apart from symptoms related to her cholelithiasis. As is normal practice in this institution, the antibiotics to be administered by the anesthesiologist are hanging on the IV pole on the patient's stretcher. The anesthesiologist notices the antibiotic that has been sent is cefazolin, despite the fact that the patient's allergy to cefazolin is clearly documented in the chart. He asks the nurse to replace the cefazolin with an alternative antibiotic. As he is about to take the patient to the operating room, one of his colleagues interrupts him to ask if he will take late call that night. A brief discussion ensues. He is now late bringing the patient into the operating room and the surgeon is making his impatience obvious. The anesthesiologist induces anesthesia and starts the antibiotic infusion.

Fifteen minutes later he notices a rash covering the patient's body. The airway pressures have increased and the patient is wheezing. The blood pressure falls precipitously. To his dismay he sees that, in his haste to get the patient anesthetized he failed to confirm that the antibiotic had been replaced and he has accidentally administered the cefazolin. He diagnoses acute anaphylaxis and initiates treatment. The patient responds and her condition stabilizes, surgery is abandoned and the patient is admitted to the ICU for further care.

"To err is human; to forgive, divine" Alexander Pope 1688–1744.

A competent anesthesiologist would instantly recognize the classic signs of anaphylaxis. Once diagnosed, prompt treatment of anaphylaxis usually results in a complete recovery.

In contrast to the medical management of this error, disclosure of the error resulting in the anaphylactic reaction is not straightforward; layers of hospital policies, legal precedents, ethical codes and personal biases complicate the correct course of action. A thorough understanding of the issues involved in disclosure of medical errors is important to every anesthesiologist.

Ethical principles involved in disclosure of medical errors

If this incident had happened prior to the modern era, it would be easy to imagine the patient being told that she had experienced a "complication" related to her anesthetic, and perhaps very little else. This reflects the paternalist approach by physicians that dominated medicine until the last half of the twentieth century, and summed up by Oliver Wendell Holmes, the dean of Harvard Medical school from 1847–1853. *"The patient has no more right to the truth than he has to all the medicine in the physician's saddlebag"*.[1] Many physicians believed it was right to deny the patient the truth for a number of seemingly good reasons.

Modern medical ethics emphasizes four guiding principles; respect for patient autonomy, beneficence, nonmaleficence, and justice. Autonomy refers to the right of an individual to make decisions about one's life and body without coercion by others. When applied to the disclosure of medical errors, autonomy refers to the patient's right to possess all the available information about their health necessary to making decisions. In our case, the patient required admission to the intensive care unit, escalation of medical care, and investigation of the anaphylactic reaction. She also needed to have her surgery rescheduled. The patient must understand all the facts related to the case in order to be able to consent to extra treatment. Respect for patient autonomy therefore requires the open and timely disclosure of all the facts, including an admission that the wrong antibiotic was delivered.

The American Medical Association (AMA) Code of Medical Ethics is clear about the ethical duty of physicians to disclose errors:

It is a fundamental ethical requirement that a physician should at all times deal honestly and openly with patients.... Situations occasionally occur in which a patient

Clinical Ethics in Anesthesiology: A Case-Based Textbook, ed. Gail A. Van Norman, Stephen Jackson, Stanley H. Rosenbaum and Susan K. Palmer. Published by Cambridge University Press. © Cambridge University Press 2011.

suffers significant medical complications that may have resulted from the physician's mistake or judgment. In these situations, the physician is ethically required to inform the patient of all the facts necessary to ensure understanding of what has occurred. Only through full disclosure is a patient able to make informed decisions regarding future medical care. ...... Concern regarding legal liability which might result following truthful disclosure should not affect the physician's honesty with a patient.[2]

Likewise, the General Medical Council of the UK has stated that doctors should:

...offer an apology and explain fully and promptly to the patient what has happened, and the likely short-term and long-term effects.[3]

In 2009, the National Health Service of the UK announced a new "Being Open" framework as the best practice guide for healthcare staff concerning communication with patients, their families and their caregivers following harm.[4]

National policies and standards for disclosure of medical errors

In 1999, The Head of the Clinical Risk Unit at the University College London reported that an estimated 40 000 patients die annually in Britain due to medical errors.[5] Shortly thereafter in the US, the Institute of Medicine published a landmark report "To Err is Human" making the startling revelation that medical errors accounted for an estimated 44 000 to 98 000 preventable deaths annually.[6] This report heralded a significant re-structuring of US healthcare systems aimed at improving patient safety. In 2001 the Joint Commission for Accreditation of Health Care Organizations (JCAHO) in the US issued the first nationwide disclosure standard that required patients to be informed about all outcomes of care, including "unanticipated outcomes." Since then, guidelines for disclosure have increasingly been used by institutions as well as pay-for-performance programs to promote safer patient care.

A systems-based approach to medical error

It is apparent that a number of problems within the system may have contributed to the error described in our case. These include the delivery of the wrong antibiotic to the patient's bedside, the distraction by a colleague, and the failure of the anesthesiologist to identify the drug prior to administration. There is also a small chance that the anaphylactic response was due to another drug administered within the same

timeframe as the cefazolin. Without investigation of the error, the flaws in the system or the true nature of the patient's allergy may not be completely revealed. A common response by patients who are the victims of medical errors is a desire that the same thing doesn't happen again to someone else. The premise of the policies put in place by the quality and safety organizations is that, by encouraging reporting, a greater openness and understanding of medical errors will develop and measures to prevent them can be determined. Hospitals have much in common with the airline and nuclear power industries which are also complex systems in which individuals are rarely solely responsible for serious errors.

In our case, the anesthesiologist clearly has an ethical duty to disclose the error to the patient. The implementation of patient safety and quality policies reinforces this duty. Disclosure respects the patient's autonomy to be fully informed about their medical care. From a systems perspective, the disclosure of errors allows healthcare systems to identify and eliminate system errors, thereby improving safety for all patients. The ethical principle of justice requires that patients be treated equally, thus patients are entitled to the truth regardless of the views of their physicians or the policies of the institution in which they receive care.

Barriers to effective error disclosure

Studies show significant discrepancies between what physicians say they would do and what they actually do when it comes to reporting medical errors and disclosing them to patients.[7] Patients report both concerns that their doctors have withheld the truth concerning medical errors, and dissatisfaction with the way in which errors are disclosed.[8]

There are many barriers to effective error disclosure. To begin with, which errors need to be disclosed? When ethical standards and policies are examined closely, they are not as clear as they might be. The AMA code of ethics refers to "significant" events and JCAHO to "unanticipated outcomes." Neither of these terms is well defined.

Fear of litigation is a major reason why physicians have avoided open error disclosure.[9] In the US, JCAHO recognizes that this "wall of silence" attributable to the medical liability system impedes the course of open disclosure and error reporting, and that these conceptions (or in many cases misconceptions) will not easily be solved without re-structuring the legal system.[10] Evidence that error disclosure may *decrease* the incidence of litigation and liability costs is largely unknown or ignored by doctors.[11] Physicians in the US greatly overestimate the percentage of adverse events that result in lawsuits. Medical malpractice lawsuits represent a prolonged period of emotional trauma, and perhaps even permanent harm to one's reputation and livelihood, and physicians are likely to attempt to avoid them.

Advocates of patient safety have called for removal of blame and shame from the discussion of medical errors, recognizing that most medical errors are the result of a systems failure involving multiple events with the physician often being the last "nail in the coffin." Patients on the other hand often want someone to blame and surveys show that the public want to see doctors punished for errors.[12]

In our scenario it is clear that a systems error caused the wrong antibiotic to be delivered to the patient and also that the interruption by a colleague distracted the anesthesiologist at a time when he needed full concentration. However, it is the anesthesiologist who must face the patient and her family, apologize and rightly or wrongly be blamed for the error.

The introduction of apology laws in many of the US has helped physicians by providing a safe harbor from admission in court for expressions of sorrow and apologies made after a medical error.[12]

A lack or perceived lack of institutional support can prevent physicians from embracing full error disclosure. In a well-publicized case, an anesthesiologist was actively discouraged from any contact with his patient after she had suffered an adverse reaction. The institution forbade contact on the grounds that this would increase the risk of litigation. Eventually, the anesthesiologist was able to communicate with his patient and much of the emotional pain, guilt, and misunderstanding on both sides were reconciled.[13]

Ethical considerations in apologizing and telling the truth

It is difficult for physicians to acknowledge their mistakes when the duty to *"first do no harm"* (nonmaleficence) is a basic tenant upon which medical training is based. A medical error violates this professional norm. The emotional impact for the physician dealing with the guilt and shame of causing a medical error is considerable and physicians will often avoid seeking help because of this.

When physicians disclose an error, feelings of guilt are often alleviated, and this may call into question the physician's motives for apologizing. Is the physician apologizing for an error out of concern for telling the truth, or is he motivated to seek forgiveness or absolution from his own feelings of guilt and shame? Berlinger and Wu have used the term "cheap grace" to describe the situation when a physician expects forgiveness for an error which harms a patient without first disclosing, apologizing for and making amends for his mistakes.[14] A similar criticism has been leveled at apology laws, where the apology may be made to "make the doctor look good in the eyes of a jury".[12]

Placing the patient's interest foremost and being truthful respects patient autonomy and upholds the ethical principles of beneficence and nonmaleficence. Beneficence results when the physician puts aside his own fear of personal harm and provides the patient with an honest explanation. Such an account helps the patient understand what has happened and allows him or her to engage in further treatment decisions fully informed. In a similar way, the principle of nonmaleficence is upheld when the doctor spares the patient harm, both physically and emotionally, that could result from not knowing about the error. The doctor also spares other patients harm if an erroneous system is identified and corrected as a result of proper error reporting.

In the end, however, the physician must understand and accept that he or she may not receive the patient's absolution from blame. Some patients and families may never be able to forgive the injury, or want any contact with those responsible for harming them.

Should the physician disclose medical errors that do not cause harm?

In the case of an obvious medical error that has caused harm, disclosure and apology on the part of the physician is the right thing to do, even though physicians may struggle to achieve this. In the case where an error has not harmed a patient the correct course of action is much less clear. Let us consider an alternative case scenario. This time the anesthesiologist notices a rash spreading up the arm, but nothing else happens and by the end of the case the rash has disappeared. What is the correct course of action for the anesthesiologist?

There are ethical arguments both for disclosing this error to the patient and for not disclosing it. These can be approached from a consequence-based perspective, or from a deontological or duty-based perspective.

In the alternative scenario the patient would have no knowledge that she received the wrong antibiotic. In a consequence-based approach, there is little reason for a patient to ask her anesthesiologist "did you give me cefazolin?" and in the absence of this question, the anesthesiologist is not guilty of lying to the patient. Voluntary disclosure of the error by the anesthesiologist could conceivably be harmful if the patient suffers emotionally from knowing that she had been placed at risk. Alternatively, one could argue that the patient may not be truly allergic to cefazolin and this serendipitous event in which she did not suffer a major reaction should trigger re-evaluation of her supposed "allergy." In this case it would be right to inform the patient and suggest further investigations. Finally, if the event were not disclosed to the patient, she may later notice that she was charged for cefazolin on her medical bill and question this. The discovery that some facts related to her case had been withheld could result in loss of confidence in the healthcare system.

The deontological, or duty-based approach is based on the works of Emmanual Kant. His main thesis was that the moral worth of an act is not related to the outcome, but whether or not it is done from a sense of duty or obligation.[15] A duty-based argument would determine that the consequences are irrelevant and the patient should be told the truth regardless of the outcome. In the case of a near miss or an error with no adverse outcomes, the patient still should be informed.

The correct procedure in the case of near misses and errors with no harm is yet to be defined in the policies and practices of institutional risk management departments. Currently, most would investigate these errors to help better understand systems issues, but may not disclose all the information to the patient.

Key points

- Adherence to established ethical principles and the strong arguments in favor of open, transparent medical error disclosure are hindered by physicians' fears and mistrust of the legal system.
- Raising awareness amongst anesthesiologists of the ethical arguments involved in error disclosure, as well as the provision of strong institutional support and training in error

disclosure, will help to improve error disclosure practices and enhance patient safety.
- The correct ethical path for physicians involved in medical errors that do not cause harm and particularly the case where an anesthesiologist delivers the wrong drug without obvious adverse effects can be debated from different ethical stand points. Currently, there is no generalized consensus as to the correct procedure in these cases.

References

1   Oliver Wendell Holmes, addressing the graduating class of Bellevue Hospital Medical College, New York, March 2, 1871.

2   American Medical Association. (1994). Code of Medical Ethics: Opinion 8.12. Council on Ethical and Judicial Affairs. Chicago, IL.

3* General Medical Council, GB. (2006). Good medical practice. London; GMC.

4* Being Open; Communicating with Patients, Their Families, and Carers Following a Patient Safety Incident. National Patient Safety Agency, London UK. November 19, 2009. Accessible on line at: http://www.nrls.npsa.nhs.uk/rsources/?entryid45=65077.

5* Blundering Hospitals 'Kill 40,000 a year'. The Times, London. August 14, 2004. http://thetimesonline.co.uk/tol/news/uk/article468980ece.

6* Koln, L.T., Corrigan, J.M. and Donaldson, M.S. (1999). To Err is Human: Building a Safer Health System. Washington, DC: National Academy Press.

7* Kaldjian, L.C., Jones, E.W., Wu, B.J., et al. (2007). Disclosing medical errors to patients: attitudes and practices of physicians and trainees. J Gen Intern Med, 22, 988–96.

8* Gallagher, T.H., Waterman, A.D., Ebers, A.G., et al. (2003). Patients' and physicians' attitudes regarding the disclosure of medical errors. JAMA, 289, 1001–7.

9* Kachalia, A., Shojania, K.G., Hofer, T.P., et al. (2003). Does full disclosure of medical errors affect malpractice liability? The jury is still out. Jt Comm J Qual Saf, 29, 503–11.

10 Joint Commission on Accreditation of Healthcare Organizations. (2005). Health Care at the Crossroads: Strategies for Improving the Medical Liability System and Preventing Patient Injury.

11* Kraman, S.S. and Hamm, G. (1999). Risk management: extreme honesty may be the best policy. Ann Intern Med, 131(12), 963–7.

12* Wei, M. (2007). Doctors, apologies, and the law: an analysis and critique of apology laws. *J Health Law*, **40**(1), 107–9.

13 "Patient and doctor reconcile for the greater good." (2006). Anesthesia Patients Safety Foundation Newletter, Spring, **21**(1),

14* Berlinger, N. and Wu, A.W. (2005). Subtracting insult from injury: addressing cultural expectations in the disclosure of medical error. *J Med Ethics*, **31**, 106–8.

15* Bernstein, M. and Brown, B. (2004). Doctors' duty to disclose error: a deontological or Kantian ethical analysis. *Can J Neurol Sci*, **31**, 169–74.

Further reading

Bismark, M.M. (2009). The power of apology. *NZ Med J*, **122**(1304), 96–106.

Center for Compassion in Health Care. http://www.compassioninhealthcare.org.

Lazare, A. (2004). *On Apology*. New York: Oxford University Press.

Medical Malpractice: an International Perspective of Tort System Reform. The Hon Justice Michael Kirby AC CMG. http://www.hcourt.gov.au/speeches/kirbyj/kirbyj_med11sep.htm.

Anesthesiologists, the state, and society

DISCOVERY LIBRARY
LEVEL 5 SWCC
DERRIFORD HOSPITAL
DERRIFORD ROAD
PLYMOUTH
PL6 8DH

Physician conscientious objection in anesthesiology practice

Cynthiane J. Morgenweck and Stephen Jackson

The Case

An anesthesiologist learns of an assignment in an isolated, off-campus location on the day of the procedure, which is a transvaginal oocyte retrieval. During conversation with the patient in the preanesthesia area, he learns that she is having pre-implantation genetic diagnostic studies of any fertilized eggs, and that these results will determine future options, which include deciding to reject and discard any that would test positive for rare inheritable diseases such as cystic fibrosis. The anesthesiologist believes that this case should not have been assigned to him as he previously had stated to his department that he has a conscientious objection to participating in certain reproductive procedures. Time is of the essence as the infertility obstetrician indicates that the timing of the retrieval must take place within the next hour.

Perhaps the most fundamental political ideal in the US is that one should be free to pursue whatever conceptions of "the good" one desires (autonomy), but subject to the limitation of avoiding acts that are harmful to others (nonmaleficence). As such, there is general acceptance of rights-of-conscience, which in this chapter we shall refer to as conscientious objection – a refusal by a physician to act in a way that is not in accord with deeply valued personal beliefs. In the scenario above, however, insistence on withdrawal from providing care not only could result in harm to the patient, but will disrupt the efficiency of institutional operational functions (with attendant adverse economic consequences), potentially incurring the wrath of unsympathetic coworkers (including those of the anesthesiology department). The potential to create not only physiologic but also psychological harm to this patient is ethically preeminent.

In this case the infertility obstetrician already has "contracted" for services with the patient, and, per routine has "arranged" for anesthesia services. However, the "contract" between patient and anesthesiologist does not take hold until the agreement between them actually has occurred. It is reasonable for the patient to expect unimpeded care by a team of physicians led by her infertility obstetrician.

The anesthesiologist in this case has unwittingly been placed in the position of being expected to provide anesthesia for a procedure that could lead to events that are in violation of his deeply held moral convictions. Perhaps the most common example of conscientious objection for anesthesiologists in the US is that of anesthetizing a patient who is having an abortion. Indeed, the federal government has promulgated healthcare workers' right-to-conscience protection laws, rules, and regulations. However, federal employment laws require the *balancing* of reasonable accommodation for employees who have religious, ethical, or moral objections to specific aspects of their jobs with the resultant hardships that would burden employers given their accommodations of the employees' beliefs. The needed delay to rectify our anesthesiologist's assignment, given the extremely tight window of opportunity for the success of this infertility process (retrieval of high quality oocytes) has the potential to violate the contract between the infertility obstetrician and the patient.

The following discussion is limited to requested medical services that have been deemed medically appropriate and to which there is legal entitlement. The focus will be on why conscientious objection (refusal) by physicians is generally considered ethical behavior; however, there are controversial caveats.

Validity of conscientious objection

In the US, citizens are permitted significant latitude in defining the personal beliefs and values they adopt for themselves. Furthermore, in developing a lifestyle

Clinical Ethics in Anesthesiology: A Case-Based Textbook, ed. Gail A. Van Norman, Stephen Jackson, Stanley H. Rosenbaum and Susan K. Palmer. Published by Cambridge University Press. © Cambridge University Press 2011.

that is congruent with their moral convictions, they need not be concerned with personal safety because their beliefs might be construed as those of a minority. When claiming conscientious objection, individuals endeavor to preserve a sense of self, their integrity or wholeness that enables their human spirit to flourish. Americans value the diversity of its citizenship and its attendant disparate convictions and lifestyles. Because respect for conscientious objection is based, at least in part on respect for personal integrity, some understanding of integrity is in order.

Personal integrity includes a set of coherent principles that have been expressed verbally (or in writing), and manifest conduct that is consistent with those stated principles. "One's words and deeds generally [should] be true to a substantive, coherent and relatively stable set of values and principles to which one is genuinely and freely committed."[1] These core values are arrived at over time – and even may change over a lifetime – as each member of society decides how to live an individually satisfying life within the framework of common social goals. Yet, there may be tension among competing principles as problems can arise that are impossible to resolve by adherence to one principle without violation of another. For individuals to retain their integrity, their values and actions ought to be relatively constant over time.

Moral distress may occur when an individual is manipulated or coerced into performance of actions contrary to core values. A person's conscience must assess whether or not such behavior is permissible within the context of those core values. If deemed impermissible, then it is reasonable to refuse to perform otherwise socially acceptable – or even expected – actions, particularly if that individual is willing to accept the consequences – even harm – of such refusal. Society has codified that an individual's core values, should they fail to coincide with established societal core values, are, nonetheless, potentially socially permissible. Witness certain of the more common types of conscientious objection, such as refusal of vaccinations and military service. Indeed, for healthcare providers, there are legal precedents and protections afforded to those who conscientiously object to participation in services to which the patient is legally entitled, therein setting the stage for ethical debate.

Concerns with conscientious objection

There are concerns with the potential abuse of conscience clauses as they could involve the inappropriate application of personal beliefs to the physician–patient relationship. Indeed, invocation of a conscience clause could serve as a subterfuge for discrimination against patients based on characteristics of the patient such as race, gender, religion, sexual orientation and so forth.

Refusal by a physician to perform a service based on conscientious objection may constitute only part of what is entailed in an objection. The generally accepted obligation of a physician after refusal is to facilitate the referral and orderly transfer of the patient to another physician willing to perform the procedure. However, the objecting physician may strongly believe that even making such a referral constitutes complicity in the objectionable procedure. Others, however, construe such conscience-based refusal to refer as patient abandonment.

The possibility always exists that referral to a qualified nonobjector may not be feasible. Referral even may create new problems: the receiving physician is physically at a considerable distance; or the service in question is of an urgent nature and further delay is harmful to the patient; or a health insurance plan refuses to reimburse the services of the receiving physician and/or institution not contracted with that plan. Recently, the Constitutional Court of the country of Columbia issued a ruling that limited the claim of conscientious objection by institutions although objection by an individual physician is to be honored.[2] The ruling stated that an institution does not have such a safe harbor, and further, it must provide a means of access for legally sanctioned services. Lynch takes a similar stance, suggesting that state licensing boards should be tasked with assuring timely patient access to physicians and services by directing areas of practice for physicians based on their conscientious objections.[3]

It is suggested that there are degrees of immorality, and in general, physicians who conscientiously object do so when they judge that the *process* in which they would participate is *sufficiently* immoral. The physician has judged that participation is immoral because the physician will facilitate the ability of the patient to engage in immoral activity. Note that the statutory conscience clause protections are directed at physicians and other healthcare workers. There is no protection for the patient's fundamental medical entitlement to the procedure: it is the patient who is powerless. Many argue that, in an emergency situation, this powerlessness creates an ethical obligation for the objecting physician to provide the services *if* there is no other physician to perform the service, referral and transfer are not possible, or delay would further imperil the patient's life.

The social contract

Becoming a physician is a voluntary act and one in which physicians enter into an informal contract with society at large. Society bestows benefits attendant to the practice of medicine in return for which the physician has an obligation to perform according to the medical profession's mores and standards. In essence, society gives physicians significant control of their work in exchange for their placing foremost the best interests of society and its citizens. Physicians as a group, therefore, decide who will be admitted to the profession, how they will be educated and credentialed, what standards of care are appropriate, and what constitutes appropriate research. There are, of course, external controls (laws), but medicine – as other professions – is given significant latitude in deciding how to conduct its work.

This social contract between society and the medical profession is characterized by a continuous discourse between parties, with corrections and redirections. Indeed, conceived as a shift toward patient autonomy within the past half century, society has urged physicians to have their patients become more fully participatory in medical decision-making. The preeminence of informed consent signifies this radical ethical shift pursuant to the demise of physician paternalism.

The issue of conscientious objection by a physician enters center stage here: although physicians do have personal core values that guide the conduct of their practice, these generally ought not take precedence over professional standards of practice and respect for patient self-determination. The professional role of a physician requires provision of care (appropriate to his/her skill set) for all who suffer, not just those with coinciding belief systems. A patient's expectation of receiving an unwavering standard of competent care from those with the expertise and license to practice is a fundamental element of the social contract. The patient–physician relationship is, in part, based upon the physician's specialized knowledge and skills, and therein places the physician in a position of power to usurp the moral convictions of the patient. In the introductory case, the power dynamic between physician and patient is skewed toward the physician, and the time pressure is so urgent that there is little time for any discussion of conflicting values, no less negotiation.

"Preventive" ethics

By the completion of one's residency, an anesthesiologist should have a thorough understanding of what procedures, if any, he/she will not perform based on conscientious objection. The knowledge should be translated into requests for policies to address conscientious objection concerns before there is a case such as the one introducing this chapter. Physicians should not choose specialties that constitute moral minefields for them. Anesthesiologists interface with many other physicians in the medical field. They are likely to encounter moral dilemmas not only in the field of reproductive biology, but also in transplant medicine, critical care medicine (especially end-of-life issues) and pain management. A practice situation should be chosen that likely would lead to few, if any, scenarios calling for conscientious objection, unless the practice is able to support and accommodate that anesthesiologist's personal values. If the lay community expects to have access to procedures that are contrary to the anesthesiologist's deeply held values, then there should be concern that the practice is not a proper fit. If an anesthesiologist chooses to invoke conscientious objection, then it ought not to be at the last moment, but rather with ample time for deliberation, discourse and planning to avoid the potential contentions and troublesome consequences pursuant to a last minute objection. The reason for such objections should be constant over time so as to preclude the loss of support from colleagues and accusations of discrimination or unwillingness to carry one's share of the workload.

It should be noted that the American Medical Association's *Principles of Medical Ethics*,[4] recognized as a basic guide to ethical conduct, are included in the American Society of Anesthesiologists' *Guidelines for the Ethical Practice of Anesthesiology*.[5] Specifically, AMA Principle VI declares:

> *A physician shall, in the provision of appropriate patient care except in emergencies, be free to choose whom to serve, with whom to associate and the environment in which to provide medical care.*

Whereas these guidelines do not address conscientious objection, conflict resolution is offered for the conscientious objector in the American Society of Anesthesiologists' *Ethical Guidelines for the Anesthesia Care of Patients with Do-Not-Resuscitate Orders or Other Directives that Limit Treatment*:

> *When an anesthesiologist finds the patient's or surgeon's limitations of intervention decisions to be irreconcilable with one's own moral views, then the anesthesiologist*

should withdraw in a nonjudgmental fashion, providing an alternative for care in a timely fashion.[6]

Key points

- Our society supports an individual's right to conscientious objection, to refuse an action that is not in accordance with one's deeply held moral convictions.
- A sense of personal integrity is based on conduct that is consistent with an expressed set of coherent principles and values.
- There are legal protections for physicians who conscientiously refuse to participate in medical services to which the patient is legally entitled.
- There is a potential for abuse of statutory conscience clauses protecting physicians should they inappropriately apply their personal moral convictions to the physician–patient relationship.
- Most ethical dilemmas raised by conscientious refusal can be prevented by forethought, communication, planning and accommodation.
- Pursuant to the social contract between society and the profession of medicine, physicians should provide appropriate care for all patients, not just those with coinciding belief systems.
- When feasible, and excepting emergencies, the refusing physician's ethical duty is to facilitate referral and orderly transfer to a competent physician willing to perform the service that was requested of the conscientious objector. Such referral and transfer do not equate to complicity.

References

1* Benjamin, M. (1990). *Splitting the Difference*. Kansas: Lawrence University Press.

2* Cook, R.J., Olaya, M.A., and Dickens, B.M. (2009). Healthcare responsibilities and conscientious objection. *Internat J Gyn and Obstet*, **104**, 249–52.

3* Lynch, H. (2008). *Conflicts of Conscience: An Institutional Compromise*. MA: MIT Press.

4 Accessible at the American Medical Association website: www.ama-assn.org.

5 Accessible at the American Society of Anesthesiologists website at: http://www.asahq.org/publicationsAndServices/standards/10.pdf.

6 Accessible at the American Society of Anesthesiologists website at:http://www.asahq.org/publicationsAndServices/standards/09.pdf.

Further reading

American Academy of Pediatrics, Committee on Bioethics. (2009). Physician refusal to provide information or treatment on the basis of claims of conscience. *Pediatrics*, **124**(6), 1689–93.

Brock, D.W. (2008). Conscientious refusal by physicians and pharmacists: who is obligated to do what, and why? *Theor Med Bioeth*, **29**, 187–200.

Cantor, J. (2009). Conscientious objection gone awry – restoring selfless professionalism in medicine. *NEJM*, **360**, 1484–5.

Davis, J.K. (2004). Conscientious refusal and a doctors' right to quit. *J Med Phil*, **29**, 75–91.

Fjellstrom, R. (2005). Respect for persons, respect for integrity. *Med Health Care Phil*, **8**, 231–42.

Lawrence, R.E. and Curlin, F.A. (2007). Clash of definitions: controversies about conscience in medicine. *AJOB*, **7**, 10–14.

May, T. and Aulisio, M.P. (2009). Personal morality and professional obligations. *Persp Bio Med*, **52**, 30–8.

Pelligrino, E.D. (2002). The physician's conscience, conscience clauses, and religious belief: a catholic perspective, *Fordham Urban Law Journal*. http://www.thefreelibrary.com/The physician's conscience, conscience clauses and religious belief:…-a097823705. (Accessed November 5, 2008).

Savulescu, J. (2007). Conscientious objection in medicine. *BMJ*, **332**, 294–7.

Sulmasy, D.P. (2008). What is conscience and why is respect for it so important? *Theor Med Bioeth*, **29**, 135–49.

Wardle, L.D. (2005). Five reasons why rights of conscience must be protected. *Linacre Quarterly*, **72**, 158–63.

The ethics of expert testimony

Louise B. Andrew

The Case

Dr. X is contacted by an attorney in a plaintiff's firm with which he has worked frequently on prior cases. The attorney requests that he provide expert testimony in a malpractice case involving a patient who died intraoperatively following pacemaker placement by an anesthesiologist during cardiac surgery. Although Dr. X is well known and respected in the specialty for his expertise in regional anesthesia and has written several respected textbooks, he is not board certified in anesthesiology. He does not practice cardiac anesthesia. He has never placed a pacemaker himself. Despite misgivings, he agrees to review the case.

After chart review, Dr. X identifies no obvious breach in the standard of care by the defendant anesthesiologist, and informs the attorney. However, after he has read selected reference materials provided by the attorney, and following a discussion during which a significant fee is discussed, he decides that he might testify that the death resulted from improper pacemaker placement.

Because judges and juries generally are not knowledgeable about medicine, the integrity and credibility of the litigation process in the United States and elsewhere depends on expert witnesses who help them to understand technicalities and decide complex cases by articulating the applicable standard of care and rendering an opinion as to whether or not it was met. To protect patients and physicians and uphold the highest standards of medical care, it is morally and ethically appropriate for anesthesiologists with sufficient expertise to testify in medical malpractice claims.

Qualifications of an expert witness

The American Society of Anesthesiologists (ASA) has established guidelines regarding expert witness testimony to guide members in providing such service.[1] The guidelines state that to qualify to act in this capacity,

> "(1) *The physician (expert witness) should have a current, valid and unrestricted license to practice medicine,*

> (2) *The physician should be board certified in anesthesiology or hold an equivalent specialist qualification*, and
> (3) *The physician should have been actively involved in the clinical practice of anesthesiology at the time of the event.*"[1]

The legal qualification of a witness as an expert in court is determined by the judge on a case-by-case basis. Judges have broad discretion for such determinations, but for practical purposes are usually limited to consideration of those "experts" brought to them by the parties to the case.

Expertise in the subject matter forming the basis of any legal case is the *sine qua non* of an ethical expert witness. Such expertise is established on the basis of: (1) **knowledge** of the field; and (2) relevant clinical **experience**. In medicine, board preparation and current certification are the best indicators of knowledge of a specialty. Relevant experience is established by a period of active clinical practice beyond training, as well as practice *during the time frame of the incident in question*. An ethical expert witness should be actively practicing within his/her field in order to be aware of the current standard of care. Holding an active and unrestricted license to practice medicine constitutes a bare minimum qualification for expert testimony.[a]

ASA guidelines for expert witness testimony

The ASA ethical guidelines include six explicit points:
(1) "*The physician's review of the medical facts should be truthful, thorough and impartial and should not exclude any relevant information to create a view favoring either the plaintiff or the defendant.*"[1]

As an expert witness, the anesthesiologist has an ethical responsibility to be truthful, thorough, and impartial when evaluating a case for adherence to the standard of care. An expert witness' primary

---

Clinical Ethics in Anesthesiology: A Case-Based Textbook, ed. Gail A. Van Norman, Stephen Jackson, Stanley H. Rosenbaum and Susan K. Palmer. Published by Cambridge University Press. © Cambridge University Press 2011.

responsibility must always be to discernment of the truth[2]. Truthfulness is a fairly self evident concept; but in expert testimony based on case analysis, truthfulness carries several other ethical obligations. One obligation is that the analysis must be thorough, including all sources of possible information, even if the information initially provided is insufficient or might be misleading in light of further relevant details. Before forming any opinion, the physician must familiarize him or herself with all aspects of the case. Every relevant medical record must be accessed, as well as imaging or other ancillary studies if potentially germane to the medical issues. The witness has an obligation to review these materials even if they are difficult to obtain and are not volunteered by the attorney requesting expert consultation. This is important – an unscrupulous or incompetent attorney may provide selective information favoring the side for which he or she is an advocate. Failure to review all potentially relevant materials can render any expert susceptible to unwitting partiality, just as selective exclusion of mitigating data, facts, or circumstances may render an expert opinion unethical for partiality.

"…the ultimate test for accuracy and impartiality is a willingness to prepare testimony that could be presented unchanged for use by either the plaintiff or defendant."[1]

This is a valid and useful concept, though it could prove difficult to apply. In some instances, two blinded experts could examine the same set of facts and circumstances and ethically render opinions that are opposite in their conclusions, thus rendering either opinion useful to one party and damning for the other.

(2) "The physician's testimony should reflect an evaluation of performance in light of generally accepted standards, reflected in relevant literature, neither condemning performance that clearly falls within generally accepted practice standards nor endorsing or condoning performance that clearly falls outside accepted medical practice."[1]

The expert witness must review time-appropriate literature to substantiate the existing standard, or to identify alternative acceptable approaches to care. Testimony should reflect knowledge of, and comparison with, applicable and generally accepted standards of care. Though not explicit in the ASA guidelines, the expert must be aware of and apply the standard of care that existed at the time of the incident giving rise to the claim, and should also take into consideration regional and even institution-specific and resource based variations in practice.

The legal principle of the medical "standard of care" is usually defined by case law or statute for each jurisdiction and entails some version of "that degree of care which would be rendered by a reasonably competent physician practicing under the same or similar circumstances."[3] In their zeal for advocacy, attorneys do not always clearly define this concept for their experts. Even the pivotal concept of "standard of care" is not well understood by many who agree to serve as expert witnesses, though most believe that they both understand it and can accurately describe the specific standard applicable in a given case. Legal scholars believe that medical expert testimony regarding what constitutes the standard of care is more apt to reflect what experts think that they and their immediate colleagues would do rather than what most physicians actually do.[4] Research suggests medical expert witnesses share with all of us the tendency to have selectively optimistic recall of how well they themselves typically handle clinical situations.[5] This means that well intended experts will tend to overestimate the applicable standard of care. As a fundamental principle, however, it is important to understand that the legal standard requires only that the physician acted reasonably under the circumstances.

An ethical witness must be careful in differentiating between a widely utilized standard of care, and ideal care that might be provided by the most astute clinician practicing under optimum circumstances. Application of an "ideal" standard (sometimes called "counsel of perfection") may be a particular hazard for clinicians whose only practice experience has been in a tertiary care facility, such as a medical school faculty, or newly graduated residents.

It is easier to define what the standard is not, than what it is. The legally required standard of care is not perfect care, or care that creates a perfect result. Although such care would presumably meet the standard, it would in many if not most instances, exceed the actual standard required under the law. The standard of care is also not necessarily what "I do in my practice, which I assume others also do." It is also not necessarily what "I was taught to do in training," what the textbooks recommend, or even what clinical policies/guidelines say it is (although these may be good indicators of things which peers believe to represent optimal care, best practices, or recommended practices according to the best available evidence). Each of these sources can provide information as to what constitutes good or excellent care for a given condition, but they do not define the legal standard of care.

An expert must be able to help the jury to understand the difference between the type of care that is most commonly rendered for a particular condition, and an equally acceptable method (the "two schools of thought" or "respectable minority" test) which is not often rendered, but is also medically valid or theoretically sound. The expert must also be able to assess and to clearly delineate the difference between reasonably competent care, and care which would be considered substandard by an average practitioner under any circumstances.

(3) "The physician should make a clear distinction between medical malpractice and adverse outcomes not necessarily related to negligent practice."

(4) "The physician should make every effort to assess the relationship of the alleged substandard practice to the patient's outcome. Deviation from a practice standard is not always causally related to a poor outcome."[1]

In a typical malpractice case, one of the most important roles of a medical expert witness is to help a judge and jury to understand the difference between maloccurrence (an adverse patient experience or outcome), and malpractice (an adverse experience or outcome that more likely than not resulted from substandard care or negligence). Causation is defined as being the "proximate cause," or that which brings about injury as a direct result, and without which the injury would not have taken place. An expert may not be asked to render an opinion as to "causation,"[b] or may be asked to render an opinion only as to causation of an adverse outcome by negligence or substandard care. If asked to render an opinion as to causation, an ethical expert must carefully consider whether the adverse outcome could have occurred in the absence of any substandard care, and be able to explain why this is or is not likely in this particular case. In addition to a thorough review of all relevant case materials for possible confounding influences, such an opinion also should be informed by personal experience, literature, and an assessment of probabilities. An expert who cannot reach a conclusion regarding the relationship of an adverse outcome to the degree of care that was provided, should ethically decline to testify as to causation.

Representation of one's personal opinion as absolute truth is misleading and unethical. Personal opinion may be proffered during expert testimony, but should be clearly designated as such. The ethical witness will recognize that with respect to medical management, in most cases differences of opinion between competent medical practitioners will exist. The ethical expert will acknowledge that the ideal course of events is almost always clearer when viewed retrospectively in light of a less than optimal outcome. Because it is impossible to avoid knowledge of the ultimate outcome of a case, an ethical expert must be vigilant in analyzing the facts of a case as if the outcome is unknown, and limit standard of care opinion testimony to the adequacy of care provided.

(5) "The physician's fee for expert testimony should relate to the time spent and in no circumstances should be contingent upon the outcome of the claim."[1]

Financial remuneration must never be the key motivation behind expert witness work. Compensation for time expended in analysis or testimony should be commensurate with compensation that would be earned during the same amount of time devoted to medical practice, and not indexed to the "market rate" for expert testimony.[b]

For a physician to earn more through work as an expert witness than as a practicing physician is morally questionable if not unethical. Expert testimony by physicians can be useful to juries, the profession, and society, but exorbitant fees charged for such review and testimony will predictably increase the cost of malpractice defense, and therefore threaten liability insurance premiums and availability, and ultimately the availability and affordability of healthcare.

Under no circumstances is it appropriate for an expert's professional remuneration to be contingent on the outcome of a case. All medical professional ethics codes and legal codes of professional responsibility prohibit this practice, because it immediately casts doubt on the objectivity of an expert witness. In general, an ethical expert would be wise to establish a fee schedule at the beginning of any case and require payment at the time service is commenced – not at the conclusion of the case – to avoid even the appearance of contingency billing and attendant bias. Experts must also acknowledge that there is an unspoken inherent contingency in every consultation for an attorney, because repeat engagement is less likely when an expert is unable to provide the opinion or the testimony sought by that attorney.[6]

(6) "The physician should be willing to submit such testimony for peer review."[1]

Ideally, medical expert testimony would be routinely peer reviewed to ensure it meets the ethical standards of medical professional societies. In some of the US expert testimony has been subject to Medical Board peer review and disciplinary action by under the authority of the state Medical Practice Act. A few states are moving towards requiring a limited state license in order to testify in the state. Although several states have issued discipline based on falsification of credentials by those acting as medical experts, none has yet successfully disciplined a medical expert for giving unethical testimony. Many professional societies, including the American Society of Anesthesiology have followed the lead of the American Association of Neurological Surgeons in reviewing the testimony of members acting as expert witnesses upon complaint by another member.[7]

The US Supreme Court has upheld the right of a professional society to discipline a member for inappropriate expert testimony in the Austin case.[6] The American Association of Neurological Surgeons suspended a member for giving improper expert witness testimony at a medical malpractice trial. Judge Posner speaking for the 7th court of appeals applauded the association for increasing the accountability of experts from its ranks. This precedent was an important victory for those professional societies that include ethics review of expert witness testimony in their policies and disciplinary procedures. A member who believes that an expert has acted unethically while giving testimony has standing to request a review of the testimony by their specialty society (if the witness is a member). Not all societies, however, have a mechanism in place to perform this function, and ethics reviews are not without attendant costs and liability to the professional society.

Medical association sanctions in the event of proven false or unethical testimony are generally limited to those affecting the expert's membership in that society. Unfortunately, not all "experts" belong to medical societies, or are even eligible for membership. Further, if the expert is from a different specialty than that of the defendant, the expert's specialty society has no obligation to respond to a nonmember complainant from another specialty. Parenthetically, there is an inherent selection bias in such reviews, rightfully noted by plaintiff's bar, that members are extremely unlikely to report questionable testimony on behalf of a defense witness.

Acting as an expert witness has become a second career for some physicians. Medical legal case reports are replete with testimony by "hired guns" who earn a significant portion or even the majority of their income from testifying in malpractice cases. Some such physicians have not practiced for years or may have restricted their practice to a very small subspecialty area, then falsify their current practice experience, or practice just enough to maintain their medical licenses. Some so-called "experts" have been barred by judges from acting as expert witnesses in some states, yet continue to do so in others. Some witnesses use past credentials or academic accomplishments as evidence of current expertise.

Although some physicians believe themselves to be eminently qualified to testify after retirement from clinical practice because of their knowledge of the basic precepts of the specialty and the breadth of their experience, the fact is, that what the courts need – education about currently prevailing standards of clinical practice – cannot honestly be provided by a person who no longer practices clinically. An ethical expert witness should be actively practicing within his field at the time of the incident involved in a claim in order to be aware of the actual applicable standard of care in effect as of that date. A retired physician might ethically be able to render opinion about causation, as opposed to the prevailing standard of care.

Some witnesses testify almost exclusively for either the defense or the plaintiff. This practice in itself calls into question the objectivity of the witness. Federal court rules now require that an expert keep detailed records about parties on whose behalf they have testified for the purpose of exposing such potential sources of bias.

Case resolution

In the introductory case, several obvious potential ethical violations are apparent. Dr. X does not meet the ASA's minimal qualification for expert witness testimony of board certification or preparation in the specialty. Although he still practices part time, it is in a subspecialty area that is far removed from the subspecialty that is the basis of the case. It is difficult to assess whether he could even know what additional data could be relevant in determining the standard of care in the case, since he may have relied upon selected references provided by the attorney to form even a basic understanding of this area of subspecialization. It could be argued that he may have allowed financial considerations to influence his willingness to provide a favorable opinion/ testimony.

Dr. X's testimony was submitted to his professional association for peer review, and he was judged to have breached the ethical guidelines and thus was disciplined by the society.

Key points

- Those who take part in expert medical testimony should make every attempt to give fully informed, truthful, non-biased opinion about the care that the patient received and the relationship between that care and the outcome of the case.
- The opinion of the expert witness should never be influenced by the outcome of the case, the party that retains the expert, or the remuneration which is offered.
- An expert should be willing for their testimony to be subjected to peer review when requested.
- The hallmark of the ethical expert witness is conscientious, objective, thorough, truthful, and impartial evaluation and testimony, signifying an unswerving dedication to the integrity of the process.

Notes

[a] Yet surprisingly, in a number of states there is no legal requirement that an expert witness testifying about the standard of care of physicians be qualified as a physician.

[b] Defined by Black's law dictionary as the fact of being the "proximate cause", or "that which produces injury as a direct result, and without which the result would not have occurred".

[c] Which is increasing dramatically in recent years, and can reportedly reach $600–1000 per hour in some specialties. Baldas, "Nonexperts taking the Stand", National Law Journal March 21, 2005 http://www.law.com/jsp/article.jsp?id=1111572309683 accessed May 19, 2009.

References

1* Guideline for Expert Witness Qualifications and Testimony. (2008). American Society of Anesthesiologistst. http://www.asahq.org/publicationsAndServices/standards/07.pdf accessed May 19, 2009 (Fig 1).

2* Bucy, P.C. (1975). The medical expert witness in malpractice suits. *JAMA*, **232**, 1352–3.

3 Shilkret v Annapolis Hospital Emergency Association, 349 A 2d 245, 249–250 (Md 1975)

4 Peters, P.G. (2002). "Empirical Evidence and Malpractice Litigation", 37 Wake Forest Law Review, 2002, 757, at 759.

5 Meadow and Sunstein, (2001). "Statistics, not Experts", **51** *Duke Law Journal* 629, at 630–31. 2001

6 Moss, S., Opinion for Sale: Confessions of an Expert Witness http://www.legalaffairs.org/issues/March-April-2003/review_marapr03_moss.html#, accessed May 19, 2009.

7 Maryland, DC, New York, and on other grounds in WA.

8 Donald C. Austin v AANS, 253F3d 967 (2001).

Further reading

Andrew, L.B. (2006). Expert witness testimony: the ethics of being a medical expert witness. *Emerg Med Clin North Am*, **24**(3), 715–31.

Baldas, T. (2005). Nonexperts taking the Stand. *National Law Journal* March 21. http://www.law.com/jsp/article.jsp?id=1111572309683 accessed May 19, 2009.

Crosby, E. (2007). Medical malpractice and anesthesiology: literature review and role of the expert witness. *Can J Anaesth*, **54**(3), 227–41.

Meadow, W. and Lantos, J.D. (1996). Expert testimony, legal reasoning, and justice. The case for adopting a data-based standard of care in allegations of medical negligence in the NICU. *Clin Perinatol*, **23**(3), 583–95.

Rabeinerson, D. and Green, Y. (2007). The problem of double loyalty: medical expert opinion and its cost. *Harefuah*, **146**(7), 539–43.

Weinstein, J.B. (1999). Expert witness testimony: a trial judge's perspective. *Neurol Clin*, **17**(2), 355–62.

45 Ethical principles regarding physician response to disasters: pandemics, natural disasters, and terrorism

Susan K. Palmer

The Case

During morning rush hour, a subway station in a major metropolitan area is rocked by a sudden explosion. The train platforms and several cars that were in the station at the time of the explosion are severely damaged, and the structural integrity of the underground system is compromised. The scene is chaotic. There is concern that the subway tunnel may collapse. The cause of the explosion is unknown – the smell of gas may indicate a potential cause, or may be the result of gas leakage after the explosion. There is concern that if this is a terrorist attack, there may be additional bombs awaiting detonation timed to kill rescuers.

A live victim cannot be extricated from one of the trains because her leg is entrapped in the wreckage. Her injuries appear otherwise not life-threatening. An anesthesiologist is requested by rescuers to provide airway support and analgesia for an immediate on-site amputation in order to free the victim.

The idea that physicians have ethical duties during mass casualty incidents is a relatively modern one. During episodes of the plague in Europe, for example, clergy and magistrates were expected to remain in the cities to minister to the sick, but physicians generally were not. Most did in fact leave the cities, arguing that they needed to live to serve the greater good by taking care of survivors.[1] Ideas about the ethical duties of physicians during pandemics, natural disasters and other mass casualty incidents have changed, now that modern medical practice can positively impact survival. But contemporary studies indicate that physicians as a group continue to be reluctant to respond to "societal" medical emergencies. In one study, 45% of surveyed physicians felt that it would be ethical to abandon their workplace in the event of an influenza pandemic.[2]

The unique skills of anesthesiologists as experts in airway management, fluid and blood resuscitation, and intraoperative anesthesia make them particularly desirable as early emergency responders. Anesthesiologists sometimes serve in pre-hospital treatment, including in-field airway management and administration of anesthesia to facilitate victim extrication,[3] in early hospital triage of victims according to available resources, and in the management of intensive care patients and patients who need immediate surgical intervention.

Physician's ethical obligations to respond in public health emergencies

General and special positive duties

Common moral theory holds that we all, by virtue of being a part of humanity, have a duty to help others in peril – particularly if we can do so without great risks to ourselves. For example, we should all prevent a toddler on the sidewalk from running out in traffic, and we should all call 911 if possible when we witness an accident. These are termed "positive" duties, since they require us to take an action, rather than to refrain from taking an action. An example of a negative duty – in which there is an ethical obligation to refrain from an action–is a general duty not to kill. Malm and colleagues[4] differentiate general positive moral duties, which morally bind all persons, from special positive moral duties, which require a special relationship between the actor and the recipient of their actions. They use the example of the relationship between a lifeguard and swimmer as a special relationship. The lifeguard has a special positive duty to rescue, based on their skills and the general expectations of their work. Such special positive duties also exist between physicians and victims of disaster who require medical care.

The special positive duties of physicians are generally argued to exist based on several considerations.

Clinical Ethics in Anesthesiology: A Case-Based Textbook, ed. Gail A. Van Norman, Stephen Jackson, Stanley H. Rosenbaum and Susan K. Palmer. Published by Cambridge University Press. © Cambridge University Press 2011.

First, physicians freely choose to enter a profession whose primary function is to serve the sick; they therefore agree to some degree of exposure to illness and the resulting personal risk. The medical profession enjoys a privileged position in society. In order to enjoy those privileges, physicians must accept certain responsibilities that go with them. Second, special skills are needed in mass casualty incidents, and physicians are members of a restricted group that have those skills. Third, physicians owe a debt to patients and to society. Not everyone can be trained to be a physician. The resources needed to teach physicians are both limited and expensive. Training every physician involves the consent/cooperation of the hundreds of patients who allow trainees to work with them. There is therefore a societal contract which obligates physicians to reciprocate by serving both patients and societal needs.[5,6]

Although physicians enter the medical profession of their own free will, it is nevertheless difficult to convincingly argue that they therefore are obliged to assume unlimited risks. Such an argument relies on an "implied consent" of all physicians to a strong duty to treat – but actual evidence that implied consent exists is lacking. Only about 55% of physicians now believe there is such a "profession-wide duty to treat patients despite risk to one's health."[7]

The idea that physicians have special abilities that increase their obligation to respond in emergencies has more traction. While people with special skills may not be ethically obliged to serve the public good all the time, communitarian principles do acquire more authority in times of emergency. As Sawicki points out:

> "As the risk of harm grows more imminent, as the gap between harm to the rescuer and harm to the public widens, and as the pool of available and qualified rescuers shrinks (particularly where state regulations preclude unlicensed individuals from developing special abilities to rescue), potential rescuers may indeed find themselves obliged to subvert their own interests for the public good."[7]

This type of argument is based on rights-based, or deontologic, theories in which one generally should act in a manner that promotes beneficence and respect for the lives and autonomy of others. Such duties, however, are not restricted to the medical profession itself.

The American Medical Association's Code of Medical Ethics states that:

> Because of their commitment to care for the sick and injured, physicians have an obligation to provide urgent medical care during disasters. This ethical obligation holds even in the face of greater than usual risks to their own safety, health or life.[8]

The AMA opinion goes on to say that physicians are a limited resource, and the physician should balance the immediate benefits to individual patients against the ability to care for future patients. Similar duties are stated by the UK's General Medical Council, which states:

> Doctors must not refuse to treat patients because their medical condition may put the doctor at risk. The balance between protecting individual doctors and their families from harm, and ensuring patients are not put at unnecessary risk is best addressed at the local level, taking into account the principle that those who place themselves at additional risk should be supported in doing so and the risks and burdens minimized as far as possible.[9]

The limits of risk

Military physicians have a duty to put the requirements of the military "mission" ahead of the interests of themselves or of individual patients. Physicians serving in the military can be ordered to assume almost any level of risk and even be expected to serve in situations where they will likely die. Civilian physicians, however, are not obligated in the way soldiers may be to take unlimited risks.

In general, risks are more acceptable if they are proportionate to the benefits expected. When HIV/AIDS was becoming epidemic, some surgeons and anesthesiologists refused to provide care for infected patients or to treat them equitably in other ways. But actual risks to healthcare providers who take care of HIV positive patients are now known to be very low. It is therefore unethical for physicians to refuse to treat HIV/AIDS patients on the basis of maintaining their own safety. On the other hand, infections with the SARS virus are not only extremely contagious, but are associated with high mortality. In order to obligate physicians to be exposed, there must be a proportionate expectation that their response will result in significantly better overall patient outcomes, and/or in significantly better societal outcomes through containment of the disease.

The ethical obligations of physicians to respond in natural disasters or terrorist attacks, as well as what manner of response can be required of them, must be balanced between the probability that such participation will improve survival for more casualties, and the risks of mortality to the physicians themselves. Risks to casualties may be obvious early on, but the benefits of intervention unknown. Assessing the risks to physicians in such situations is complicated; routes of contamination during an epidemic and toxic exposure during natural or man-made disasters may be unknown, at least initially. The means of reducing risks to healthcare workers may not be fully understood, and the equipment to reduce such risks not readily available.

Supererogatory actions

In general, it is not an ethical obligation to risk one's own life to save another. Acts involving such risks are usually termed "supererogatory"– literally "payment beyond that which is owed or asked." Many examples of supererogatory – or heroic – acts can be found among physicians responding to emergencies.[10] Tse Yuen-man was the first physician volunteer in the SARS epidemic in Hong Kong in 2003 to die of SARS. She had volunteered knowing that SARS is highly contagious and very deadly. Anesthesiologists have been early responders in stabilizing patients in earthquakes and terrorist bombings, even at times providing on-site anesthesia when amputations are required for victim extrication. Structural instability, possible toxic contamination, and the risk of being injured or killed in aftershocks of an earthquake or additional terrorist bombs detonated in order to kill the rescuers present imminent danger for early responders.

What does society owe to physicians in mass casualty situations?

Society and hospitals have interests in having competent, seasoned and responsive physicians, and therefore have obligations to physicians, e.g., to provide physicians with personal protection, training and logistical support to minimize their risk while maximizing the potential benefit of physicians' service to patients. Dr. Tse Yuen-man, for example, did not have protective gloves to wear when she responded to an emergency resuscitation of a SARS patient. The Asian Human Rights Commission offered the following words of condolence, and appreciation for Dr. Yuen-man's sacrifice, and called upon healthcare authorities to recognize their own obligations to physicians responding to emergencies:

> The right to life is at the centre of all human rights, and all efforts of the community should be geared toward its protection and promotion…The people in the medical profession, particularly those that work to save life, are at the centre of safeguarding people's right to life. They become living witnesses of the commitment of human beings to the life of others, living symbols of the tremendous respect with which the supremacy of life and its dignity are upheld.

> … It is perhaps pertinent for the community and Hong Kong healthcare authorities to ask some poignant questions, however, about their commitment to people that work on the front line to safeguard our right to life. Is adequate care being taken to safeguard their lives by providing the necessary protection for them in a timely manner, for instance? This is a vexing question that needs to be answered if our appreciation of their efforts is to make any sense.[11]

Emergency response workers have rights to adequate rest, updated information, and to participate in decision-making throughout the crisis. This not only assures their well-being, but enhances their ability to perform. Society has obligations to provide adequate housing and other basic needs for emergency responders.

Healthcare workers are on "the front lines" and should be among the first to receive effective preventative treatment, such as vaccines in the event of pandemics or bioterrorism situations. Additionally, society has obligations to provide physicians made ill, injured or disabled during emergency response with appropriate medical care and social support, much as it has an obligation to provide such things for wounded soldiers.

Case resolution

The situation in the introductory case presents extreme potential risk to rescuers. An anesthesiologist who responds performs an act that is "above and beyond the call of duty," i.e., one that cannot be required of him or her. No rules, moral or legislative, can obligate a civilian to risk sacrificing their life for another.

On the other hand, the broader context of this emergency will require responses that do not necessarily place physicians at great personal risk. Anesthesiologists will be needed at the hospital, both to triage and to care for patients who may require immediate surgical intervention. Reporting for duty at the local healthcare facility may present an individual healthcare provider with personal challenges, such as making alternative arrangements to fulfill family obligations, as well as personal discomfort, such as prolonged work hours to manage multiple casualties. The "special" positive duties incurred by entering the medical profession and acquiring special skills impose greater obligations of response. Even if unwilling to go into the subway to help extricate the trapped victim, the anesthesiologist is ethically obliged to respond to the general call for help and report for duty.

Key points

- Ethical obligations of physicians to respond to mass casualty incidents have arisen in modern times, as medical care has developed the potential to improve outcomes of casualties.
- The unique skills of anesthesiologists make them valuable in early emergency response – for in-the-field management of casualties, triage, and intensive care unit and operating room management of victims.
- Everyone has general positive moral duties to help others in peril, particularly if there is low personal risk in doing so.
- Special positive moral duties occur when certain "relationships" exist between the actor and the recipient of action: one such relationship is the physician–patient relationship.
- Physician ethical duties in disaster are based in part on the special skills they acquire that are needed in emergency situations. Those duties are strengthened by the restricted pool of qualified responders, due to the limitations on who can be trained in the medical profession.
- Physicians are not ethically obliged to risk their lives in emergency situations, but do have ethical duties to respond and perform non-life-threatening duties.
- Society has obligations to physician emergency responders, such as providing appropriate protective equipment, first line therapies such as vaccines, and treatment when illness or injury results from emergency response actions.

References

1 Wallis, P. (2006). Plagues, morality and the place of medicine in early modern England. *Eng Hist Rev*, **CXXI** (490), 1–24.

2 Ehrenstein, B., Hanses, F., and Salzberger, B. (2006). Influenza pandemic and professional duty: family or patients first? A survey of hospital employees. *BMC Public Health*, **311**.

3 Mahoney, P.F. and Carney, C.J. (1996). Entrapment, extrication, and immobilization. *Eur J Emer Med*, **3**, 244–6.

4* Malm, H., May, T., Francis, L.P., *et al.* (2008). Ethics, pandemics, and the duty to treat. *Am J Bioeth*, **8**(8), 4–19.

5 Anantham, D., McHugh, W., O'Neill, S., and Forrow, L. (2008). Clinical review: influenza pandemic – physicians and their obligations. *Crit Care*, **12**, 217–21.

6 Bostick, N., Levine, M., and Sade, R. (2008). Ethical obligations of physicians participating in public health quarantine and isolation measures. *Public Health Rep*, **123**, 3–8.

7* Sawicki, N.N. (2008). Without consent: moral imperatives, special abilities, and the duty to treat. *Am J Bioeth*, **8**(8), 33–5.

8* American Medical Association. Opinion 9.067 – Physician Obligation in Disaster Preparedness and Response. Adopted June, 2004. AMA. Council on Ethical and Judicial Affairs. Chicago, Il. http://www.ama-assn.org/ama/pub/physician-resources/medical-ethics/code-medical-ethics.shtml.

9* General Medical Council. (2009). Good Medical Practice. Pandemic Influenza: Responsibilities of Doctors in a National Pandemic. London, General Medical Council.

10 Tai, D.Y. (2006). SARS plague; duty of care, or medical heroism? *Ann Acad Med Singapore*, **35**(5), 374–8.

11 A Statement of the Asian Human Rights Commission Offering Condolences and Deep Appreciation for the Life and Work of Dr. Tse Yuen-man, 2003.

Further reading

Simonds, A.K. and Sokol, D.K. (2009). Lives on the line? Ethics and practicalities of duty of care in pandemics and disasters. *Eur Respir J*, **34**, 3003–9.

Trotter, G. (2007). *The Ethics of Coercion in Mass Casualty Medicine*. Baltimore: The Johns Hopkins University Press.

Triage in civilian mass casualty situations

Susan K. Palmer

The Case

A small community hospital located several hundred miles from any other hospital gets word that it is about to receive 100 casualties from a F-5 tornado that touched down five miles away. All elective surgeries are cancelled, and surgeons are encouraged to quickly complete ongoing procedures. An anesthesiologist is assigned to perform "front door triage" – deciding which casualties go directly to the OR, which can wait for treatment, and which can probably not be saved. At least 20 casualties are expected to need critical care or urgent surgery. There are five operating rooms. The ICU consists of eight beds, and is full. The local blood supply consists of 20 units of RBCs, including only four O negative units. Resupply of blood and other critical provisions is several hours away.

The American Medical Association's Code of Medical Ethics states:

Individual physicians should take appropriate advance measures to ensure their ability to provide medical services at the time of disasters, including the acquisition and maintenance of relevant knowledge.[1]

In medical triage, a "disaster" is defined as an incident in which local response resources are overwhelmed by patient needs. Recent terrorist attacks, catastrophic earthquakes, and potential global pandemics have resulted in more discussion and effort towards planning for the next mass casualty situation.

General principles of civilian triage should be familiar to all physicians. Isolated instances of mass casualties can happen in a region with only one small hospital, and any physician may be called upon to act as a triage officer. Anesthesiologists in particular have special knowledge useful in triage – airway assessment and management, fluid and blood resuscitation, intensive care expertise and knowledge of surgical treatment and local operating room capabilities.

Principles of civilian versus military triage

Military triage is an example of a situation in which limited medical resources must be allocated among multiple casualties. The goals of combat medicine are to return the greatest number of soldiers to combat, and then to preserve life. Seriously wounded soldiers may be quickly stabilized, but then wait while attention turns to returning less seriously wounded soldiers to the battlefield. (For a discussion of military triage principles, see Chapter 47.) Combat triage principles do not appropriately address civilian mass casualty situations in which survival, not combat-readiness, is the main goal of medical treatment.

Ethical principles of civilian triage

Consequentialism

Traditional medical ethics teaches that a physician should put their patients' interests ahead of his or her own interests or preferences and also ahead of the interests of any other patients. In mass casualty situations traditional patient-centered ethical principles of medicine may have to yield temporarily to the consequentialist (or utilitarian) principle of "doing the most good for the greatest number." Consequentialism was described by the British philosopher and socialist, Jeremy Benthamand, and was further developed by James Mill and his son John Stuart Mill. Consequentialism does not value an individual as much as the collective group of people affected in a mass casualty situation. Individuals may even be viewed as a "means to an end" when applying consequentialist principles in practice. In the words of Jonsen and Edwards,

This [disaster] is one of the few places where a "utilitarian rule" governs medicine; the greater good of the greater

---

Clinical Ethics in Anesthesiology: A Case-Based Textbook, ed. Gail A. Van Norman, Stephen Jackson, Stanley H. Rosenbaum and Susan K. Palmer. Published by Cambridge University Press. © Cambridge University Press 2011.

Table 46.1. Catagories and color-coding for casualties in civilian disasters

Priority	Color-code (for tagging casualties)	General description of injury category	Specific examples
(1)Emergent	Red	Critical; may survive with simple life-saving measures. **Allocated to immediate care**	Airway obstruction, hemorrhage, cardiorespiratory failure, shock
(2) Urgent	Yellow	Likely to survive if care is provided within hours **Allocated to delayed care, next priority**	Penetrating abd wound, severe eye injury, fractures, avascular limb
(3)Nonurgent	Green	"Walking wounded." Injuries generally minor and can be delayed **Allocated to delayed care, low priority**	Lacerations, contusion, superficial or partial thickness burns < 20% body surface area, uncomplicated fractures
(4) Catastrophic or dead (sometimes divided into 2 groups to identify those in need of comfort care	Blue (dying) Black (dead)	Catastrophically wounded patients who are unlikely to survive if they don't receive care within minutes, or patients who have already died **Allocated to comfort care only if still alive**.	Head injury – Glasgow Coma Scale < 8, burns > 85% of body surface area, multisystem trauma, signs of impending death

number rather than the particular good of the patients at hand. This rule is justified only because of the clear necessity of general public welfare in a crisis.[2]

Justice

Patients' trust in the medical profession is based heavily on the belief that physicians will do what is best for them individually. Utilitarian decision-making has the potential to erode that trust, if it is perceived that such decisions are made capriciously or are based on subjective judgments. Therefore, decisions about which patients will receive limited medical care resources in a disaster must be based on thoughtful criteria that are agreed upon and transparent to the community of patients. A number of models of medical triage in civilian mass casualty situations are available. For one example of triage criteria, see Table 46.1.

The principle of justice dictates that criteria for triage of civilian patients must be based on their medical condition and not on their social connections. Ethically acceptable criteria for withholding or withdrawing care from patients could include the likelihood of benefit from medical care, the urgency of need for care, and the availability of the resources needed to care for a particular patient. Unacceptable criteria might include

social worth, patient contribution to their illness/injury, or the patient's ability to pay for care. No patient group should receive special consideration in a disaster situation, other than that dictated by their physiology – *including children.*

Such principles of justice may be difficult to strictly follow, however, since judgments of social worth are nearly inevitable sometimes. For example, if some of the survivors of a tsunami are healthcare workers with minor injuries, they might be given priority for treatment because of their value in then being able to help others. Physicians might be given the first doses of protective vaccine in a pandemic, so that they will not become infected and will be able to care for those who are. Such decisions amount to prioritization based on social worth, but may be justified in this very restricted context if the individual's abilities are indispensable to the larger goal of *this* disaster's containment. The decisions should be strictly limited to only those skills that are essential to the successful management of the disaster, and not to general social assessments.[3]

The risks of consequentialism

When physicians are forced into mass casualty situations where they must temporarily abandon the usual ethical principles of medicine, then they must recognize that what they are doing is distinctly different from what would be acceptable in the normal course of patient care. Consequentialism, especially when it is not recognized as distinctly different from usual medical ethics, can subvert the patient-centered values that form the bedrock of medical professionalism.

A historical example of the subversion of patient-centered ethical values by consequentialist arguments can be found in the "Nazification" of the medical profession in pre-WWII Germany.[4] In a decades-long process, German physicians were gradually convinced to adopt consequentialist principles in medical decision-making in order to serve the interests of the "state" as the highest "good" and to bring the "greatest happiness" to the greatest number of people. The process began with the replacement of academic physicians at universities with patriotic doctors who were not qualified as teachers or researchers and were less likely to question the shift in ethical decision-making. Physicians were promoted to positions of power on the basis of their political beliefs, and became increasingly involved in judgments regarding the "social worth" of certain groups of patients. They were then recruited to research "humane" methods of killing persons whose social worth was questioned. Consequentialist-type reasoning was offered to convince physicians that they were doing what was best for the "greatest number" of Germans. Ultimately, refusal by physicians to participate in these activities was branded as "unpatriotic," and therefore harmful to society.

Consequentialism may be a legitimate ethical framework in which to make decisions regarding how resources should be allocated when mass casualties overwhelm the traditional delivery of medical care, but is not the ethical framework applied to usual medical care.

Lifeboat Ethics

Once initial triage is performed to decide which patients do *not* need immediate care (the walking wounded, and the dead or near-dead), another set of decisions face providers in facilities to which the survivors are evacuated. During public health disasters, hospitals perform as "lifeboats," with finite capacity to "surge" to meet the medical needs of arriving casualties. The extent of a hospital's ability to "surge in place" depends on ability to acutely increase staff, the current status of critical supplies, the number of available beds,

and the capacity to "create" available beds, among other things.

One consideration is the re-allocation of hospital beds from *current* inpatients to *future* ones, in a process sometimes called "reverse triage." In reverse triage, patients who are capable of being cared for in lower acuity beds or at home are discharged to make room for incoming casualties.

The primary principle in disaster triage is utilitarian in aiming to provide the most benefit for the most people. Therefore reassignment of resources away from existing patients must meet a test of proportionality – there should be at least as much, and preferably significantly more potential benefit expected for the incoming casualties, than there is potential for harm to those hospital patients who are reassigned. Kraus and colleagues describe such considerations as "lifeboat ethics." The needs of all – those in the lifeboats and those still in the water – are treated equally.[5]

Lifeboat ethics create concerns about breach of expectations to existing patients. Inpatients expect that they are benefiting from the hospitalization, and may therefore be harmed by early discharge. Some argue that in a public health disaster, all patients are equal, and therefore the priority of *any existing* patient, in the lifeboat or outside of it, is re-triaged in the setting of the mass casualty event. By this reasoning, it might be ethical to balance the likelihood that discontinuing "futile" care to an inpatient and reallocating resources to a "more salvageable" casualty will result in greater benefits than continuing critical care to a moribund patient while the casualty is denied the resource. Thus, a terminally ill ICU patient might be transferred to comfort care measures – in much the same way as a "black" listed pre-morbid casualty might be – so that another injured patient whose survival is more likely can occupy the bed.

As with other forms of triage, "lifeboat" triage should be transparent, and based on empirical data and community approval. In promoting disaster preparedness, hospital administrators who consider developing lifeboat triage policies should do so with considerable community input.

Case resolution

Several measures have already been taken to prepare for the arriving casualties. An assessment of the current status of all operating rooms has been made, and the operating rooms are being freed as soon as possible to accept casualties. All available staff have been contacted and asked to report to the hospital. The hospital, in other words, is preparing to "surge" as much as possible. The available blood has been inventoried, as well as an assessment of when resupply is likely to be possible. All of this information is helpful to the triage officer in allocating resources.

When casualties arrive, all patients who do not need immediate attention, either because they are not seriously injured, or because they are not expected to survive their injuries, should wait for resource-intensive treatment. Seriously and critically injured patients who have a potential to survive will receive first intensive treatment. The anesthesiologist should continue to reassess casualties even after they arrive, to "re-triage" if they later fit a different triage category, or as supplies arrive and more resources become available and can be extended to them. An assessment should also be made regarding how many hospital beds are available, and whether any inpatients can be allocated to lower acuity beds, or discharged home.

The recent earthquakes in Haiti and Chile underscore the need for physician and hospital preparedness should a natural disaster strike. Merin and colleagues describe the process of inventorying and managing limited resource, including the formation of triage consult committees to aid in difficult on the ground decision-making. Knowledgeable and prepared physicians are desperately needed in times of mass casualties, to have the best chance of providing life-saving care to as many people as possible.[6]

Key points

- During mass casualty situations, the goals of medical management change from those focusing on individual patient benefit, to more utilitarian principles of "doing the most good for the most people."
- Civilian casualty triage differs from military triage. In military triage, a primary goal is returning the less severely wounded to combat. In civilian triage the goal is overall survival. Thus, victims not expected to survive may be allocated to lower treatment priority than those who have survivable injuries.
- Consequentialism is not philosophically supportable as an ethical basis for the best medical care because it approves of using

individual patients as a means to achieve certain ends for others.
- Triage in mass casualty events should be based on principles of justice that treat all patients equally, and from the perspective of their medical condition rather than social worth.
- However, "social worth" may be applicable in very limited interpretations, when the particular skills of the individual are critical to managing the disaster itself. One example is allocation of vaccines to physicians in pandemics so that they remain well and continue to treat victims.
- "Lifeboat" ethics may lead to decisions to reallocate resources away from existing hospital patients in order to provide capacity to treat disaster victims.
- Triage should be based on ethically sound principles, should be transparent, should include public input, and should be developed *before disaster strikes.*

References

1 American Medical Association Code of Medical Ethics, Opinion 9.067. Physician obligations in disaster preparedness and response. Adopted June, 2004. AMA, Chicago, IL.

2 Jonsen, A. and Edwards, K. Resource allocation in *Ethics in Medicine*, University of Washington School of Medicine. http://eduserv.hscer.washington.edu/bioethics/topics/resall.thml.

3* Beauchamp, T.L. and Childress, J.F. (1994). Justice in *Principles of Biomedical Ethics*, 4th edn. NY: Oxford University Press, pp. 386–7.

4* Lifton, R. J. (1986). *The Nazi Doctors, Medical Killing and the Psychology of Genocide.* New York, NY: Basic Books.

5* Kraus, C.K., Levy, F., and Gabor, K. (2007). Lifeboat ethics; considerations in the discharge of inpatients for the creation of hospital surge capacity. *Disaster Med Public Health Prep*, **1**(1), 51–6.

6* Merin, O., Nashman, A., Levy, G., *et al.* (2010). The Israeli field hospital in Haiti – ethical dilemmas in early disaster triage. *New Eng J Med*, published online, March 3.

Further reading

Code of Medical Ethics of the American Medical Association. (2006). Council on Ethical and Judicial Affairs, current opinions with annotations 2006–2007 edition. AMA, USA.

Devereaux, A.V., Dichter, J.R., Christian, M.D., *et al.* (2008). Definitive care for the critically ill during a disaster: a framework for allocation of scarce resources in mass critical care. *Chest*, **133**, 51S–66S.

Moreno, J.D. (2004). *In the Wake of Terror. Medicine and Morality in a Time of Crisis*. The Cambridge, MA: MIT Press.

Trotter, G. (2007). *The Ethics of Coercion in Mass Casualty Medicine*. Baltimore: The Johns Hopkins University Press.

VA Office of Public Health and Environmental Hazards: www.vethealth.cio.med.va.gov/

Veterans Health Administration – Central Office:Pandemic influenza in general, www.pandemicflu.gov.

National Center for Ethics in HealthCare.www.ethics.va.gov.

47

Triage and treatment of wounded during armed conflict

Craig D. McClain and David B. Waisel

The Case

The triage physician at a forward clearing station receives two wounded enemy enlisted men, an injured local villager, and a wounded friendly soldier. The enemy soldiers appear to have serious but not life-threatening internal bleeding and may require blood transfusion. The triage physician estimates that short operations will stabilize both enemy soldiers. It is unlikely they have any useful military intelligence. The villager's open femur fracture will require surgical treatment and a blood transfusion under normal circumstances. He has a hematocrit of 25% and a compression dressing has effectively limited his rate of bleeding. The friendly soldier has a vascular injury in his groin. He is conscious, mildly hypotensive and his hematocrit is 18%. The triage physician is concerned that this operation will consume extensive resources both during the operation and postoperatively. Many additional casualties will arrive within the hour. The triage physician estimates that treating all four patients will deplete the unit's blood supply, and she is aware that no further personnel or material resources are expected.

"It is forbidden to kill; therefore all murderers are punished unless they kill in large numbers and to the sound of trumpets." (Voltaire)

Military medicine intertwines the military and medical professions. Under most circumstances, the military physician serves primarily as a physician, and to a lesser extent as a member of the military. However, on occasion, the two positions can battle each other for ascendency. In Greek mythology the sons of Asclepius were both healers and warriors. However, in modern times, military physicians do not take up arms to confront the enemy unless their own lives – or those of their patients – are under threat. In fact, many of the ethical challenges met by the modern military physician are not encountered in civilian settings, and as such, it *may not* always be appropriate – or practicable – to apply the principles of civilian medical ethics to military medicine.

The underlying discrepancy between civilian and military medical ethics can be attributed to their respective goals and how they are to be achieved. Civilian physicians, in most circumstances, concentrate on primary medical goals, while military physicians must adhere to the organizational objective of defeating the enemy. As such, military physicians must occasionally subordinate other values to achieve defeat of the enemy.

This is the origin of the core ethical quandary with which military physicians must wrestle: finding a balance between giving absolute priority to the principle of military necessity – and its attendant obligations as a military officer – with that of lending moral weight to their patients' interests according to the traditional principles of civilian medical ethics. Indeed, military physicians may have to choose to sacrifice their patients' autonomy and best interests when required to fulfill the military mission of protecting their society. Physicians trained within modern medical ethics in which an individual patient's rights are paramount may have difficulty balancing those views with their duty to place the needs of the military before those of his/her patients.

Triage is a system of sorting patients according to need when resources are insufficient for all wounded to be treated. Military medical ethics becomes even more complex and challenging in the arena of armed conflict when triage of the wounded involves friendly soldiers, "enlisted" enemy soldiers, and local civilians.

International guidelines for ethical conduct of physicians engaged in armed conflict

In response to wartime outrages, international organizations codified the conduct of armed conflict. Statements from the Geneva Conventions,[a] International Committee of the Red Cross, the United

---

Clinical Ethics in Anesthesiology: A Case-Based Textbook, ed. Gail A. Van Norman, Stephen Jackson, Stanley H. Rosenbaum and Susan K. Palmer. Published by Cambridge University Press. © Cambridge University Press 2011.

Nations, and the US military[1] have proposed that war can be conducted in an orderly fashion by adhering to certain guidelines. The World Medical Association's (WMA's) resolution entitled "Regulations in Times of Armed Conflict" typifies these statements[2*]:

> Medical ethics in times of armed conflict is identical to medical ethics in times of peace, as stated in the International Code of Medical Ethics of the WMA. If, in performing their professional duty, physicians have conflicting loyalties, then their primary obligation is to their patients; in all their professional activities, physicians should adhere to international conventions on human rights, international humanitarian law and WMA declarations on medical ethics.
>
> The primary task of the medical profession is to preserve health and save life. Hence it is deemed unethical for physicians to … give advice or perform prophylactic, diagnostic or therapeutic procedures that are not justifiable for the patient's health care.

While codifying wartime behavior sounds ironic, these principles are accepted by most of the international community. Indeed, modern bioethical priority of respect for autonomy is promoted by the WMA's prohibition against performing procedures that would not benefit the soldier-patient. Both independence from controlling influence and capacity for intentional action are essential for making an informed choice regarding medical treatment.

During state-sponsored armed conflict, however, the goals and needs of the state often supersede the rights of individuals. Combatants, by definition, are members of a state-controlled military force actively participating in armed conflict. By joining the military, soldiers have willingly accepted some level of controlling influence from the state, particularly during combat. Using this standard, it may be necessary for individuals to make willing or unwilling sacrifices – including that of their health and survival – for the benefit of the state.

Triage

Triage is the dynamic process of prioritizing treatment for casualties in a resource-poor environment. Tables 47.1 and 47.2 illustrate the complexity and imprecision of triage. Table 47.1 describes theoretical and practical triage categorization. Table 47.2 describes the multiple known and unknown factors that affect the otherwise discrete categorization of the wounded. But this oversimplification is belied by the demand for in-the-moment functional use of these categories.[b]

The goals of combat medicine are to return the greatest possible number of wounded soldiers to combat and to preserve life. These sometimes conflicting goals necessitate tough decisions. Faced with an impending attack, physicians may try to quickly stabilize critically wounded soldiers while focusing most resources on returning *the less seriously wounded* soldiers to fighting. If speedily returning soldiers to combat is less essential, then combat physicians may devote most of their resources to treating the critically wounded.

Soldiers may receive care during triage that they would not receive in a resource-rich environment. For example, rather than performing limb salvage surgery on a soldier with a neurovascular injury, the physician may amputate the arm in order to conserve time and other resources. In his article, Gross crystallizes the sacrifices soldiers accept in regard to triage:

> … (military) medical personnel bear an obligation to salvage soldiers and return as many to duty as quickly as possible. Salvage speaks to a specific and objective measure of quality of life distinct from the patient's own subjective evaluation. Salvageable soldiers may not invoke quality of life to refuse treatment, however painful or onerous, if it will return them to military duty. Those beyond salvage, on the other hand, may not appeal to any right to life to secure medical care when resources are scarce.[3]

Clashing demands of patient and state may cause cognitive dissonance in the physician, requiring mindful attention to balancing loyalty to the state with loyalty to the patient.

Enemy non-combatants

Enemy combatants pose a direct and dangerous threat to the security and stability of the state. In war, active enemy combatants have no intrinsic right to life or medical care. Wounded enemies are no longer a significant threat and are reclassified as non-combatants, thereby regaining their rights to life, medical care and humane treatment. The Geneva Convention states, "All wounded, sick and shipwrecked, to whichever Party they belong, shall be respected and protected…shall be treated humanely and shall receive, to the fullest possible extent and with the least possible delay, the medical care and attention required by their condition. There shall be no distinction between them on any other grounds."[1]

There is a theoretical and practical basis for treating wounded enemy non-combatants the same as wounded friendly soldiers. It is consistent with the training of physicians that all patients are equally deserving of treatment. Supporting this belief may

Table 47.1. Traditional wartime triage categories

Traditional	Practical

Immediate
• Lifesaving intervention
• Brief
• High chances of survival
• Examples
  • Respiratory obstruction
  • Pneumothorax
  • Amputation
  • Unstable casualties with chest or abdominal injuries
	Critical
	• Urgent intervention needed to avoid death or major disability
	• Examples
	  • Airway obstruction / compromise (actual or potential)
	  • Uncontrolled bleeding
	  • Shock
	  • Systolic BP < 90 mm Hg
	  • Decreased mental status without head injury
	  • Unstable penetrating or blunt injuries of the trunk, neck, head, and pelvis
	  • Threatened loss of limb or eyesight
	  • Multiple long-bone fractures

Delayed
• Can delay surgery without increasing risk
• Time-consuming surgery
• Sustaining treatment required (e.g. IV fluids, splinting, antibiotics, gastric decompression, and pain relief)
• Examples
  • Large muscle wounds
  • Fractures of major bones
  • Abdominal and thoracic wounds
  • Burns less than 50% of total body surface area
	Noncritical
	• May require surgery
	• Does not require emergent attention
	• Lacks significant potential for loss of life, limb, or eyesight
	• Examples
	  • Single long-bone fractures
	  • Closed fractures
	  • Soft tissue injuries without significant bleeding
	  • Facial fractures without airway compromise

Minimal
• Treatable by non-medical personal
• Examples
  • Minor lacerations and abrasions
  • Fractures of small bones
  • Minor burns	

Comfort Care
• Survival unlikely in the best of circumstances
• Provide comfort care
• Examples
  • Unresponsive patients with penetrating head wounds
  • High spinal cord injuries
  • Mutilating explosive wounds involving multiple anatomical sites and organs
  • Second and third degree burns in excess of 60% total body surface area
  • Profound shock with multiple injuries
  • Agonal respiration
	Comfort Care
	• Survival unlikely given the situation and resource constraints
	• Examples
	  • No vital signs or signs of life, regardless of mechanism of injury
	  • Transcranial gunshot wound
	  • Open pelvic injuries with uncontrolled bleeding; in shock with decreased mental status
	  • Massive burns

The traditional column represents the standard wartime triage. The practical column suggests a more functional approach to triage.

Table 47.2. Factors influencing discrete categorization of the wounded

- The tactical situation and mission
- Current supply of consumable resources and anticipated resupply, if any
- Current status of static resources and capabilities: the number of operating rooms, holding and ward capacity and diagnostic equipment
- Opportunity costs of individual casualties, i.e. one overwhelming patient can limit available resources (particularly operating room tables, which is often the choke point) for other patients
- Evacuation intervals of wounded to a main treatment facility; e.g. shorter evacuation intervals may lead to more treatment for more complex patients, because they will not consume as many resources post-operatively
- The status of personnel resource
  - Professional capability (type and experience of individual physician/ nurse/medic)
  - Perishable resources
    - Emotional stability of personnel
    - Sleep status of personnel
  - Stress (degrades individual and unit capability)

help protect (or at least not breach) the internal morality of military physicians, whose behavior by virtue of formal and informal authority influences others. Treating enemy non-combatants the same as wounded friendly soldiers emphasizes the enemy's humanity and may prevent abuses rooted in the dehumanization of the enemy. Practically, physicians hope that following this agreement will incent their enemies to do the same.

Civilian non-combatants

Civilian non-combatants are those taking no active part in hostilities such as the local civilians, aid workers, displaced persons, and media. Similar to enemy non-combatants, civilian noncombatants are to be triaged akin to friendly soldiers. Noncombatants may have involuntarily diminished autonomy due to the hegemony of the armed conflict. Despite the humanitarian imperative and the public relations boon of treating civilian noncombatants, access to care may be hindered in a resource-poor environment.

Principled triaging

Principled triaging is arduous. It would be easy for honorable physicians to be unconsciously influenced during triage. One can also imagine physicians consciously overcorrecting to inappropriately prioritize enemy noncombatants out of a fear of being unfair. On the other hand, it takes courageous physicians to choose appropriately to spend limited resources on enemy noncombatants instead of countrymen.

The case emphasizes the murkiness of triage. One could imagine prioritizing the friendly soldier given his more tenuous state and the realization that resources may diminish after the others receive care and other wounded arrive. On the other hand, repairing a vascular injury could be time and material consuming and more pressing demands eventually may require intraoperative abandonment and re-categorization of the soldier to expectant.

If all the wounded men were treated as equals, then one could imagine starting with the patients with internal bleeding (on the theory that an easily fixable problem now may turn into a more costly problem later), temporizing the femur fracture and delaying work on the patient with the vascular wound until the next wave of wounded and more resources arrive.

Key points

- During state-sponsored armed conflict, military physicians will be placed in situations where they need to triage honorably.
- Knowledge of some of the ethical underpinnings of the decision-making process would aid in making these difficult decisions in a tense situation.
- Close examination of the nature of the differences between bioethical principles in peacetime as well as wartime will ultimately lead to a better understanding of the difficulties faced by physicians during armed conflict.

Notes

a   Rules relating to the conduct of combatants and the protection of prisoners of war, 1988 extract from "Basic Rules of the Geneva Conventions and their Additional Protocols"; Geneva: ICRC, 2nd edn.

b   Rules relating to the conduct of combatants and the protection of prisoners of war, extract from "Basic rules of the Geneva Conventions and their Additional Protocols"; ICRC, Geneva, 1988; 2nd edn.

References

1* Beam, T. and Howe, E. (2003) A proposed ethic for military medicine. *Military Medical Ethics: Volume 2.* Peligrino, E.G., Hartle, A.E. and Howe, E.G., eds. Department of Defense, Borden Institute, Washington, DC, USA.

2* The World Medical Association Regulations in Times of Armed Conflict. Originally adopted by the 10th World Medical Assembly, Havana, Cuba, October 1956, most recently amended by The WMA General Assembly, Tokyo 2004 and editorially revised at the 173rd Council Session, Divonne-les-Bains, France, May 2006.

3* Gross, M.L. (2004). Bioethics and Armed Conflict: Mapping the Moral Dimensions of Medicine and War. *Hastings Cen Rep*, **34**(6), 22–30.

Further reading

Emergency War Surgery (2004). 3rd United States Revision. Department of Defense, United States of America.

International Dual Loyalty Working Group (2003). Dual Loyalty & Human Rights in Health Professional Practice. Physicians for Human Rights 2003.

Repine, T.B., Lisagor, P., and Cohen, D.J. (2005). The dynamics and ethics of triage: rationing care in hard times. *Mil Med*, **170**, 505–9.

Rubenstein, L.S. (2004). Medicine and War. *Hastings Cen Rep*, **34**(6), 3.

Singh, J.A. (2003). American physicians and dual loyalty obligations in the "war on terror." *BMC Med Ethics*, **4**, E4.

48

Physician facilitation of torture and coercive interrogation

David B. Waisel

The Case

A suspect informs police that he has buried a 5 year-old girl in a box with a limited air supply. Standard interrogation techniques have failed to ascertain the girl's location and it is believed she may have only several hours to live. A judge authorizes torturing the suspect to obtain the girl's location. The proposed method of torture is to have an anesthesiologist administer a paralytic drug to the awake prisoner, and then allow the prisoner to experience periods of awake paralysis without respiratory support. This will result in acute hypercarbia, severe dyspnea, and an experience of awake suffocation. After a period of time, time the anesthesiologist will be instructed to ventilate him with a bag and mask, reverse the paralytic, and allow him to answer questions. The technique will leave no lasting physical disfigurement or disabilities.

This type of scenario, known as the "ticking time bomb scenario" is often proposed as one in which torture might be justified. Some authors suggest that in cases of "ticking time bomb scenarios," not only is torture possibly justified, but that it should be regulated by judicial warrant and oversight.[1]

Torture is the deliberate infliction of mental and physical suffering in order to overcome resistance or to sufficiently disorient prisoners so that the torturer can intimidate, extract information, and obtain confessions. Methods of physical torture include, but are by no means limited to, beating, choking, stressful positioning, "simulated drowning"[a] and use of electric shock. Methods of psychological torture involve sensory manipulation, sleep deprivation, exploitation of phobias, and humiliation. Torture is performed during peace and wartime – by state policy or by individual decision. "Participation in torture" is not necessarily confined to administration of the coercive technique itself. Historically, medical personnel have participated in torture by evaluating prisoners for interrogation, monitoring coercive interrogation, allowing interrogators access to medical records of the prisoners

to develop their interrogative approaches, falsifying medical records and death certificates, and failing to provide even basic healthcare.[2]

All mainstream medical ethicists unwaveringly reject torture as an affront to the fundamental and absolute right of all humans to dignity. We shall consider the morally impermissible nature of torture (as well as of coercive interrogation), the ethical prohibition of physician participation in torture, and the dilemma of dual loyalties facing physicians requested or mandated to participate in such universally condemned activities.

International statements banning torture

Arguments prohibiting torture are straightforward and powerful. Perhaps the most potent argument is the psychological, emotional, cultural and legal prohibition to treat people inhumanely. For that reason, a number of agreements and statements ban torture.[3] For example, the 1984 Convention Against Torture and Other Cruel, Inhuman or Degrading Treatment or Punishment from the United Nations[4] states:

> Torture and other cruel, inhuman or degrading treatment or punishment are particularly serious violations of human rights and, as such, are strictly condemned by international law.

The Convention declared that no "exceptional circumstances" and no legal authority may supersede this absolute prohibition.

For long periods of history, torture was legal, and physician participation was common. Following revelations about atrocities during World War II, Western nations condemned torture through documents such as the Geneva Conventions and statements from the international medical tribunal at Nuremberg. In 1982, the United Nations reiterated the foundational ethical

Clinical Ethics in Anesthesiology: A Case-Based Textbook, ed. Gail A. Van Norman, Stephen Jackson, Stanley H. Rosenbaum and Susan K. Palmer. Published by Cambridge University Press. © Cambridge University Press 2011.

medical principle of nonmaleficence (*primum non nocere* – first do no harm), imploring physicians to adhere to this dictum when requested – or ordered – to participate in medical interventions that are not intended to be beneficial:

> It is a great contravention of medical ethics, as well as an offence under applicable international instruments, for health personnel, particularly physicians, to engage, actively or passively, in acts which constitute participation in, complicity in, incitement to, or attempts to commit torture or other cruel, inhuman or degrading treatment or punishment.[5]

The World Medical Association has repeatedly made declarations against physician participation in torture as well as in other cruel, inhumane or degrading practices. In particular, it iterated that:

> Medical ethics in times of armed conflict is identical to medical ethics in times of peace … [and that] … if, in performing their professional duty, physicians have conflicting [dual] loyalties, their primary obligation is to their patients.

The American Medical Association lends even further support by calling upon physicians to support victims of torture, reject the use of torture, and endeavor to change situations in which torture is practiced.[6]

Treaties and statements prohibiting torture encourage states not to torture so that their enemies also will not torture. For example, the prohibition on gas warfare was effective in World War II because each side feared that initiating gas warfare would result in a similar enemy response. The moral clarity provided by statements may enable states to refrain from torture regardless of enemy actions. In addition, torture rents the fabric of both the torturer and the community. If torture were to become acceptable within society, it may become psychologically easier to permit other immoral acts.

Some commentators suggest that torture *may be* acceptable under certain conditions,[7] but that torture should be a last resort only after other less intrusive measures have failed. They further declare that interrogators would need robust reasons for believing that the prisoner has the desired information, and that such information must have immediate benefits for reducing or preventing imminent harm. Under these specific conditions, they contend, torture *may be* worth its associated harms. However, these authors further opine that torture should not be used to force confessions or to uncover unspecified, future crimes. Other gross considerations may include the likelihood that the information is accurate and the potential benefits such as lives saved from the information.

No studies confirm or deny the relative accuracy of torture in extracting accurate information, or how often information obtained from torture has saved lives. Many experienced interrogators believe that torture is less likely to lead to *accurate* information than other techniques such as relationship building. If the rate of success is relevant in deciding whether to torture, however, this implies that the decision to torture should be based on risks and benefits. From an ethics point of view, if torture is wrong because it is an affront to human rights and dignity, then it is always wrong, regardless of the rate of success.

Returning to the case example at the beginning of this chapter, we find that the kidnapped girl in the box is an example of a scenario that fulfills many of these aforementioned requirements. The confessed perpetrator has provided sufficient evidence to prove his participation and knowledge of the crime (to help rule out coerced confession), less invasive methods have failed, and time-sensitive results will immediately benefit the kidnapped girl. Presumably acting in good faith, interrogators desired to avoid torture, but feel compelled by their obligation to help the girl. Importantly, the judge, a formal authority operating within her jurisdiction of protecting others, has approved proceeding, so there is no legal impediment. False leads will not cause a misallocation of limited resources that otherwise might expose society to other harms, and the information can be quickly confirmed or disproven.

While there may be no *tangible* losses in this case, there may be meaningful societal losses. Torturing that leads to rescuing the girl may nudge society toward being more accepting of torture. If society were to choose to sanction torture, then the policy and process ideally would be wholly transparent, inviting public discussion and review. But, no matter what precautions are taken, permitting torture – even under limited circumstances – likely will lead to abuses. Moreover, a declaration removing the taboo of the unethical nature of torture would give other countries (and terrorists) a public relation's safe harbor to perform torture.[b]

Should physicians participate in torture?

The American Medical Association (AMA) Opinion on Torture states, "Physicians must oppose and must not participate in torture for any reason."[8] The argument, in part, is that torture is antithetical to the physician's primary responsibility to help patients as they define help. Moreover, the AMA's Code of Medical Ethics states, "Physicians may treat prisoners or detainees if doing so is in their best interest, but physicians should not treat individuals to verify their health so that torture can begin or continue." This "best interest" phrase has laid the basis for a distinct minority of commentators who believe that traditional medical values mandate at least minimal physician participation in hostile interrogation even though this theoretically could prepare the prisoners to undergo further hostile interrogation. However, the AMA condemns coercive interrogation as well as torture.

Countervailing the argument that physicals should only act in the patients interest is that number of physicians work for the public good and do not prioritize helping individual patients. Consider, for example, the specialties of forensic psychiatry, public health and occupational health in which physicians often incorporate an investigative component when providing services to the public. In this sense, it has been suggested that legally sanctioned torture is similar in that it would claim that it serves the public good. This specious argument ignores the critical factual difference that forensic psychiatrists and public health and occupational health physicians do not directly physically or psychologically harm individual patients, either. Furthermore, although physicians may make it easier to accomplish torture, their participation is in fact not necessary for torture to happen. Torture can be accomplished in many other ways.[9]

The military physician

A newly deployed physician must decide whether to post physician assistants and medics behind a one-way mirror during interrogations. A military police commander tells the physician that "the way this worked with the unit here before was: We'd capture a guy; the medic would screen him and ensure he was fit for interrogation. If he had questions he'd check with the supervising doctor. The medic would get his screening signed by the doc. After that, the medic would watch over the interrogation from behind the glass."[10]

In this scenario, coercive interrogation is designed to find general information, not specific, time-sensitive information. Moreover, there would be a limited ability to immediately validate the confession, leading to a much higher likelihood of wasting resources while pursuing false leads.

The US military has stated that they perform coercive interrogation but not torture. Military conflicts usually lead to the detention and interrogation of adversaries, but whether hostile "stress and duress" tactics are tantamount to torture is debatable. The military further argues that the physicians assisting in devising or performing coercive interrogation strategies do not have doctor–patient relationships with the prisoners because other physicians not participating in coercive interrogation provide the medical care for the prisoners. In fact, they argue, physicians participating in coercive interrogation are using medical skills outside of functioning in the role of a physician. Many consider this interpretation as a dubious one, arguing that physicians are, indeed, acting as physicians by virtue of using medical knowledge and skills in their interaction with the prisoners.

Military physicians are faced with balancing what is simplistically known as *"dual loyalty"* when deciding whether they have an obligation to participate in coercive interrogation as part of their military and societal obligation.[11] Military medicine is a mingling of the military and the medical professions. Under most circumstances, the military physician serves primarily as a physician, and to a lesser degree as a member of the military. However, on occasion, the two positions can be contradictory. On one hand, military physicians have obligations to fellow soldiers, the military and the nation's military units to perform what is necessary to achieve the goals of the military and their country. On the other hand, these physicians have an obligation to honor personal values and beliefs as well as their obligation to society of not harming the image of the physician. To advise military physicians, commentators mostly declare that one of the two obligations has absolute hegemony over the other. While dogma may be helpful to some physicians, others appreciate having a process to resolve these dilemmas.

The International Dual Loyalty Working Group (IDLWG) guidelines call for education of physicians to recognize dual loyalty situations involving human rights and international law. They suggest that an independent group should set standards for behavior in dual loyalty situations, and, additionally, that a formal appeals process and whistle-blower protections be instituted. Their proposals center on the premise that population-based interventions of standards through oversight and statements of professional organizations will change behavior and provide support for the individual physician.

Notwithstanding the recommendations of the IDLWG, commentators generally insist that military and civilian physicians must hew to the same standards of ethical behavior because medical ethics are universal.[12] In addition, they argue, the military benefits by adhering to civilian standards because it is more consistent with the mindsets of physicians. Both arguments, however, have been challenged. While possibly true in theory, in reality medical ethics are not universal. And given that the unique experiences and obligations of military physicians are not often encountered in civilian settings, the ethical principles of the civilian physician *may not* always be appropriate – or practicable – to apply to military medical standards.

A danger in excusing the military physician lies in the possibility that torture for the purposes of the state may be viewed without the same critical eye as torture by law enforcement agencies within a state. Furthermore, participation in torture leads to degradation of the physician, whether civilian or military, by allowing him or her to become "socialized to atrocity."[13]

As Annas stated:

> Preventing torture is everyone's business – but three professions seem to be especially well suited to prevent torture: medicine, law and the military. Each profession has particular obligations. Physicians have the obligations of the universally recognized and respected role of healers. Lawyers have the obligations to respect and uphold the law, including international humanitarian law. And military officers have the obligation to follow the international laws of war, including the Geneva Conventions.[14]

Physician participation in torture harms the integrity of the medical profession and societal trust in physicians, and physicians must consider the societal consequences of such behavior. Statements by organized medicine provide some reflection of the potential for such public harm. The ethical analysis of statements written during peacetime is often superior to the impromptu analysis made in the heat of battle. Physicians under considerable stress may want to consider the limitations of their ability to perform ethical analysis and may want to defer to such statements.

Key points

- Every treaty, international agreement, national policy, and medical association code of ethics declares that torture is not morally permissible and that physicians should not be involved in coercive interrogations.
- Commentators disagree about distinctions between torture and coercive interrogation.

- There is similar disagreement about distinctions between when a physician is acting as a physician and when a military officer, who happens to be a physician, is not acting as a physician.
- Nearly all commentators prohibit any physician participation in any aspect of coercive interrogation or torture.
- Dual loyalty decisions by physicians about torture and interrogation are emotionally charged and highly stressful, and should not be made by the individual in the moment, but rather based on central policies with fervent oversight.

Notes

a It should be noted that in this usage, "simulated drowning" refers to the creation of a sensation of drowning, often through the submersion in and aspiration of water.

b Author's note: If a judge were to come to me as a physician and ask me to torture a confessed suspect in order to try to save the little girl's life in a time-limited situation, then I would find it difficult to refuse to participate. If the girl were a child I knew, then I suspect that I might even find it quite easy to torture the suspect. While emotions in the heat of the moment are understandable, such emotionally based behaviors are precisely why society prohibits vigilante justice. I want to convey that we should *not* leave emotional, stressful, and even dual loyalty decisions about torture or coercive interrogation to the individual (in this case, a physician) in the moment. These decisions should be based on central policies guarded with fervent oversight.

References

1 Dershowitz, A.M. (2002). *Why Terrorism Works: Understanding the Threat, Responding to the Challenge.* New Haven, CT: Yale University Press

2 Miles, S.H. (2004). Abu Ghraib: its legacy for military medicine. *Lancet*, **364**, 725–9

3* World Medical Association Declaration Concerning Support for Medical Doctors Refusing to Participate in, or to Condone, the Use of Torture or Other Forms of Cruel, Inhuman or Degrading Treatment. 1997.

4 Convention against Torture and Other Cruel, Inhuman or Degrading Treatment or Punishment. United Nations. 1984.

5 United Nations General Assembly resolution 37/194, Principle 2. 111th plenary session, 18 December 1982 www.un.org/documents/ga/res/37/a37r194.htm

6 Council on Ethical and Judicial Affairs, American Medical Association. E-2.067-Torture.

7* Kennedy, R.G. (2003). Can interrogatory torture be morally legitimate? Presented at JSCOPE 2003: A Joint Services Conference on Professional Ethics

8 Council on Ethical and Judicial Affairs, American Medical Association. E-2.067-Torture.

9* Benatar, S.R. and Upshur, R.E. (2008). Dual loyalty of physicians in the military and in civilian life. *Am J Public Health*, **98**, 2161–7.

10* Singh, J.A. (2003). American physicians and dual loyalty obligations in the "war on terror." *BMC Med Ethics*, **4**, E4.

11 International Dual Loyalty Working Group. Dual Loyalty and Human Rights in Health Professional Practice: Proposed Guidelines and Institutional Mechanisms. New York and Cape Town, South Africa: Physicians for Human Rights and the School of Public Health and Primary Health Care, University of Cape Town, Health Sciences Faculty; 2002.

12* Annas, G.J. (2008). Military medical ethics – physician first, last, always. *N Engl J Med*, **359**, 1087–90.

13* Lifton, R.J. (2004). Doctors and torture. *N Engl J Med*, **351**, 415–6.

14 Annas, G.J. (2005). Unspeakably cruel – torture, medical ethics and the law. *New Eng J Med*, **352**: 2127–32

Further reading

Bloche, M.G. and Marks, J.H. (2005). When doctors go to war. *N Engl J Med*, **352**, 3–6.

Silove, D.M., and Rees, S.J. (2010). Interrogating the role of mental health professionals in assessing torture. *BMJ*, **340**, c124.

Walzer, M. (2006). *Just and Unjust Wars: A Moral Argument with Historical Allusions*. 3rd ed. New York: Basic Books

DISCOVERY LIBRARY
LEVEL 5 SWCC
DERRIFORD HOSPITAL
DERRIFORD ROAD
PLYMOUTH
PL6 8DH

Physician participation in executions

Gail A. Van Norman

The Case

RB, a 53-year-old US prison inmate is scheduled for execution by lethal injection. His crime is heinous: the abduction, rape, and stabbing death of a 14-year-old girl. There is no doubt of his guilt. DNA profiling confirms he is the murderer.

On execution day, after several hours' administrative delay, the execution team commences placement of intravenous catheters, which is complicated by the prisoner's long history of IV heroin use. The session drags on for more than 2 hours. Members of the prison team take turns, making more than two dozen unsuccessful insertions. After the only successful acquisition of a vein, the IV infiltrates. Team members take multiple breaks due to stress. The prisoner at times appears to be crying, and offers to "help" the IV team, requesting at one point to place his own IV. He moves tourniquets, attempting to locate veins himself.

Eventually, all attempts are terminated and the exhausted execution team retires for the day. The prisoner is returned to his cell with a promise that his execution will be resumed one day the following week. Internet commentary regarding the botched execution includes a renewed call for anesthesiologists to provide execution services.

In the US, physician organizations have consistently held that physician participation in executions is unethical, yet up to 41% of physicians state they would agree to participate in executions.[1] Physician involvement in euthanasia and executions concerns anesthesiologists in particular; their skills appear to make them ideal candidates for duties that involve killing. To date, there are no reported cases of disciplinary action against a physician or expulsion from a professional society for such involvement.

Medicine, retribution, and executions

For much of human history, executions have been designed to extract humiliation, remorse and dread in addition to the life of the prisoner. Ritual and even "religious" overtones were intentionally incorporated into the execution process by the state in order to unite the community in virtue. Until several hundred years ago, executions also often incorporated protracted torture (drawing and quartering, impaling, breaking on the wheel), intended to exact retribution from the prisoner, and to inspire horror as a means of criminal deterrence.

Since 1608, around 20 000 judicial executions have been carried out in territories now known as the US,[2] which remains one of the very few Westernized countries that still wields the death penalty. Until the mid-nineteenth century, US executions were conducted as public spectacles. With the development of "mechanistic" forms of execution such as electrocution and the gas chamber, the public spectacle all but disappeared, and the concept of execution acquired a detached and almost "civilized" tone.

Recent execution methods evolved largely at the hands of physicians, who developed increasingly "humane" methods of killing, including the guillotine (Drs. Antoine Louis and Joseph Ignace-Gillotin), hanging (Dr. Samuel Haughton) and the gas chamber (Dr. Allen McLean Hamilton). The inventor of the electric chair, to be complete, was a dentist. When macabre aspects of many modern execution methods rendered them repugnant to public sensibilities, Jay Chapman, a medical examiner, and Dr. Stanley Deutsch, an anesthesiologist, introduced a recipe for "humane" executions via intravenous injection of a cocktail consisting of a hypnotic, a paralytic agent, and high-dose potassium. This concoction was first used in 1982 and has become the preferred method of execution in most of the US. With lethal injection, capital punishment has acquired a sterile, almost benign, medical veneer, and physicians have increasingly been seen by judicial authorities to be its logical administrators.

Clinical Ethics in Anesthesiology: A Case-Based Textbook, ed. Gail A. Van Norman, Stephen Jackson, Stanley H. Rosenbaum and Susan K. Palmer. Published by Cambridge University Press. © Cambridge University Press 2011.

In weighing whether physicians should ethically be involved in executions, we should consider several questions: (1) Is it consistent to accept that physician aid-in-dying may be within the scope of professional integrity, but that physician participation in executions is not; (2) does respect for autonomy support physician participation in executions; (3) do harms outweigh the benefits if physicians become executioners; and (4) should the moral acceptability of physician involvement in executions take into account the moral acceptability of the death penalty itself – in other words, can actions ever be legitimately separated from the context in which they are carried out?

Physicians, the Hippocratic Oath, and the question of killing

Ethical arguments against physician participation in killing usually begin with a recitation of one of the many versions of the Hippocratic Oath: "I will neither give a deadly drug to anybody if asked for it, nor give advice to that effect."[3] Interestingly, this is not an argument based in principles of beneficence or nonmaleficence, but one centered in *professionalism* – an argument that killing violates behavioral standards that distinguish physicians from other professionals.

The ancient oath must now be reconciled against a modern culture. Physicians participate in abortions, physician-assisted suicide, and in some cases even euthanasia. We no longer restrict teaching the discipline of medicine to only our teachers' sons. Some of us have become surgeons All of these were forbidden by the Hippocratic Oath. In the context of modern medicine, why is the Hippocratic Oath still so compelling?

Margaret Mead observed that the Hippocratic Oath, apart from being one of the first statements of moral conduct for physicians, represented a breakthrough from primitive concepts in which physicians and sorcerers were one and the same.

> He with the power to kill had the power to cure … He with the power to cure would necessarily have the power to kill….With the Greeks, the distinction was made clear. One profession, the followers of Asclepius, were to be dedicated completely to life…regardless of rank, age or intellect – the life of a slave, the life of the Emperor, the life of a foreign man, the life of a defective child.[4]

The Oath of Hippocrates is compelling, because it describes the emergence of the modern physician

from the chrysalis of an ancient shaman. It represents, quite literally, the defining moment of The Physician. Any challenge to the principles of that oath therefore *redefines what it means to be a physician*, and should not be undertaken without solemn consideration.

Autonomy, beneficence, and nonmaleficence

Arguments for physician involvement in execution often invoke principles of beneficence (relieving or preventing suffering during execution) and respect for autonomy (of a prisoner who requests death by lethal injection). Arguments against invoke principles of nonmaleficence (harms to persons and the profession) and professionalism (erosion of trust in physicians and corruption of the physician in the execution process).

Beneficence

Anesthesiologists Truog and Waisel use the principle of beneficence to argue that physician participation in execution is acceptable because it prevents prisoners' suffering.[5] But Caplan points out that announcing a duty to alleviate the suffering of condemned prisoners is nonsensical if we don't also acknowledge a duty to minimize their suffering prior to execution.[6] In order to accept a beneficence argument even in the narrow context of preventing suffering only during the execution, we must first believe two critical assumptions: (1) that suffering is indeed prevented or relieved by lethal injection; and (2) that such relief or prevention can only be accomplished by physicians, and that therefore physicians' professional skills are uniquely *necessary* to humane executions.

As with other methods of execution invented by well-meaning physicians, lethal injection has its own set of complications that cause considerable documented physical suffering in a substantial number of cases. Ironically, these complications are familiar to most anesthesiologists because they also occur during anesthesia care: complications of obtaining IV access, unintended awareness, and suffocation due to respiratory muscle paralysis in the absence of adequate airway support.

Many condemned prisoners have poor options for intravenous (IV) access because of prior drug abuse, obesity, and terror. Attempts to establish IV access have sometimes persisted for hours, and at times have had to be terminated because of lack of success, with the prisoner thereafter returning to his cell to dread future execution attempts. At least one study demonstrated that, in 43% of executed prisoners, inadequate blood levels of the hypnotic were achieved to guarantee unconsciousness throughout the duration of the execution.[7] A legal review in California showed that a majority of prisoners were not apneic when the paralytic agent was administered,[8] raising questions about the depth of anesthesia achieved. Many prisoners may have regained consciousness after administration of the paralytic agent, and it is likely that at least some have suffered an agonizing death of suffocation while being paralyzed and aware. It is worthy of note that the American Veterinary Medical Association considers the administration of paralytic agents during animal euthanasia to be unethical because it might cause or mask *suffering*.[9]

Both legal and medical authorities have argued that "botched" executions are proof that physicians are needed to prevent these complications. But there is no evidence that many if not most "botched" executions would not also occur in the hands of physicians, particularly since similar complications occur in the course of anesthetic administration. Physicians do not have a monopoly on skills in accessing veins and administering IV substances, and lethal doses of the agents involved are not a "trade secret." Inadequate training or experience among non-physicians can be remedied by appropriate training, and is therefore not a compelling argument for physician involvement. The special training of anesthesiologists is not needed, nor even appropriate, if the goal is to produce unconsciousness *and subsequent death*.

Clearly, current execution methods cannot be guaranteed to be "humane." But suppose we *could* eliminate all of the complications of lethal injection – would that be sufficient to vacate ethical objections to physician participation in executions? Oral administration of lethal medicinal cocktails has been closely studied and is highly effective as well as virtually complication free in places where physician-assisted suicide is legal. Can we eliminate ethical objections to physician participation in executions by simply using the same method that is considered ethically and legally acceptable by many at the end-of-life due to disease? Or are there important ethical distinctions between physician-assisted suicide and participation in state-sponsored executions that transcend methodology?

Respect for autonomy at end of life

Physicians now embrace the promotion of the comfort and dignity of patients during the dying process – even if such comfort measures might hasten death. But in order for physicians to use their skills to enable death and yet not violate the professional distinctions that set physicians apart, there must be clear, compelling, and distinguishing ethical criteria that tell us when and why such actions are acceptable.

Brody and others suggest that the (rare) legitimacy of a physician's role in physician aid-in-dying or euthanasia has two critical elements, both of which must be preserved in order that the physician does not violate the integrity of his or her professional ethic: (1) the request for aid-in-dying must be autonomous; and (2) the physician must have no realistic means to reduce or relieve the suffering from which the patient seeks release.[10]

Some argue that participation in lethal injection fulfills a prisoner's "autonomous" request for aid-in-dying, analogous to patients' requests for physician-assisted suicide. But this argument confuses the presence of a "choice" for the presence of "autonomy." Many choices are made in the presence of manipulation and coercion, but are then not "autonomous," because autonomy requires absence of coercion or manipulation. Picture a robbery victim, for example, who is told to hand over her purse or be killed. Presumably, she considers both options to be bad and would not choose between them if she were not forced to do so. The robber coerces her and makes a choice, but her choice is not an autonomous one.

A dying patient differs from the robbery victim in that no one is intentionally "forcing" the choice. Strictly speaking, disease cannot "force" or "manipulate." Disease is merely a set of circumstances, within the framework of which human beings make choices, such as whether to pursue or forgo therapy. However, a prisoner choosing between methods of execution *is* being forced to do so by the state, which represents human intentions. The prisoner can't simply "not choose," because refusal to make a choice results in "default" to an execution method that is predetermined. In this case, the prisoner is more like the robbery victim than a patient. The "choice" does not represent an act of autonomy and is not ethically analogous to an end-of-life decision by a dying patient. In fact, when prisoners *seek* the death penalty, it is usually argued that they suffer from limited capacity due to mental illness and therefore they cannot be autonomous.

Nonmaleficence – are physicians harmed by participation in executions?

Moral disengagement among participants in executions

Moral disengagement is a process by which individuals "turn off" aspects of moral self-regulation while participating in activities that may violate some of their internal moral standards. Mechanisms of disengagement occur at four sites in an action: (1) characterization of the action (the "locus of behavior"); (2) minimizing the responsibility of the actor (the "agent" of the action); (3) minimizing the outcomes of the action; and (4) recharacterization of the recipient of the action. Some specific mechanisms include moral justification, minimizing consequences, dehumanization of victims, and displacement or diffusion of responsibility (Table 49.1).

Moral disengagement plays a facilitative role in injurious conduct by individuals and groups, and is systematically used to manage adverse psychological consequences to the participants as well as to maintain loyalty. Examples of situations in which moral disengagement is used include antisocial pursuits (crime), international terrorism, and support for military action in international conflicts. The penal system formally and intentionally incorporates methods of moral disengagement (such as diffusion of responsibility) to decrease guilt among participants in executions and to enable members of the execution team to carry out future executions (Table 49.2).

A study of moral disengagement during executions among prison guards, support personnel (persons providing support and spiritual guidance to the prisoner and family members) and the actual executioners at several US penitentiaries found moral disengagement at all levels.[11] Executioners were found to have the highest levels of moral disengagement, and support personnel the lowest. Most disturbing was the fact that participation in more executions not only progressively inured executioners to their actions, but had even more marked effects on support personnel, converting them from "moral engagers" to "moral disengagers." Behaviors of moral disengagement that were demonstrated in the study, such as demonizing and dehumanizing the prisoner and deflecting personal responsibility to others would appear to be particularly antithetical to the professional ethics and demeanor of physicians.

Concerns regarding the moral legitimacy of the death penalty

While physician professional organizations have carefully avoided making pronouncements about the morality of the death penalty itself, ethicists are not as silent on the issue. In the words of Caplan, when physicians participate in executions that are carried out "capriciously" or for "immoral reasons", even if their personal motivation is one of mercy, *"[they] grant such systems ethical legitimacy and are complicit in the unethical killing of sometimes helpless, hapless, and vulnerable persons."*[12] Physicians, in other words, have an obligation to examine the morality of a process before becoming a part of it.

How is the death penalty applied? Globally, the death penalty has been all but eliminated in Western nations, and it is prohibited throughout the European Union. The five countries carrying out the most executions in the world in 2008 were China, Iran, Saudi Arabia, Pakistan and the US. In addition to "heinous crimes," the death penalty is imposed for reasons as varied as tax fraud, political protest, bribery, homosexuality, adultery, minor drug offenses, and the importation of alcohol. Six nations permit the execution of children (defined as persons under 18 years of age).[13]

Capital punishment is unevenly applied across race and social groups in the US.[14] Almost all studies demonstrate that the death penalty does not deter crime.[15] Capital punishment is more expensive in the US than lifelong incarceration, largely due to a protracted and costly appeals process. This fact has fueled objectionable proposals to curtail existing judicial "safeguards" – the appeals process – to cut such costs.[16] There is no evidence that it provides emotional "closure" to victims' families.[17] To date, 139 condemned US prisoners have been freed from death row by DNA or other evidence, suggesting that innocent victims have almost certainly been wrongly executed by the state.[18] Finally, the death penalty in the US is seen by many to be an impediment to foreign relations.[19]

Professional statements

The American Medical Association (AMA) states that physician participation in executions is unethical. Physician participation includes, but is not limited to:

> *Prescribing or administering tranquilizers and other psychotropic agents and medications that are part of*

Table 49.1. Mechanisms of moral disengagement

Locus of moral disengagement	Mechanisms of moral disengagement and examples of reasoning applied in capital punishment
Locus of behavior (characterizing the action)	*Moral justification* • Deters crime • Provides closure to victims and their families • Is justified by religious precepts ("an eye for an eye") • Is necessary for law and order to prevail and for society to survive *Euphemistic language* • "Capital punishment is just the legal penalty for murder." *Exonerative (or advantageous) comparisons* • Lethal injection is more humane than a murder • The murderer's victims did not have the benefit of a trial
Locus of the agent (diffusing responsibility of the person or persons carrying out the action)	• Sentencing requirements forced the jury to impose the death penalty • The decision involved 12 jurors, and no one juror is responsible • The criminal will still have the decision reviewed on appeal, therefore the jury is not ultimately the decision-maker • I am not the one who made the decision, it is just my job to carry out the sentence
Locus of the outcomes (minimizing or mischaracterizing the outcomes of the action)	• The death penalty is humane and the murdered doesn't suffer • The murderer suffered less than the victims
Locus of the recipient (characterizing the recipient as deserving of the action)	• The murderer is to blame for being put to death • Murderers forfeit their rights to be treated as human beings

Moral disengagement occurs at several "loci" in an action, in order to prevent the actors from experiencing self-condemnation.

Table 49.2. Fractionalization of responsibility during executions to diffuse responsibility

• Lethal injection "recipe" is determined by someone who will not be involved in injection

• The lethal cocktail is drawn up by someone who will not be involved in injection

• Guards who care for the prisoner awaiting execution are not involved in the death chamber activities

• Tasks such as tying straps on the prisoner, taking vital signs, and finding sites of intravenous cannulation are all assigned to different persons, none of whom will be involved in injection of lethal drugs

• Person involved in ordering the execution to commence does not inject the drugs

• Person involved in checking vital signs did not inject the drugs

• In many cases, physicians are allowed to "confirm" death, but not "declare" death, to avoid the appearance of ordering an execution if the prisoner is still alive and requires another dose

• Multiple drug lines run from the prisoner to a blind screen: several persons "inject" drugs from behind the screen, but none knows which of their lines is connected to the prisoner's IV. This is analogous to firing squads, in which several executioners will have weapons, but not all contain live ammunition. No one is entirely sure of whether their bullet contributes to the prisoner's death.

(Note: not all institutions have identical execution processes, so these examples may not be universal) *the execution procedure; monitoring vital signs on site or remotely (including monitoring electrocardiograms); attending or observing an execution as a physician; and rendering of technical advice regarding execution. In the case where the method of execution is lethal injection, the following actions by the physician would also constitute physician participation in execution: selecting injection sites; starting intravenous lines as a port for a lethal injection device; prescribing, preparing, administering, or supervising injection drugs or their doses or types; inspecting, testing, or maintaining lethal injection devices; and consulting with or supervising lethal injection personnel.*[20]

The American Society of Anesthesiologists (ASA) also states that capital punishment in any form is not the practice of medicine, and agrees with the AMA's position on physician involvement in capital punishment.[21]

In February of 2010, the American Board of Anesthesiology announced that an anesthesiologist's participation in an execution by lethal injection is inconsistent with the ABA's Professional Standing Policy, and diplomats of the ABA who participate in lethal injection may be subject to disciplinary action including revocation of their ABA diplomate status.[22]

Key points

- Physician professional organizations consistently state that it is unethical for physicians to be involved in executions.
- Arguments for physician participation in lethal injection usually rely on principles of beneficence (relieving suffering) and respect for autonomy (of the prisoner).
- Lethal injection is plagued by complications that cause physical suffering in a substantial number of cases.
- Arguments that lethal injection respects a prisoner's "autonomy" are flawed, in that they confuse "choice" with "autonomy."
- Physician aid-in-dying for patients suffering from medical disease, is ethically distinct from execution of condemned prisoners. Dying patients suffer from adverse circumstances, and are not manipulated by an intentional third party. Condemned prisoners, on the other hand are being coerced by human actors.

- Participation in executions leads to moral disengagement by members of the execution team; methods of moral disengagement such as dehumanizing the prisoner or deflecting responsibility for actions, are antithetical to the professional ethics of physicians.
- The morality of participation in executions cannot be divorced from the morality of capital punishment. Global characteristics suggest that the death penalty is applied capriciously, unequally, and does not fulfill the public's expectations for security and emotional closure.
- Anesthesiologists who participate in lethal injection in the US now risk professional sanctions.

References

1 Farber, N.J., Aboff, B.M, Weiner, J., *et al.* (2001). Physicians' willingness to participate in the process of lethal injection for capital punishment. *Ann Intern Med*, **135**, 884–8.

2 Espy, M.W. and Smykla, J.O. (2003). *Executions in the United States, 1608–1991: The Espy file*. 2002. Retrieved from The Inter-University Consortium for Political and Social Research. http://www.icpsr.umich.edu/icpsrweb/ICPSR/studies/8451?archive=ICPSR&q=espy

3 The Hippocratic Oath. http://en.wikipedia.org/wiki/Hippocratic_Oath.

4 Levine, M. (1972). Personal communication quoted in *Psychiatry and Ethics*, New York. George Braziller, p324.

5* Gawande, A., Denno, D.W., Truog, R. and Waisel, D. (2008). Physicians and execution – highlights form a discussion of lethal injection. *New Eng J Med*, **385**, 448–51.

6* Caplan, A.L. (2007). Should physicians participate in capital punishment? *Mayo Clin Proc*, **82**(9), 1047–8.

7 Koniaris, L.G., Zimmers, T.A., Lubarsky, D.A., and Sheldon, J.P, (2005). Inadequate anaeshtesia in lethal injection for execution. *Lancet*, **365**(9468), 1412–14.

8 Gawande, A. (2006). When law and ethics collide – why physicians participate in executions. *New Eng J Med*, **354**, 1221–9.

9 American Veterinary Medical Association Guidelines on Euthanasia. June 2007. http://www.avma.org/issues/animal_welfare/euthanasia.pdf.

10* Brody, H. and Wardlaw, M. (2008). Two gorillas in the death penalty room. *Am J Bioethics*, **8**(10), 53–4.

11* Osofsky, M., Bandura, A., and Zimbardo, P. (2005). The role of moral disengagement in the execution process. *Law Human Behav*, **29**(4), 371–93.

12 Caplan, A. L. (2007). Should physicians participate in capital punishment? *Mayo Clin Proc*, **82**(9), 1074–8.

13 The Death Penalty Information Center. http://www.deathpenaltyinfo.org/.

14 Phillips, S. (2008). Race disparities in the capital of capital punishment. *Houston Law Rev*, **45**(3), 807–40.

15 Radelet, M.L. and LaCock, T. (2009). Recent developments: do executions lower homicide rates? The views of leading criminologists. *J Criminal Law Criminology*, **99**(2), 489–508.

16 In the Senate of the United States; 109th Congress, 1st Session. 2005. S1088. "Streamlined Procedures Act of 2005."

17 Goldberg, M. (2003). The 'closure' myth. Salon.com. January 21, 2003. http://dir.salon.com/news/feature/2003/01/21/closure/index.html.

18 The Death Penalty Information Center. http://www.deathpenaltyinfo.org/innocence-list-those-freed-death-row, accessed Feb 15, 2010.

19 Warren, M. (2004). Death, dissent, and diplomacy: the US death penalty as an obstacle to foreign relations. *Wm and Mary Bill Rights J*, **13**, 309–38.

20 American Medical Association Code of Medical Ethics. Opinion 2.06. Capital Punishment. http://www.ama-assn.org/ama/pub/physician-resources/medical-ethics/code-medical-ethics/opinion206.shtml.

21 American Society of Anesthesiologists' Statement on Physician Nonparticipation in Legally Authorized Executions. Approved by House of Delegates October 18, 2006. http://www.asahq.org/publicationsAndServices/standards/41.pdf.

22 Anesthesiologists and capital punishment; professional standing. February 2010, American Board of Anesthesiology. Raleigh, NC. http://www.theaba.org/Home/notices#punishment.

Further reading

Annas, G.J. (2008). Toxic tinkering – lethal injection execution and the Constitution. *New Eng J Med*, **359**, 1512–18.

Freedman, A.M. and Halpern, A.L. (1996). The erosion of ethics and morality in medicine: physician participation in legal executions in the United States. *NY Law Sch Rev*, **41**, 169–88.

Osofsky, M. and Osofsky, H. (2002). The psychological experience of security officers who work with executions. *Psychiatry*, **65**(4), 358–70.

Ragon, S. (1994). A doctor's dilemma: resolving the conflicts between physician participation in executions and the AMA's code of medical ethics. *U. Dayton Law Rev*, **20**, 997–1008.

Wilkinson, D.J. and Douglas, T. (2008). Consequentialism and the death penalty. *Am J Bioethics*, **8**(10), 56–8.

Index

DISCOVERY LIBRARY
LEVEL 5 SWCC
DERRIFORD HOSPITAL
DERRIFORD ROAD
PLYMOUTH
PL6 8DH